MEDICAL TERMINOLOGY
Mastering the Basics

Cindy Destafano, BS, RT(R)
Instructor
Consolidated School of Business
Lancaster, Pennsylvania

Fran Federman, MSEd
Instructor/Educational Consultant
York, Pennsylvania

Publisher
The Goodheart-Willcox Company, Inc.
Tinley Park, Illinois
www.g-w.com

D1319435

Instructor's Edition Contents

Instructional Package

Medical Terminology: Mastering the Basics uses clear, accessible language to help beginning students develop a solid understanding of the building blocks of medical language. The more than 200 colorful, richly detailed illustrations captivate students' interest and reinforce their understanding of important, related concepts such as basic anatomy and physiology, pathology, diagnostics, and treatments.

To enhance your students' ability to succeed in what can be a challenging course for beginners, the textbook is supplemented by a variety of engaging study aids, including interactive games and activities, audio pronunciations of key medical terms, and audio recordings of patient chart notes that simulate the real-world experience of analyzing and interpreting medical records dictated by physicians. The robust teaching package offers ample assessment opportunities to help you gauge student comprehension and determine grades. For ease of grading, answers have been provided in this instructor's edition as well as in the online instructor's resources.

The information that follows will help you become familiar with the textbook and supplemental resources in the teaching package. In addition to the student textbook, the *Medical Terminology: Mastering the Basics* teaching package includes

- the instructor's edition;
- an online course;
- instructor's resources;
- instructor's presentations for PowerPoint®;
- the ExamView® Assessment Suite;
- a companion website; and
- a mobile site.

All of the printed products in the teaching package are also available in a digital format, giving you the flexibility to teach *Medical Terminology: Mastering the Basics* in a variety of formats—online, with traditional print materials, or using a blended approach.

Student Text

Students using *Medical Terminology: Mastering the Basics* will find the write-in text engaging, accessible, and easy to navigate. The authors have created a text that meets the needs of beginning medical terminology students, as well as students of diverse academic backgrounds and ability levels. Without compromising factual accuracy, the authors have succeeded in elucidating concepts through engaging, student-friendly language that facilitates comprehension. Students' conceptual understanding is further reinforced by the richly detailed, full-color drawings and diagrams developed by artists with advanced education in medical illustration.

Chapter Organization

The student-friendly organization of *Medical Terminology: Mastering the Basics* has been designed by the authors to promote comprehension and retention. Each chapter of the text is organized into sections that make the material more manageable for the beginning student and appropriate for a variety of class formats. The chapter material is divided into a series of discrete topics, logically arranged beneath headings that not only facilitate comprehension but also make it easier to locate during lesson reviews. Furthermore, the sections within each chapter are self-contained, making them perfect for independent study.

Each chapter of *Medical Terminology: Mastering the Basics* begins with a list of objectives that can be used to guide instructional planning, as well as a brief outline of chapter contents. The chapter-opening Intern Experience feature—designed to capture students' interest by drawing them into a real-world healthcare scenario—is followed by a succinct overview of anatomy and physiology that gives beginning medical terminology students a basic understanding of anatomical and physiological concepts. This broad overview of anatomy and physiology enables students to contextualize the medical language that they encounter in the text.

Key medical terms throughout each chapter are clearly defined, and medical word parts (prefixes, combining forms, and suffixes) are presented with literal definitions to promote comprehension and retention. Clear, concise descriptions are given of diseases and disorders related to the body system covered in the chapter, along with student-friendly discussions of diagnostic tests, procedures, and therapeutic treatments. Dynamic, full-color illustrations, diagrams, and photography help reinforce students' understanding of concepts related to pathology, diagnostics, and treatments.

Medical records activities that simulate authentic content are a cornerstone feature of the textbook. Students have multiple opportunities in each chapter to analyze and interpret patient chart notes in a variety of authentic formats, from the standard SOAP format (Subjective-Objective-Assessment-Plan) to emergency department records. These opportunities to practice working with patient medical records allow students to relate classroom learning to the practical experiences they will encounter in a real-world healthcare environment.

Learning Activities and Study Aids

The *Medical Terminology: Mastering the Basics* textbook program features a variety of learning activities and study aids to help students master the subject matter. Beyond the exercises in the textbook, students can practice and reinforce their medical terminology skills with engaging digital media activities that include e-flash cards; anatomical diagram-labeling activities; spelling, matching, and multiple-choice exercises; and games that make learning fun, such as crossword puzzles.

Medical word parts in the textbook are color-coded to assist students in identifying prefixes, combining forms, and suffixes. The text provides linguistic support through phonetic spellings of key medical terms, and students can strengthen their pronunciation skills by listening to audio recordings of key medical terms at the G-W Medical Terminology Companion Website.

Vocabulary

To help students master the extensive new vocabulary of an introductory medical terminology course, and to help interested students prepare for a career in the healthcare industry, the *Medical Terminology: Mastering the Basics* textbook program includes a variety of strategies and features that emphasize content vocabulary acquisition.

Because the number of new terms pertaining to each body system in a beginning medical terminology course can be overwhelming to students, key medical terms are presented in boldface type and defined or explained when they are introduced in the chapter. Phonetic spellings have been provided for terms that are difficult to pronounce. Secondary medical terms are represented in italics and are defined or explained upon their introduction in the chapter. This distinction between key terms and secondary terms helps students prioritize and focus on the most essential terminology in the text, while recognizing other important terms that contribute to a solid knowledge and understanding of the concepts encompassed within medical terminology: anatomy and physiology, pathological conditions, and diagnostic and treatment methods.

The companion website includes multiple features to help students study and learn key medical terms. For example, when students access the Audio Glossary, they will hear the correct pronunciation of each key term. The audio pronunciations help students master medical terms that can be challenging to pronounce. In addition, the companion website features interactive e-flash cards, games, and puzzles that students can use to practice identifying, spelling, and pronouncing key medical terms. At the mobile website, students can use the e-flash cards to test their knowledge of medical word parts and key anatomy and physiology vocabulary from the textbook.

Assessments

Each chapter of *Medical Terminology: Mastering the Basics* includes multiple assessment opportunities for gauging student progress and mastery of the material. A unique "scorecard" feature allows students to obtain immediate feedback on their performance by calculating the number of items correctly answered in each assessment. The simple, self-scoring rubric is perfect for independent study.

A Cumulative Review feature appears at regular intervals throughout the text. This assessment feature allows students to check their mastery of the medical word elements within a particular chapter range before they advance to a new chapter. The Cumulative Review is organized as follows:

Chapters 2–4: Integumentary, Digestive, and Musculoskeletal Systems

Chapters 5–7: Lymphatic and Immune Systems, Special Sensory Organs (Eye and Ear), and Nervous System

Chapters 8–10: Male and Female Reproductive Systems, Respiratory System, and Cardiovascular System

Chapters 11–12: Endocrine System and Urinary System

Finally, a Chapter Review at the conclusion of each chapter presents a summary of word elements and a variety of fun, challenging activities for skill-building practice. Students can access the G-W Medical Terminology Companion Website or the G-W Medical Terminology Mobile Site for More Practice activities and games to reinforce their skills and assess their mastery of the medical terminology they have learned in the chapter.

G-W Online

The G-W Online course provides instructors and students with the opportunity to extend learning beyond the classroom. The processes of teaching and learning medical terminology are made more efficient through a host of robust digital features including the advanced gradebook, prebuilt assessments, reports for measuring and tracking learning progress, and tools that allow students and instructors to communicate.

The Medical Terminology Online Course can be accessed by visiting www.g-wonline.com.

Instructor's Edition

This instructor's edition of the textbook is included in the teaching package for *Medical Terminology: Mastering the Basics*. The instructor's edition contains the full student text plus additional pages of resources to help you successfully plan and teach this course. A sample instructional pacing chart offers a recommended schedule for a 15-week course; this pacing chart can be modified for courses of other lengths. For ease of grading, answers have been printed directly in the student assessments in this instructor's edition.

Instructor's Resources

The instructor's resources include everything you need to use *Medical Terminology: Mastering the Basics* in your classroom. A variety of materials are provided to help you make the most of every aspect of the teaching package, including

- the instructor's edition of the text in digital format;
- a sample instructional pacing chart for a 15-week course, which can be modified for courses of other lengths and formats;
- answer keys for the assessments in the student edition; and
- an easy-to-edit, customizable lesson-plan template and sample lesson plan in Microsoft Word®.

Pacing Chart

The authors are cognizant of institutional and instructor concerns and expectations regarding curriculum and scheduling accommodations. In classrooms across the United States, a variety of instructional pacing schedules are used to deliver course content. This textbook allows flexibility in accommodating time and resource constraints. Instructors can choose among a variety of activities to meet their scheduling needs. A sample Instructional Pacing Chart with a recommended timeline for delivery of *Medical Terminology: Mastering the Basics* content appears near the end of this front matter and in the instructor's resources that accompany this program.

Lesson Plans

Sample lesson plans have been supplied (near the end of this front matter and in the Instructor's Resources) to help you develop and implement daily classroom lessons for the *Medical Terminology: Mastering the Basics* program. The lesson plans, which provide an outline for instructional presentation, may be modified based on your unique classroom needs and teaching style. We encourage you to use these lesson plans as a springboard for tailoring them to meet your specific curriculum needs.

Each lesson plan offers multiple recommendations for using special instructional features and assessment activities. The suggestions in these lesson plans are merely guidelines; you may choose to make modifications.

Instructor's Presentations for PowerPoint®

The Instructor's Presentations for PowerPoint® are a highly useful and convenient tool for lesson presentation. These slides help you teach and visually reinforce the key terms and concepts from each chapter of *Medical Terminology: Mastering the Basics*. The content of the slides corresponds to the narrative in the student edition chapters. Each PowerPoint presentation includes key figures from each lesson.

ExamView® Assessment Suite

The ExamView® Assessment Suite allows you to quickly and easily create and print tests from a test bank consisting of hundreds of questions. The ExamView software components include the ExamView Test Generator, ExamView Test Manager, and ExamView Test Player.

The ExamView Assessment Suite allows you to generate tests containing randomly selected questions. Alternatively, you may choose specific questions from the test bank, and can even add your own questions to create customized tests. The ExamView Assessment Suite offers the convenient option of generating multiple versions of the same test for use during different class periods.

Automatically generated answer keys simplify grading. In addition, you can manage your class roster, administer and score online tests, and automatically score paper tests.

Tests that you create with the ExamView Assessment Suite may be published for LAN-based testing, or they may be packaged for online testing using WebCT (a Blackboard learning system) or ANGEL Learning Management Suite. The ExamView software products are compatible with interactive whiteboard technology.

G-W Learning Companion Website

The *Medical Terminology: Mastering the Basics* companion website features extensive resources for learning and review. To help students learn challenging vocabulary, an audio glossary provides pronunciations of key medical terms in the textbook, plus a printed definition for each term.

To reinforce their learning, students can practice medical terminology using an abundance of interactive tools, including e-flash cards, anatomical diagram-labeling activities, matching exercises, crossword puzzles, and spelling challenges. Once students have completed any of these assessments on the companion website, they can e-mail their answers to themselves or directly to their instructor for grading and evaluation.

The G-W Learning Companion Website can be accessed by visiting www.g-wlearning.com/healthsciences/.

G-W Learning Mobile Site

The G-W Learning Mobile Site is a convenient study tool that gives students the flexibility to practice their medical terminology skills on the go. The mobile site is easy to read, easy to use, and fine-tuned for quick access. For *Medical Terminology: Mastering the Basics*, the G-W Learning Mobile Site contains e-flash card exercises that allow students to practice identifying medical word parts and their meanings and key anatomy and physiology terms and definitions from the text. If students do not have a smartphone, they can access these features by visiting the G-W Learning Companion Website using an Internet browser, such as Microsoft® Internet Explorer® or Mozilla® Firefox®.

The G-W Learning Mobile Site can be accessed by visiting www.m.g-wlearning.com.

Instructional Pacing Chart

The following pacing chart offers suggestions for dividing the chapter content of *Medical Terminology: Mastering the Basics* over a 15-week course schedule. This pacing chart can be modified for other course schedules (for example, 12 weeks or 18 weeks).

Week	Activity(ies)
Week 1:	• Meet one another; introduce the Medical Terminology course, review class rules and expectations • Introduce the textbook, Medical Terminology: Mastering the Basics • Begin **Chapter 1: Introduction to Medical Terminology**
Week 2:	• Complete Chapter 1 • Begin **Chapter 2: The Integumentary System**
Week 3:	• Complete Chapter 2 • Review and test students on Chapter 1
Week 4:	• Complete **Chapter 3: The Digestive System**
Week 5:	• Review and quiz students on Chapters 2–3 • Complete **Chapter 4: The Musculoskeletal System**
Week 6:	• Review and quiz students on Chapter 4 • Do Cumulative Review of Chapters 2–4
Week 7:	• Test students on Chapters 2–4 • Complete **Chapter 5: The Lymphatic and Immune Systems**
Week 8:	• Complete **Chapter 6: Special Sensory Organs: Eye and Ear**
Week 9:	• Review and quiz students on Chapters 5–6 • Complete **Chapter 7: The Nervous System**
Week 10:	• Do Cumulative Review of Chapters 5–7 • Complete **Chapter 8: The Male and Female Reproductive Systems**
Week 11:	• Review and quiz students on Chapter 8 • Begin **Chapter 9: The Respiratory System**
Week 12:	• Complete Chapter 9 • Complete **Chapter 10: The Cardiovascular System**
Week 13:	• Review and quiz students on Chapters 9–10 • Complete **Chapter 11: The Endocrine System**
Week 14:	• Complete **Chapter 12: The Urinary System** • Do Cumulative Review of Chapters 11–12 • Let's celebrate all your hard work!
Week 15:	• Review and quiz students on Chapters 11–12 • Review Chapters 6–12 • Final examination

Lesson Plan

To assist instructors in planning for delivery of *Medical Terminology: Mastering the Basics* course content, a lesson-plan template and a sample lesson plan are provided below.

Lesson-Plan Template

INSTRUCTOR NAME: _____   **SUBJECT/COURSE:** _____

Week, Cycle, or Date: _____   **UNIT OF STUDY:** _____

OBJECTIVES	Depending on the requirements and the time period of the lesson plan (daily, unit, weekly), list the learning objectives.
NATIONAL STANDARDS*	List applicable national standards for subject-matter content.
TEACHING ACTIVITIES	List teaching activities for the lesson-plan time period.
ACTIVITIES for ENGAGEMENT	List student activities for the lesson-plan time period.
ASSESSMENT of STUDENT LEARNING	List assessments for the lesson-plan time period.
MATERIALS/TECHNOLOGY	List materials/technology for the lesson-plan time period.

*If applicable to your course/institution

Sample Lesson Plan

INSTRUCTOR NAME: Jane Doe   **SUBJECT/COURSE:** Medical Terminology

Week, Cycle, or Date: Week 4   **UNIT OF STUDY:** Digestive System

OBJECTIVES	1. Label an anatomical diagram of the digestive system. 2. Dissect and define common medical terminology related to the digestive system. 3. Build terms used to describe digestive system diseases and disorders, diagnostic procedures, and therapeutic treatments. 4. Pronounce and spell common medical terminology related to the digestive system. 5. Understand that the processes of building and dissecting a medical term based on its prefix, word root, and suffix enable you to analyze an extremely large number of medical terms beyond those presented in this chapter. 6. Interpret the meaning of abbreviations associated with the digestive system. 7. Interpret medical records containing terminology and abbreviations related to the digestive system.

(Continued on next page)

NATIONAL HEALTHCARE FOUNDATION STANDARDS AND ACCOUNTABILITY CRITERIA*	1.21 Research common diseases and disorders of each body system. 1.22 Research emerging diseases and disorders. 2.15 Apply speaking and active listening skills. 2.21 Use root words, prefixes, and suffixes to communicate information. 2.22 Use medical abbreviations to communicate information.
TEACHING ACTIVITIES	• Discuss overview of digestive system anatomy and physiology. • Discuss vocabulary words/terminology and pronunciations. • Give practice in both pronunciation and understanding the terms through student activities. • Discuss word elements of the digestive system. • Build medical terms of the digestive system. • Discuss diseases, disorders, procedures, and treatments of the digestive system. • Discuss clinical documents and have students analyze them. **Suggested Guest Speaker/Field Trip:** **Integumentary System**—Dermatologist/Participate in skin cancer screening offered through the American Cancer Society **Digestive System**—Gastroenterologist **Musculoskeletal System**—Orthopedist **Lymphatic and Immune Systems**—Immunologist **Special Sensory Organs (Eye and Ear)**—School nurse for vision or hearing test **Nervous System**—Psychiatric nurse **Reproductive System**—Obstetrician/Gynecologist **Respiratory System**—Representative from American Lung Association **Cardiovascular System**—Cardiologist/Observe stress test; participate in blood drive **Urinary System**—Urologist

(Continued on next page)

*Example provided for illustrative purposes. Standards listed above may not apply to your course/institution.

ACTIVITIES for ENGAGEMENT	E-Flash Card activity: Anatomy and Physiology Vocabulary—page 91
	Identifying Major Organs of the Digestive System (labeling an anatomical diagram)—page 92
	Matching Anatomy and Physiology Vocabulary—page 93
	E-Flash Card Activity: Word Elements—pages 94–96
	Matching Prefixes, Combining Forms, and Suffixes—pages 97–99
	Audio Activity: Pronounce It—page 103
	Audio Activity: Spell It—pages 103–104
	Break It Down—pages 104–106
	Build It—pages 107–109
	Multiple Choice: Diseases and Disorders—page 118
	Multiple Choice: Procedures and Treatments—pages 118–119
	Identifying Abbreviations—page 119
	Analyzing patient chart notes—pages 120–123
	Chapter Review—pages 124–131
ASSESSMENT of STUDENT LEARNING	• Assessment is an ongoing process. The instructor circulates through the classroom, observing and identifying those students who have problems with assignments.
	• Quiz on Chapter 2 and Chapter 3
	• Class participation
MATERIALS/TECHNOLOGY	• *Medical Terminology: Mastering the Basics* by Cindy Destafano and Fran Federman
	• Goodheart-Willcox Medical Terminology Companion Website
	• Goodheart-Willcox Medical Terminology Mobile Site

Best Practices for Using Smartphones in the Classroom

Medical Terminology: Mastering the Basics comes with student access to a mobile site. The mobile site includes e-flash cards of key medical terms with definitions. This feature can be accessed using a smartphone or a computer.

Smartphones, if used appropriately, can be a valuable teaching tool. Before you begin to use them in your class, you may want to establish guidelines for students on appropriate smartphone usage, including sharing of information, smartphone safety, and expectations for how the phones will be used in class. Following are some guidelines to help you with this discussion.

- Explain that all mobile activities (photos, text messages, and online posts) are part of a student's digital "footprint." That is, each time they use a smartphone or a computer to post photos, send e-mail or text messages, or share an update on a social media website, for example, they continue to build a permanent, "online trail" of digital activity that cannot be retracted.

- Encourage students to know the financial details of their mobile plan. Students may know all the features of their smartphones, but not what those features cost.

- Communicate your expectations concerning limitations on the ways in which smartphones may be used during class time. As an instructor, you are accustomed to students being distracted by activities such as sending and receiving text messages, checking content on social media websites, and posting their responses to this content. Reinforce the rule that smartphone usage in the classroom will be limited to activities that enhance and reinforce learning.

Alternatives should exist for students who do not have access to smartphones, such as using cooperative learning, differentiating assignments based on smartphone functions, or using alternative methods to access the content. All information available through the G-W Learning Mobile Site can be accessed using an Internet browser on the G-W Learning Companion Website.

G-W Learning Mobile Site: www.m.g-wlearning.com

G-W Learning Companion Website: www.g-wlearning.com/healthsciences/

Helping Students Recognize and Value Diversity

Your students will enter a rapidly changing workplace, both from the standpoint of the kinds of technology they will use and the degree of diversity they will encounter in the work environment. Today's workforce is made up of people who represent many different views, experiences, and backgrounds. The workforce is aging, too, as the ranks of mature workers swell. Because of these trends, young workers must learn how to interact with a variety of people who are considerably unlike them.

Appreciating and understanding diversity is an ongoing process. The earlier and more frequently that young people are exposed to diversity, the better able they will be to bridge cultural differences. If your students are exposed to different cultures within your classroom, the process of understanding cultural differences can begin. This is the best preparation for success in a diverse society. In addition, instructors have found the following strategies for teaching diversity helpful:

- Actively promote a spirit of openness, consideration, respect, and tolerance in the classroom.

- Use cooperative learning activities whenever possible and ensure that group roles are rotated so everyone has leadership opportunities.

- When grouping students, make sure that the racial, ethnic, and gender composition of each group is as diverse as possible.

- If a difficult classroom situation arises involving a diversity issue, ask for a time-out and have everyone write down their thoughts and opinions about the incident. This allows everyone to cool down and allows you to plan a response.

- Arrange for guest speakers who represent diversity in gender, age, race, and ethnicity.

- Have students change seats occasionally throughout the course and introduce themselves to their new "neighbors" so they become acquainted with all of their classmates.

- Several times throughout the course, ask students to make anonymous, written evaluations of the class. Have them report any problems that may not be obvious.

A Note from the Authors

Welcome to *Medical Terminology: Mastering the Basics*! As an instructor, you know the excitement and dreams of your students as they prepare to embark on a career in the allied health profession. The objective of this instructor's edition is to inspire and assist both you and your students in making those dreams a reality.

In developing *Medical Terminology: Mastering the Basics*, our goal was to present medical terminology using a streamlined approach that is not intimidating to beginning students and that allows them to have fun in the process of learning. As currently active educators with more than 30 years' experience in the classroom, we understand the pressures and time constraints placed upon you, the instructor. Thus, careful attention was given to student comprehension, readiness, and difficulty level as we prepared the scope, depth, and sequence of the contents of each chapter in this book.

This textbook has been written and designed to help beginning students develop the fundamental knowledge and skills they need to read, write, and speak the language of medicine. Unlike other medical terminology textbooks, *Medical Terminology: Mastering the Basics* does not emphasize learning medical terminology as a means to understanding anatomy and physiology. Rather, this book contextualizes basic anatomy and physiology concepts to help students develop fluency in reading, writing, and speaking the language of medicine.

This highly accessible, user-friendly textbook employs a systematic, student-driven approach to learning in which the instructor assumes the role of a coach, facilitating the learning process. *Medical Terminology: Mastering the Basics* is supported by an abundance of in-text and online, interactive exercises to help students develop competence in using medical language. A unique, self-scoring rubric allows students to evaluate their own progress as they work through the material in the text. This streamlined, integrated approach fosters mastery and confidence as students prepare for advanced study and/or employment in the allied health field.

Simply put, the mission of *Medical Terminology: Mastering the Basics* is as follows: After students have successfully completed this program, their ability to analyze, dissect, and build medical terms will enable them to figure out the meaning of virtually any new medical term that they encounter!

Cindy Destafano, BS, RT(R)

Fran Federman, MSEd

A Dynamic, Streamlined Approach to Mastering the Language of Healthcare

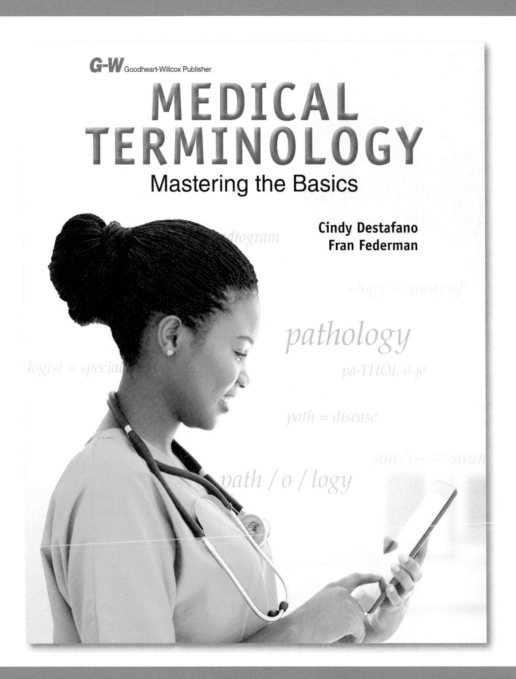

G-W Goodheart-Willcox Publisher

MEDICAL TERMINOLOGY
Mastering the Basics

Cindy Destafano
Fran Federman

-logy = study of

pathology

pă-THŎL-ō-jē

path = disease

son/o- = soun

path / o / logy

A student-friendly program that builds essential knowledge and skills for academic and career success

Written and Designed for

Medical Terminology: Mastering the Basics supports student learning with the following dynamic features:

Intern Experience

Each chapter opens with an engaging, real-world scenario in which a healthcare intern interacts with a patient who has a medical problem related to the body system covered in the chapter. As students continue to read the chapter, they learn medical terminology word elements that help them understand the patient's health condition.

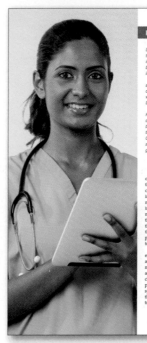

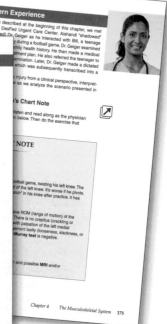

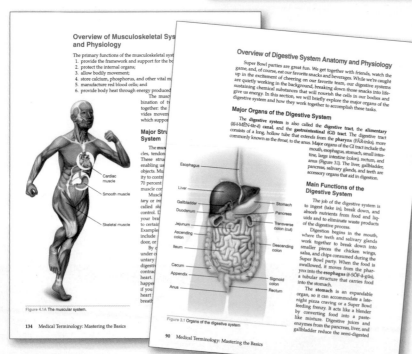

Overview of Anatomy and Physiology

Each chapter presents a basic overview of major anatomical structures and physiological functions. Assessment activities, both in the textbook and online, include labeling an anatomical diagram and matching key anatomy and physiology terms with their definitions.

Beginning Students

Word Elements

Prefixes, combining forms, and suffixes common to the body system are presented in easy-to-read charts. At the G-W Medical Terminology Companion Website or the G-W Medical Terminology Mobile Site, students can practice using e-flash cards to reinforce their knowledge and understanding of medical word elements and their meanings.

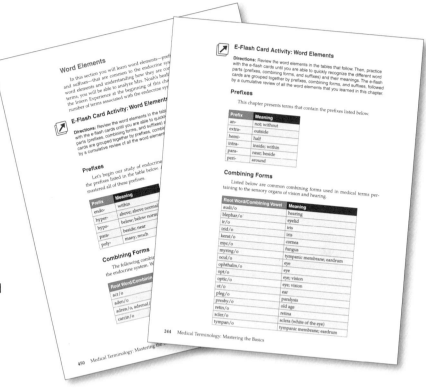

Word Elements

In this section you will learn word elements—prefixes and suffixes—that are common to the endocrine system. Understanding how they are combined... word elements and understanding how they are combined... terms, you will be able to analyze Mrs. Noah's health... the Intern Experience at the beginning of the endocrine system... number of terms associated with the endocrine system.

E-Flash Card Activity: Word Elements

Directions: Review the word elements in the table with the e-flash cards until you are able to quickly parts (prefixes, combining forms, and suffixes) and cards are grouped together by prefixes, combining by a cumulative review of all the word elements...

Prefixes

Let's begin our study of endocrine... the prefixes listed in the table below... mastered all of these prefixes.

Prefix	Meaning
endo-	within
hyper-	above; above normal
hypo-	below; below norm...
para-	beside; near
poly-	many; much

Combining Forms

The following combini... the endocrine system. W...

Root Word/Combin...
acr/o
aden/o
adren/o, adrenal/...
carcin/o

450 Medical Terminology: Mastering the Basics

E-Flash Card Activity: Word Elements

Directions: Review the word elements in the tables that follow. Then, practice with the e-flash cards until you are able to quickly recognize the different word parts (prefixes, combining forms, and suffixes) and their meanings. The e-flash cards are grouped together by prefixes, combining forms, and suffixes, followed by a cumulative review of all the word elements that you learned in this chapter.

Prefixes

This chapter presents terms that contain the prefixes listed below.

Prefix	Meaning
an-	not; without
extra-	outside
hemi-	half
intra-	inside; within
para-	near; beside
peri-	around

Combining Forms

Listed below are common combining forms used in medical terms pertaining to the sensory organs of vision and hearing.

Root Word/Combining Vowel	Meaning
audi/o	hearing
blephar/o	eyelid
ir/o	iris
irid/o	iris
kerat/o	cornea
myc/o	fungus
myring/o	tympanic membrane; eardrum
ocul/o	eye
ophthalm/o	eye
opt/o	eye
optic/o	eye; vision
ot/o	eye; vision
pleg/o	ear
presby/o	paralysis
retin/o	old age
scler/o	retina
tympan/o	sclera (white of the eye)
	tympanic membrane; eardrum

244 Medical Terminology: Mastering the Basics

Breaking Down and Building Medical Terms

Students are introduced to common medical terms related to anatomy and physiology, diagnostic tests and procedures, diseases and disorders, and therapeutic treatments. Each term is accompanied by a phonetic spelling and is dissected into its component word parts. The meaning of each word part is provided, along with the definition of the medical term.

Breaking Down and Building Digestive System Terms

Now that you have mastered the prefixes, combining forms, and suffixes for digestive system terminology, you have the ability to dissect and build a large number of medical terms related to this system.

Below is a list of common medical terms related to the study, diagnosis, and treatment of the digestive system. For each term, a dissection has been provided, along with the meaning of each word element and the definition of the term as a whole.

Term	Dissection	Word Part/Meaning	Term Definition
Note: For simplification, combining vowels have been omitted from the Word Part/Meaning column.			
1. **aphagia** (ă-FĀ-jē-ă)	a/phagia	a = not; without phagia = condition of eating or swallowing	condition of without swallowing
2. **carcinoma** (kăr-sĭ-NŌ-mă)	carcin/oma	carcin = cancerous; cancer oma = tumor; mass	cancerous tumor or mass
3. **celiectomy** (sē-lē-ĒK-tō-mē)	celi/ectomy	celi = abdomen ectomy = surgical removal; excision	excision of the abdomen
4. **cholecystitis** (KŌ-lē-sis-TĪ-tĭs)	cholecyst/itis	cholecyst = gallbladder itis = inflammation	inflammation of the gallbladder
5. **cholelithiasis** (KŌ-lē-li-THĪ-ă-sĭs)	chol/e/lith/iasis	chol = bile; gall lith = stone iasis = abnormal condition	abnormal condition of gallstones
6. **colitis** (kō-LĪ-tĭs)	col/itis	col = colon itis = inflammation	inflammation of the colon
7. **colonoscopy** (kō-lŏn-ŎS-kō-pē)	colon/o/scopy	colon = colon scopy = process of observing	process of observing the colon
8. **colostomy** (kō-LŎS-tō-mē)	col/o/stomy	col = colon stomy = new opening	new opening in the colon
9. **diarrhea** (dī-ă-RĒ-ă)	dia/rrhea	dia = through rrhea = flow; discharge	flow through
10. **diverticulitis** (DĪ-věr-tĭk-ū-LĪ-tĭs)	diverticul/itis	diverticul = diverticulum itis = inflammation	inflammation of the diverticulum
11. **diverticulosis** (dī-věr-tĭk-ū-LŌ-sĭs)	diverticul/osis	diverticul = diverticulum osis = abnormal condition	abnormal condition of the diverticulum

Prefixes = Green   Root Words = Red   Suffixes = Blue

100 Medical Terminology: Mastering the Basics

	Word Part/Meaning	Term Definition
...oden/al	duoden = duodenum al = pertaining to	pertaining to the duodenum
.../enter/y	dys = painful; difficult enter = intestine y = condition; process	painful condition of the intestines
...peps/ia	dys = painful; difficult peps = digestion ia = condition	condition of painful or difficult digestion
...hagia	dys = painful; difficult phagia = condition of eating or swallowing	condition of painful or difficult swallowing
...r/ic	enter = intestine itis = inflammation	inflammation of the intestines
	epi = upon; above gastr = stomach ic = pertaining to	pertaining to (the area) above the stomach
...eal	esophag = esophagus eal = pertaining to	pertaining to the esophagus
...o/gastr/o/ ...scopy	esophag = esophagus gastr = stomach duoden = duodenum scopy = process of observing	process of observing the esophagus, stomach, and duodenum
	gastr = stomach itis = inflammation	inflammation of the stomach
...r/o/logist	gastr = stomach dynia = pain	pain in the stomach
...o/logy	gastr = stomach enter = intestines logist = specialist in the study and treatment of	specialist in the study and treatment of the stomach and intestines
...eal	gastr = stomach enter = intestines logy = study of	study of the stomach and intestines
	gastr = stomach esophag = esophagus eal = pertaining to	pertaining to the stomach and esophagus
	gingiv = gums itis = inflammation	inflammation of the gums
	gloss = tongue algia = pain	pain in the tongue

Chapter 3   The Digestive System   101

Medical Terminology: Mastering the Basics

Captivating, Full-Color Illustrations

Diseases and Disorders

Richly detailed illustrations and clinical photography, including radiographs, reinforce students' understanding of the major characteristics of common diseases and disorders related to the body system covered in each chapter.

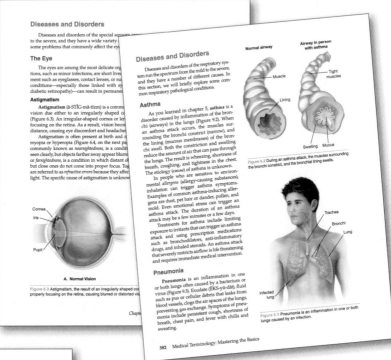

Procedures and Treatments

Sophisticated diagrams and real-life photography help students understand the basic technological concepts behind common diagnostic tests and procedures and therapeutic treatments.

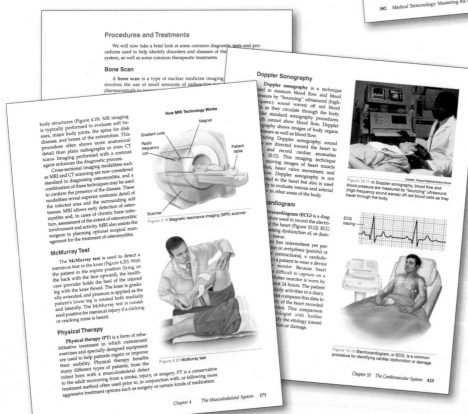

Authentic Clinical Content with Real-World Relevance

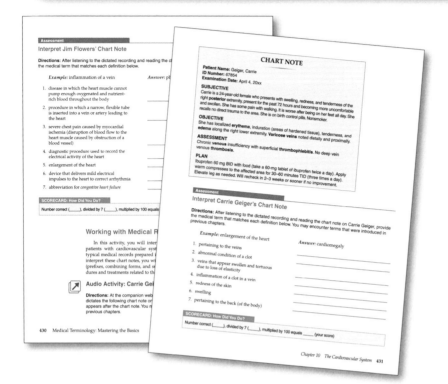

Working with Medical Records

Medical record activities offer a uniquely valuable opportunity for students to interact with authentic clinical content—the kind they will encounter in a real-world healthcare setting. As students read each patient chart note, they can listen as a "physician" dictates the contents at the G-W Medical Terminology Companion Website or the G-W Medical Terminology Mobile Site. Assessments challenge students to interpret terms and abbreviations in the medical record.

Assessment Activities

A variety of exercises throughout *Medical Terminology: Mastering the Basics* give students ample opportunities to learn, practice, and expand their medical terminology knowledge and skills. Students will find interactive versions of many of these exercises at the G-W Medical Terminology Companion Website and the G-W Medical Terminology Mobile Site. For additional skill-building practice and reinforcement, *More Practice* activities and games are available at the companion and mobile sites.

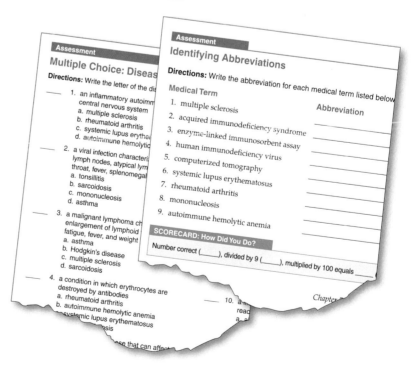

Dynamic Digital Media Offerings

Companion Website

The easy-to-navigate companion website contains a variety of engaging, interactive games and activities to reinforce students' understanding of how medical terminology works. Skill-building activities include interactive labeling of anatomical diagrams, spelling and pronunciation practice, dissecting and building exercises, and interpreting medical terms and abbreviations in patient chart notes dictated by a "physician." Students can e-mail answers to themselves or directly to their instructor for grading.

www.g-wlearning.com/healthsciences

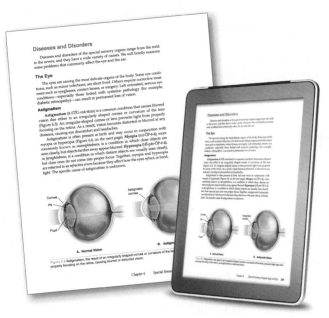

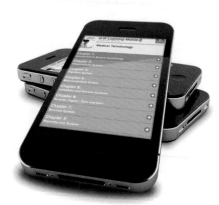

Mobile Site

Practice activities at the mobile site give students the flexibility to study medical terminology on the go. E-flash cards allow students to quiz themselves on medical word parts and their meanings.

www.m.g-wlearning.com

G-W Online

The G-W Online course delivers the same dynamic print content in a digital format. Teaching and learning medical terminology is more efficient with a host of robust digital features including a gradebook, prebuilt assessments, reports for measuring learning progress, and tools that allow students and teachers to communicate.

www.g-wonline.com

MEDICAL TERMINOLOGY
Mastering the Basics

Cindy Destafano, BS, RT(R)
Instructor
Consolidated School of Business
Lancaster, Pennsylvania

Fran Federman, MSEd
Instructor/Educational Consultant
York, Pennsylvania

Publisher
The Goodheart-Willcox Company, Inc.
Tinley Park, Illinois
www.g-w.com

About the Authors

Cindy Destafano is an Instructor at the Consolidated School of Business in Lancaster, Pennsylvania, where she teaches courses in a variety of allied health subjects, including medical terminology, anatomy and physiology, law and ethics for medical careers, medical coding, and medical transcription. Previously she was the Program Coordinator for the Medical Administrative Assistant degree program, for which she developed and wrote the curriculum. Before joining the Consolidated School of Business, she served as the Program Director for the Radiologic Technology degree program at Lancaster Regional Medical Center and taught courses in Medical Imaging. Destafano is the coauthor of *Essentials of Medical Transcription*, *Advanced Medical Transcription*, and *The Mentor Program Workbook*. She is a member of the American Society of Radiologic Technology, the American Registry of Radiologic Technology, and the American Academy of Professional Coders. A graduate of Elizabethtown College with a Bachelor of Science in Business Administration, Destafano is a Registered Radiologic Technologist and a certified Insurance and Coding Specialist.

Fran Federman is a Business Instructor and Educational Consultant in York, Pennsylvania. She teaches courses in the Microsoft® Office software suite, business principles, entrepreneurship, accounting, and medical billing and reimbursement. She has also developed the curricula for a variety of subjects including business management, personal finance, and sports marketing. After earning a Bachelor of Science degree in Business Education from the City University of New York (CUNY), Federman obtained a teaching certificate and launched her career as a Business Education Instructor. She was a Curriculum Director for the Consolidated School of Business, where she assisted in the development and coordination of internship/cooperative programs. She holds a Master of Science degree in Education from Virginia Tech and completed additional postgraduate coursework at Gratz College. Federman is the author or coauthor of several books and journal articles, including *Essentials of Medical Transcription*, *Advanced Medical Transcription*, *The Mentor Program Workbook*, and *The Role of the Business Teacher in Guidance*.

Contributors

Goodheart-Willcox Publisher would like to thank Body Scientific International, LLC, for the exquisitely rendered illustrations that appear throughout this text.

Reviewers

Goodheart-Willcox Publisher would also like to thank the following instructors who reviewed selected manuscript chapters and provided valuable input into the development of this textbook program.

Muriel Adams
Instructor
Prince George's Community College
Largo, MD

Emily Bedsted
Instructor
Anoka-Hennepin School District
Anoka, MN

Jane Best
Instructor
Chesapeake Public Schools
Chesapeake, VA

Amy Bledsoe
Instructor
Spokane Community College
Spokane, WA

Deborah Clarke
Instructor
Littleton Public Schools
Littleton, CO

Molly Day, RRT, RCP, BS Ed
Allied Health Instructor
Bainbridge State College
Bainbridge, GA

Tina Evans, PhD
Associate Professor of Health Sciences
Pennsylvania College of Technology
Williamsport, PA

Coleen Kumar, RN, MS
Professor of Nursing
Kingsborough Community College
Brooklyn, NY

Dr. Amy Lemkuil
Health and Safety Instructor
Madison Area Technical College
Madison, WI

Joan Lynch, RN, MS, MA
Medical Terminology Instructor
Academy of Allied Health and Science
Neptune, NJ

Veronique Parker
Health Professions Program Director
Phoenix College
Phoenix, AZ

Maryanna Perry
Instructor
Franklin Technology Center
Joplin, MO

Laura Sargent, MA, RN
Medical Terminology Instructor
Academy of Allied Health and Science
Neptune, NJ

Leslie Watson, BBA, RT
Associate Instructor
Virginia Western Community College
Roanoke, VA

Heidi Weingart
Medical Assisting Program Director
Santa Fe Community College
Santa Fe, NM

Zada Wicker
Director of Health Information Technology
Brunswick Community College
Bolivia, NC

Sonya Young-Riemer, MS, RMA, LCMT
Instructor
North Central Michigan College
Petoskey, MI

Contents in Brief

Contents

Goodheart-Willcox Publisher Welcomes Your Comments

Goodheart-Willcox Publisher, a leader in career and technical education since 1921, is developing fresh print and digital products for Health and Health Sciences courses. This *Medical Terminology: Mastering the Basics* textbook program is one of many titles in these subject areas that Goodheart-Willcox publishes. Other titles include *Introduction to Anatomy and Physiology* and *Essential Skills for Health Career Success*. Be on the lookout for our grade-appropriate, accessible programs for courses such as *Essential Health*, *Comprehensive Health*, and *Medical Law and Ethics*.

If you teach a Health and Wellness class or any other course in Health or Health Sciences at the high school or postsecondary level, and you have been unable to find a suitable text for your students, please let us know. We are eager to develop high-quality, innovative products that fill unmet needs in the educational market. Your suggestions may lead to the development of digital or print materials that benefit teachers and students across the country.

With each new product, our goal at Goodheart-Willcox Publisher is to deliver superior educational materials that effectively meet the ever changing, increasingly diverse needs of students and teachers. To that end, we welcome your comments and suggestions on the *Medical Terminology: Mastering the Basics* student textbook and its supplemental components.

Please send your comments and suggestions to the managing editor of our Health and Health Sciences Editorial Department. You can send an e-mail to healthsciences@g-w.com, or write to

Managing Editor—HHS

Goodheart-Willcox Publisher

18604 West Creek Drive, Tinley Park, IL 60477-6243

Chapter 1

Introduction to Medical Terminology

Chapter Organization

- Brief Overview of Medical Terminology
- Analyzing and Defining Medical Terms
- Medical Word Parts
- Breaking Down and Building Medical Terms
- Building Plural Forms
- Pronouncing Medical Terms
- Spelling Medical Terms
- Overview of Anatomical Positions, Planes, Directions, and Locations
- Body Cavities
- Common Medical Abbreviations for Anatomical Terms of Position, Direction, and Location
- Body Systems
- Mastering Medical Terminology
- Chapter Review

Chapter Objectives

After completing this chapter, you will be able to

1. describe the origins of medical language;
2. identify the four basic word parts that form many medical terms;
3. describe characteristics of prefixes, combining forms, and suffixes;
4. explain the differences between prefixes, suffixes, root words, and combining vowels;
5. understand that the processes of building and dissecting a medical term based on its prefix, root word, and suffix enable you to analyze an extremely large number of medical terms beyond those presented in this chapter;
6. pronounce and spell medical terms introduced in this chapter;
7. recognize common Latin and Greek singular nouns and form their plurals;
8. identify the anatomical planes of the human body;
9. identify major anatomical positions, locations, and directions; and
10. identify the eleven body systems and cite their primary functions.

You will see this icon ⬈ at various points throughout this chapter. The icon indicates that you will find interactive activities and games on the Medical Terminology Companion Website. These activities and games will help you learn, practice, and expand your medical terminology knowledge and skills. Some of these activities are also available on the Medical Terminology Mobile Website.

 Companion Website
www.g-wlearning.com/healthsciences

 Mobile Site
www.m.g-wlearning.com/5800

Before you begin this chapter...

Welcome to medical terminology! Why are you taking this class? Perhaps your school catalog states that you must take this course if you want to pursue a career in the healthcare profession. But why is it necessary to begin with medical terminology? Why not just start with coursework in anatomy and physiology or dive right into the study of diseases and disorders?

Whether your goal is a career in nursing, medical assisting, physical therapy, pharmacology, or any other medical profession, it all begins with an understanding of medical terminology, the language of medicine. When you are at work, the medical community— your coworkers and other healthcare professionals with whom you will have daily contact—will expect you to "speak the language." Being able to speak this language means that you can read and interpret medical documents and correctly write, spell, and pronounce medical terms.

The ability to understand and correctly use medical terminology is essential to your success in the healthcare field. Besides having an outstanding GPA and an excellent attendance record, you need to "walk the talk." This is why you are taking a medical terminology class. Now, let's get started!

Good Luck!

Cindy Destafano and Fran Federman

Brief Overview of Medical Terminology

Learning medical terminology is similar to learning a foreign language. To succeed in any allied health or medical profession, you must understand the language upon which it is founded. Just as a person unfamiliar with Spanish would have difficulty pursuing a career if he or she lived in a country where Spanish is the primary language, so, too, will the healthcare employee who doesn't understand the language of medicine.

Medical Terminology: Mastering the Basics will give you a solid foundation in the language of the healthcare profession. And it will help you learn this language in a straightforward, engaging, and fun manner.

To master the basics of medical terminology, you will

- memorize word parts: prefixes, root words, and suffixes;
- analyze, dissect, and build medical terms from word parts;
- understand word parts as they relate to diseases and disorders of the different body systems, as well as common diagnostic procedures and therapeutic treatments; and
- reinforce your knowledge, skills, and self-confidence by completing exercises in this textbook and interactive activities and games at the Medical Terminology Companion Website or Medical Terminology Mobile Site.

The language of medicine is derived primarily from Latin and Greek words, and some terms come directly from modern languages such as French and German (Figure 1.1). Many terms can be represented as abbreviations or acronyms, providing valuable shortcuts to communication among healthcare professionals. Some medical terms take the form of eponyms. (An *eponym* is a person after whom a discovery, invention, or other notable achievement has been named.) Furthermore, some medical terms are not built from word parts—that is, they cannot be divided into a prefix, root word, and suffix. For these words, you will need to use a medical dictionary to learn the correct spelling and definition of each term.

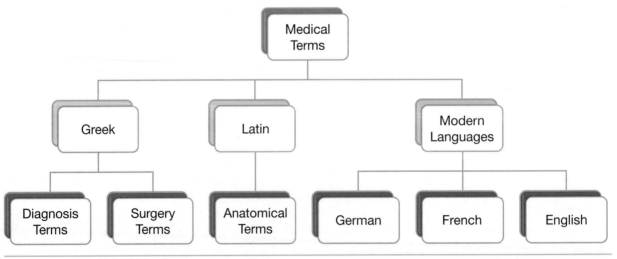

Figure 1.1 Linguistic sources of medical terminology

Medical terminology is a dynamic, fluid, and ever-evolving discipline in which terms are created to describe pioneering surgical procedures, cutting-edge technological innovations, and newly discovered pathological conditions. As a result, new medical terms are constantly being absorbed into the vast body of knowledge that is medical terminology.

A large number of medical terms are built from word parts. There are four types of word parts in medical terminology:

Word Part	Definition
Prefix	A single letter or a group of letters placed before a root word (or series of root words). The prefix shows a particular relationship, such as prepositional or adverbial. In general, most prefixes in medical terminology are used in everyday speech.
Root Word	The word part (or parts) that provides the main meaning of a medical term.
Suffix	A single letter or a group of letters added to the end of a root word (or series of root words). The suffix indicates the grammatical function of the medical term (noun, adjective, verb, or adverb).
Combining Vowel	A vowel that links together word parts for ease of pronunciation. Usually, the combining vowel is **o**, but occasionally it will be **a**, **e**, **i**, or **u**.

Together, a root word and combining vowel are called a **combining form**. For simplicity, each root word introduced in this textbook is presented with its combining vowel.

Word parts may be combined in any of several different ways to build a medical term:

- Prefix, root word, and suffix
- Prefix, root word, combining vowel, and suffix
- Prefix and root word
- Prefix and suffix
- Root word, combining vowel, and suffix
- Root word and suffix

Some medical terms contain more than one prefix, root word, and suffix.

Learning medical terminology requires the memorization of root words, prefixes, and suffixes. Although this process may seem challenging, this textbook provides plenty of skill-building exercises and digital resources to help you learn the material. At the Medical Terminology Companion Website, you will find e-flash cards, audio recordings, puzzles, games, and other activities to reinforce your skills and make learning fun. Got a smartphone? Access the Medical Terminology Mobile Site, where you can practice using e-flash cards to reinforce and test your knowledge of medical word parts and key anatomy and physiology vocabulary.

Follow the processes described in this textbook. Read the material, practice using the e-flash cards (or make your own flash cards), and do some of the digital exercises on a daily basis. Don't wait until the day before a test to study. It doesn't work. Mastering the basics of medical terminology requires a commitment of time and effort. Repetition is a key factor in memorizing medical word parts and their meanings.

To simplify the learning process, we will look at a medical term and then break it down into its word parts. Once you understand how to dissect the term into its word parts, we will put it back together and discuss its meaning and correct pronunciation.

Analyzing and Defining Medical Terms

Let's analyze a medical term and its word parts by following a basic guideline that will help you develop important skills in mastering the basics of medical terminology. You will learn how to dissect a medical term into its individual word parts and then reconstruct those word parts to determine the meaning of the term as a whole.

At this point, don't worry that you don't know the meanings of the word parts; just pay attention to the *process* of analyzing the term. You will be able to use this process (breaking down a word into its prefix, root word, and suffix) to understand a medical term that you have never seen before. We will illustrate the process using the four medical terms below:

- *gastrology*
- *gastroenterology*
- *intragastric*
- *gastrectomy*

EXAMPLE 1

The medical term *gastrology* is defined as "the study of the stomach." This term contains a combining form (root word plus combining vowel) and a suffix.

Follow these steps to analyze the medical term *gastrology*:

1. Divide the term into its word parts. Note that a slash is used to separate each word part.

Medical Term	Dissection
gastrology	gastr/o/logy

2. Define each word part.

Word Part	Type of Word Part	Meaning of Word Part
gastr/o	root word + combining vowel = combining form	gastr = stomach o = combining vowel
logy	suffix	logy = study of

3. Arrange the word parts in the correct order. To figure out the meaning of a medical term, begin with the suffix. Then go back to the beginning of the term and work your way across.

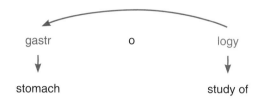

| gastr | o | logy |
| stomach | | study of |

gastrology = the study of the stomach

EXAMPLE 2

The medical term *gastroenterology* means "the study of the stomach and the intestines." (Typically, the combining form **enter/o** is used to refer to the small intestine.) This term contains two root words, two combining vowels, and a suffix.

Follow these steps to analyze the medical term *gastroenterology*:

1. Divide the term into its word parts by placing a slash between each word part.

Medical Term	Dissection
gastroenterology	gastr/o/enter/o/logy

2. Define each word part.

Word Part	Type of Word Part	Meaning of Word Part
gastr/o	root word + combining vowel = combining form	gastr = stomach o = combining vowel
enter/o	root word + combining vowel = combining form	enter = intestines o = combining vowel
logy	suffix	logy = study of

3. Arrange the word parts in the correct order. Begin with the suffix; then go back to the beginning of the term and work your way across.

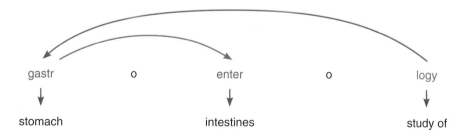

| gastr | o | enter | o | logy |
| stomach | | intestines | | study of |

gastroenterology = the study of the stomach and intestines

EXAMPLE 3

The medical term *intragastric* means "pertaining to within the stomach." This term contains a prefix, a root word, and a suffix. It does not require any combining vowels.

Follow these steps to analyze the medical term *intragastric*:

1. Divide the term into its word parts by placing a slash between each word part.

Medical Term	Dissection
intragastric	intra/gastr/ic

2. Define each word part.

Word Part	Type of Word Part	Meaning of Word Part
intra	prefix	intra = within
gastr	root word	gastr = stomach
ic	suffix	ic = pertaining to

3. Arrange the word parts in the correct order.

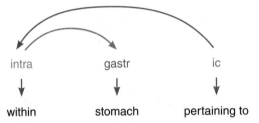

intragastric = pertaining to within the stomach

EXAMPLE 4

Gastrectomy is defined as "the excision (surgical removal) of the stomach." This term contains a root word and a suffix. It does not require a combining vowel.

Follow these steps to analyze the medical term *gastrectomy*:

1. Divide the term into its word parts by placing a slash between each word part.

Medical Term	Dissection
gastrectomy	gastr/ectomy

2. Define each word part.

Word Part	Type of Word Part	Meaning of Word Part
gastr	root word	gastr = stomach
ectomy	suffix	ectomy = excision or surgical removal

3. Arrange the word parts in the correct order.

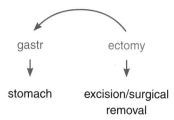

gastr ectomy

↓ ↓

stomach · excision/surgical removal

gastrectomy = the excision or surgical removal of the stomach

Medical Word Parts

Now that you understand how a medical term is built from prefixes, root words, and suffixes, we will discuss each of these word parts in more detail.

Prefixes

A **prefix** is a single letter or group of letters that appears at the beginning of a medical term before the root word(s). When written by itself, a prefix is usually followed by a hyphen.

Medical prefixes often express information about diseases or abnormal conditions; anatomical position, location, or direction; measurement; time; number; and color. Adding or changing a prefix changes the meaning of the medical term.

As you progress through this textbook, you will see that many of the same prefixes are used in medical terms relating to multiple body systems. You will also find that a large number of medical terms do not contain a prefix.

Following are some common prefixes that denote number, quantity, position, location, and direction in medical terminology.

Prefixes that Indicate Number

Prefix	Meaning
bi-	two
di-	two; double
quad-	four
tri-	three
uni-	one

Prefixes that Indicate Quantity, Size, or Magnitude

Prefix	Meaning
hemi-	half
hyper-	above normal
hypo-	below normal
poly-	many; much

Prefixes that Indicate Position, Direction, or Location

Prefix	Meaning
ab-	away from
ad-	toward
endo-	within
hypo-	below
inter-	between
intra-	within
para-	near; beside
peri-	around
post-	after
pre-	before
sub-	beneath; below
trans-	through; across

Root Words and Combining Forms

A **root word** is the foundation of most medical terms and gives the essential meaning of the term. Most medical terms are derived from Greek or Latin. These were the languages of the early scholars who discovered many of the concepts that make up the core knowledge base of biology and medicine. The ancient Greeks were the first to study medicine and to formulate a systematized vocabulary. When the Roman Empire began to displace Greek civilization, the Roman scholars adopted many of the medical terms that had been developed by the Greeks. The ancient Romans modified many other Greek medical terms to conform to the alphabet and grammar of the Latin language.

All medical terms have one or more root words. The root word often indicates a body part, but it may also denote an anatomical or physiological quality or condition. If a medical term contains more than one root word, those root words are typically joined by a combining vowel. Together, a root word and a combining vowel are called a **combining form**.

In most medical terms, a **combining vowel** is placed between word parts to facilitate pronunciation of the term. Take, for example, the word *gastroenterology*:

gastr/o/enter/o/logy

The combining vowel **o** is inserted after the root words **gastr** and **enter**, both of which end in a consonant, to make pronunciation of the term easier. The combining vowels do not change the meanings of the root words.

Some medical terms do not contain a combining vowel. The word *gastrectomy* is an example. It is composed of a root word and a suffix:

gastr/ectomy

General Rules for Use of Combining Vowels

Following are a few general rules concerning the use of combining vowels in medical terms.

1. A combining vowel is not used between a prefix and a root word (a/pnea) or a prefix combined with a suffix (quadri/plegic).
2. A combining vowel may be used between two root words (electr/o/cardi/o/gram) or between a root word and a suffix (angi/o/plasty).
3. The combining vowel is usually the letter **o**. In some medical terms, however, the combining vowel may be **a**, **e**, **i**, or **u**.

Suffixes

A **suffix** is a single letter or group of letters added to the end of a prefix, root word, or combining form. A suffix modifies the meaning of the word part to which it is added. When written by itself, a suffix is preceded by a hyphen.

Following is an example of the way in which a suffix modifies the word part to which it is added. In this example, the suffix is attached to a root word.

Word Part	Type of Word Part	Meaning of Word Part
muscul/o	combining form	muscle
-ar	suffix	pertaining to

muscul/o + ar = muscular

The term *muscular* means "pertaining to muscle."

Suffixes modify medical terms by denoting information about diseases or abnormal conditions, surgical procedures, diagnostic procedures, medical specialties, or healthcare specialties and practitioners. Suffixes are not associated with one particular body system or medical specialty; as you will see, the same suffixes are used in many medical terms. In addition, different suffixes may have the same meaning. For example, the suffixes **-ac**, **-al**, **-ar**, and **-ary** all mean "pertaining to." Not all medical terms have a suffix.

Following are some common suffixes used in medical terminology.

Suffixes Associated with Diseases and Disorders

Suffix	Meaning
-ac	pertaining to
-al	pertaining to
-algia	pain
-cele	hernia; swelling; protrusion
-ectasis	dilatation; dilation; expansion
-edema	swelling
-emia	blood condition
-ia	condition
-iasis	abnormal condition
-itis	inflammation
-malacia	softening
-megaly	large; enlargement
-oma	tumor; mass
-osis	abnormal condition
-pathy	disease
-penia	deficiency; abnormal reduction
-rrhexis	rupture
-trophy	development

Suffixes Associated with Diagnostic Procedures

Suffix	Meaning
-gram	record; image
-graph	instrument used to record an image
-graphy	process of recording an image
-meter	instrument used to measure
-metry	process of measuring
-scope	instrument used to observe
-scopy	process of observing

Suffixes Associated with Surgical Procedures

Suffix	Meaning
-centesis	surgical puncture (to remove fluid)
-ectomy	surgical removal; excision
-lysis	breakdown; loosening; dissolving
-pexy	surgical fixation
-plasty	surgical repair
-rrhaphy	suture
-stomy	new opening (created surgically)
-tomy	incision; cut into
-tripsy	crushing

General Rules for Use of Suffixes

Following are some general rules concerning the use of suffixes in medical terms.

1. **If a suffix begins with a consonant:** Insert a combining vowel between the root word and the suffix.

   Examples:

   A. The term *melanocyte* is made up of the root word melan (which means "black") and the suffix -cyte (which means "cell"). The suffix -cyte begins with a consonant; therefore, we insert a combining vowel between the root word and the suffix:

   $$melan/o/cyte = \text{cell that is black (black cell)}$$

   B. The term *colonoscopy* consists of the root word colon ("large intestine or colon") and the suffix -scopy ("process of observing"). The suffix -scopy begins with a consonant, so we insert a combining vowel between the root word and the suffix:

   $$colon/o/scopy = \text{process of observing the large intestine or colon}$$

   C. The term *pathologist* consists of the root word path ("disease") and the suffix -logist ("specialist in the study and treatment of"). The suffix -logist begins with a consonant, so a combining vowel is inserted between the root word and the suffix:

   $$path/o/logist = \text{specialist in the study and treatment of disease}$$

2. **If a suffix begins with a vowel:** Attach the suffix directly to the root word. A combining vowel is not needed.

   Examples:

   A. The term *onychosis* is made up of the root word onych (which means "nail") and the suffix -osis (which means "abnormal condition").

The suffix -osis begins with a vowel; therefore, a combining vowel does not need to be added. The suffix is attached directly to the root word:

onych/osis = abnormal condition of a nail

B. The term *melanoma* consists of the root word melan ("black") and the suffix -oma ("tumor or mass"). Because the suffix -oma begins with a vowel, we attach it to the suffix without inserting a combining vowel:

melan/oma = tumor that is black (black tumor)

C. The medical term *bronchitis* consists of the root word bronch ("bronchial tube or bronchus") and the suffix -itis ("inflammation"). The suffix -itis begins with a vowel, so it is attached directly to the suffix:

bronch/itis = inflammation of the bronchial tube or bronchus

Breaking Down and Building Medical Terms

You have learned the process of analyzing the parts of a medical term to decode its meaning. You have learned that prefixes, combining forms (root words plus combining vowels), and suffixes are meaningful word parts in medical terminology. Whether you want to understand television shows with medical content, comprehend what your doctor is saying to you, or prepare for a career in the healthcare field, the ability to recognize and understand these word parts is key to mastering medical terminology.

Once you have mastered the meanings of the medical word parts presented throughout this textbook, you will have the ability to understand a vast number of medical terms. Medical terminology is logical and systematic: Simply by analyzing and breaking down a term into the word parts that comprise it, you can decode the meaning of a medical term that you have never seen or heard before.

Breaking Down Medical Terms: Summary of Steps

When you encounter an unfamiliar medical term, don't panic. You can decode the meaning of any medical term by following these simple steps:

1. Divide the medical term into its word parts: prefix, combining form(s), and suffix.

2. Define each word part.

3. Arrange the word parts in the correct order. Begin with the suffix; then go back to the beginning of the term and work your way across to figure out its meaning.

Break It Down

Directions: Study the prefixes, combining forms, and suffixes in the charts that follow until you are familiar with each word part and its meaning. Then do the exercise that appears after the charts.

Prefix	Meaning
brady-	slow
endo-	within
epi-	upon
para-	near; beside
supra-	above
tachy-	fast

Combining Form (Root Word plus Combining Vowel)	Meaning
cardi/o	heart
dermat/o	skin
gastr/o	stomach
myc/o	fungus
neur/o	nerve
ophthalm/o	eye
pharyng/o	throat

Suffix	Meaning
-al	pertaining to
-ia	condition
-ic	pertaining to
-itis	inflammation
-logist	specialist in the study and treatment of
-logy	study of
-tic	pertaining to

Break It Down

Directions: Using the prefixes, combining forms, and suffixes shown on the preceding page, dissect each medical term into its component word parts. Write the meaning of each word part in the blanks provided. If a term does not contain a combining vowel, write "None." Finally, write the definition of each term.

Medical Term	Prefix	Root Word	Combining Vowel	Suffix
1. cardiologist		cardi	o	logist

Definition: specialist in the study and treatment of the heart

2. ophthalmology		ophthalm	o	logy

Definition: study of the eye

3. paraneural	para	neur	None	al

Definition: pertaining to the area near the nerves

4. epigastric	epi	gastr	None	ic

Definition: pertaining to the area upon the stomach

5. suprapharyngeal	supra	pharyng	None	eal

Definition: pertaining to the area above the throat

6. bradycardia	brady	card	None	ia

Definition: condition of a slow heartbeat

Medical Term	Prefix	Root Word	Combining Vowel	Suffix
7. endocarditis	endo	card	None	itis

Definition: inflammation of the inner layer of the heart

Medical Term	Prefix	Root Word	Combining Vowel	Suffix
8. tachycardia	tachy	card	None	ia

Definition: condition of a fast heartbeat

Medical Term	Prefix	Root Word	Combining Vowel	Suffix
9. dermatology		dermat	o	logy

Definition: study of the skin

Medical Term	Prefix	Root Word	Combining Vowel	Suffix
10. mycotic		myc	o	tic

Definition: pertaining to fungus

SCORECARD: How Did You Do?

Number correct (_____), divided by 10 (_____), multiplied by 100 equals _____ (your score)

Building Medical Terms: Summary of Steps

The process of building a medical term is almost the reverse of breaking it down. You can construct any medical term by following these steps:

1. Choose the word parts (prefix, root word or words, and suffix) that you need to build the medical term.
2. Place the word parts in the correct order.
3. Remember that the first word in the definition of a medical term usually is its suffix.

Build It

Directions: Study the prefixes, combining forms, and suffixes in the charts that follow until you are familiar with each word part and its meaning. Then do the exercise that appears after the charts.

Prefix	Meaning
intra-	within
peri-	around
poly-	many

Combining Form (Root Word plus Combining Vowel)	Meaning
aden/o	gland
angi/o	blood vessel
cardi/o	heart
crani/o	skull
dermat/o	skin
enter/o	intestines (usually the small intestine)
gastr/o	stomach
neur/o	nerve
pulmon/o	lung

Suffix	Meaning
-al	pertaining to
-asthenia	weakness
-ectomy	surgical removal; excision
-gram	record; image
-itis	inflammation
-logist	specialist in the study and treatment of
-logy	study of
-oma	tumor; mass
-tomy	incision; cut into

Build It

Directions: Build medical terms using the prefixes, combining forms, and suffixes shown on the preceding page. Fill in each blank with a word part that matches each definition provided. Use the key directly below as a guide to completing this exercise.

P (Prefixes) = Green
RW (Root Words) = Red
S (Suffixes) = Blue
CV (Combining Vowel) = Purple

1. surgical removal or excision of a blood vessel

angi	ectomy
RW	S

2. inflammation of the stomach

gastr	itis
RW	S

3. pertaining to around the heart

peri	cardi	al
P	RW	S

4. record of blood vessels

angi	o	gram
RW	CV	S

5. specialist in the study and treatment of the stomach and intestines

gastr	o	enter	o	logist
RW	CV	RW	CV	S

6. tumor of the gland

aden	oma
RW	S

7. inflammation of many nerves

poly	neur	itis
P	RW	S

8. specialist in the study and treatment of the skin

dermat	o	logist
RW	CV	S

9. incision to the skull

crani	o	tomy
RW	CV	S

10. inflammation of the skin

dermat	itis
RW	S

11. pertaining to within the skull

intra	crani	al
P	RW	S

12. weakness of the nerve

neur	asthenia
RW	S

13. study of the lung

pulmon	o	logy
RW	CV	S

14. specialist in the study and treatment of the heart

cardi	o	logist
RW	CV	S

SCORECARD: How Did You Do?

Number correct (_____), divided by 14 (_____), multiplied by 100 equals _____ (your score)

Building Plural Forms

As you have learned, most medical terms are composed of Latin or Greek word parts; therefore, some of the rules for building plural nouns in medical terminology differ from those in everyday English. You will, however, notice some similarities because many words in the English language have retained their original Latin and Greek forms. Whenever you are in doubt about how to represent the plural form of a medical term, consult a medical dictionary.

Following are some general rules for changing a singular noun to a plural noun in medical terminology.

General Rules for Building Plurals	Examples	
	Singular	Plural
1. If the noun ends in **s**, add **es**.	sinus virus	sinuses viruses
2. If the noun ends in **a**, add **e**.	pleura vertebra	pleurae vertebrae
3. If the noun ends in **ax**, drop the **x** and add **ces**.	anthrax thorax	anthraces thoraces
4. If the noun ends in **ex**, drop the **ex** and add **ices**.	cortex index	cortices indices
5. If the noun ends in **is**, drop the **is** and add **es**.	diagnosis metastasis	diagnoses metastases
6. If the noun ends in **ix**, drop the **x** and add **ces**.	appendix helix	appendices helices
7. If the noun ends in **ma**, add **ta**.	sarcoma stigma	sarcomata stigmata
8. If the noun ends in **on**, drop the **on** and add **a**.	ganglion spermatozoon	ganglia spermatozoa
9. If the noun ends in **um**, drop the **um** and add **a**.	bacterium ovum	bacteria ova
10. If the noun ends in **us**, drop the **us** and add **i**.	alveolus fungus	alveoli fungi
11. If the noun ends in **x**, drop the **x** and add **ges**.	larynx phalanx	larynges phalanges
12. If the noun ends in **y**, drop the **y** and add **ies**.	biopsy deformity	biopsies deformities

Building Plural Forms

Directions: Fill in each blank with the missing singular or plural form of the medical term.

1. bursa   bursae
2. diverticulum   diverticula
3. adenoma   adenomata
4. ganglion   ganglia
5. index   indices
6. diagnosis   diagnoses
7. alveolus   alveoli
8. bacterium   bacteria
9. bronchus   bronchi
10. phalanx   phalanges
11. nucleus   nuclei
12. apex   apices

SCORECARD: How Did You Do?

Number correct (_____), divided by 12 (_____), multiplied by 100 equals _____ (your score)

Pronouncing Medical Terms

Throughout this textbook, a phonetic spelling (pronunciation) is provided in parentheses for each new medical term that is introduced. Each pronunciation contains diacritical marks, or accent marks. These diacritical marks appear above vowels and provide guidance in pronouncing the vowel sounds in a term. The **macron** (ˉ), for example, is used to indicate a long vowel sound (ā, ē, ī, ō, ū). The **breve** (˘) is used to indicate a short vowel sound (ă, ĕ, ĭ, ŏ, ŭ). Nearly all vowel sounds in the medical terms presented in this textbook are shown with diacritical marks. The only exception is terms that contain the **r**-controlled vowel sound "**or**." There is only one way to pronounce this **r**-controlled vowel sound; therefore, a diacritical mark does not appear above the "**o**," as illustrated in the following examples:

anteroposterior	(ĂN-tĕr-ō-pōs-TĒR-ē-or)
oropharynx	(or-ō-phăr-ĭngks)
osteoporosis	(ŎS-tē-ō-por-Ō-sĭs)

Besides diacritical marks, which indicate the correct way to pronounce the vowel sounds in a medical term, uppercase and lowercase letters are used in phonetic spellings to show syllabic emphasis. A syllable represented in uppercase letters indicates primary emphasis on that syllable. A syllable represented in lowercase letters indicates lack of emphasis on that syllable. For the purposes of this introductory textbook, no distinction is made between primary and secondary syllabic emphasis.

Take, for example, the medical term *osteoporosis*. The pronunciation of this term is as follows:

ŎS	tē	ō	por	Ō	sĭs

Uppercase letter =				Uppercase letter =	
Syllable is emphasized				Syllable is emphasized	
during pronunciation.				during pronunciation.	

Pronunciation of medical terms may seem challenging at first, but with practice, your skill and confidence will grow. When you encounter a new medical term, the acts of reading it, writing it, and pronouncing it correctly will help you form an accurate visual and aural memory for the term.

To hear the correct pronunciations of key medical terms throughout this book, visit the Medical Terminology Companion Website (www.g-wlearning.com/healthsciences).

The ability to pronounce medical terms correctly is not only essential to effective communication in the medical profession but also crucial to patient safety and care. Medical terms are often difficult to pronounce; however, the rules for pronunciation, like the rules for building plural forms, are fairly systematic.

There are 26 letters in the alphabet that in various combinations produce 60 different sounds. Certain letter combinations and vocal sounds are attributed to letters based on their placement within a medical term, as illustrated below.

General Rules of Medical Terminology Pronunciation	Examples
1. In the letter combinations **ae**, **nd**, and **oe**, the second vowel is pronounced.	bursae roentgen
2. The letter combination **ch** is sometimes pronounced like the letter **k**.	cholera
3. When the letter combination **pn** appears at the beginning of a medical term, the **p** is silent; only the **n** is pronounced.	pneumonia
4. When the letter combination **pn** appears in the middle of a medical term, both letters are pronounced.	dyspnea
5. When the letter combination **ps** appears at the beginning of a medical term, the **p** is silent; only the **s** is pronounced.	psychology
6. When the letter **i** appears at the end of a medical term, it has the "long i" vowel sound as in *eye*. Note: Some terms that end in **i** may also be pronounced with the variant "long e" vowel sound. When in doubt about the correct pronunciation of a term, consult a medical dictionary.	bronchi
7. When **e** and **es** are the final letter(s) of a medical term, the letter(s) are pronounced as separate syllables.	syncope nares

For guidance in pronouncing medical terms, the best resource is a medical dictionary.

Spelling Medical Terms

Correct spelling of medical terms is very important. A spelling error that changes just one or two letters can change the entire meaning of a term. Some medical terms are spelled similarly but have very different meanings, for example, **arteriosclerosis** and **atherosclerosis**. The first term, *arteriosclerosis*, means "hardening of the arteries." The second term, *atherosclerosis*, means "accumulation of fatty plaques within blood vessels."

As a professional in the medical community, you will enter information into patients' electronic health records on a daily basis. Correctly spelled medical terms are critical to patient care. Furthermore, chart notes, history and physical examination reports, operative reports, and other types of health records are considered legal documents. Therefore, accuracy is essential.

Overview of Anatomical Positions, Planes, Directions, and Locations

Healthcare professionals use specific terms to describe anatomical positions, directions, and locations. These terms are important for a variety of reasons. Before a patient undergoes surgery, for example, the doctor must accurately record the precise location of the part of the body on which the surgical procedure is to be performed.

In this section, we will briefly explore key terms used by medical professionals to communicate information about anatomical positions, planes, directions, and locations.

Anatomical Position

When describing body positions or using directional terms, healthcare professionals visualize the patient in anatomical position, the standard frame of reference for communicating information about positions, planes, directions, and locations in the human body.

In **anatomical position**, a person is standing upright with the legs together, feet pointing forward, arms at the sides, palms facing forward, and head facing forward (Figure 1.2). When you view the patient from the anatomical position, everything that you "see" makes up the **anterior** (**ventral**) or *front surface* of the body. When the patient turns around, what you see is the **posterior** (**dorsal**) or *back surface* of the body.

The terms *anterior* and *ventral* are synonyms that mean "the front of the body." Likewise, the terms *posterior* and *dorsal* are synonyms that mean "the back of the body." *Anterior/ventral* is the opposite of *posterior/dorsal*.

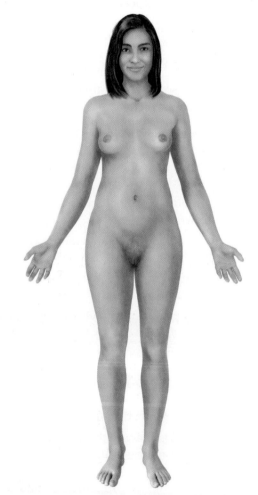

Figure 1.2 Anatomical position

Anatomical position is a reference point that must be remembered. It is the point of origin for understanding anatomical positions, planes, directions, and locations.

Anatomical Planes

In biology and medicine, the human body is divided into imaginary planes or sections that are used as reference points when describing body parts and organs. The human body can be divided into sections along three different planes: the frontal plane (also called the *coronal plane*), the sagittal plane, and the transverse plane.

The **sagittal plane** divides the body into left and right sections. A **midsagittal plane** or *median plane* divides the body into equal right and left halves (Figure 1.3).

The **frontal plane** or *coronal plane* divides the body into front (*anterior/ventral*) and back (*posterior/dorsal*) sections (Figure 1.4).

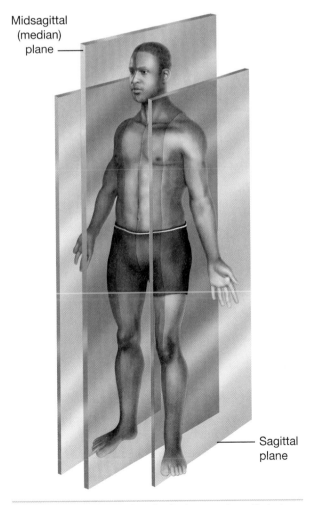

Figure 1.3 Midsagittal (median) plane and sagittal plane

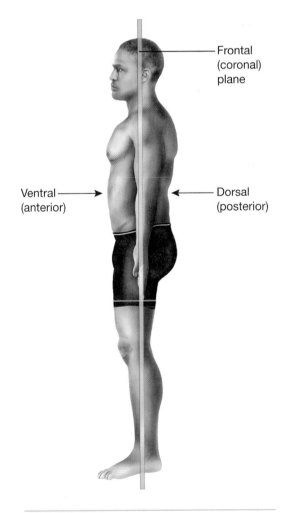

Figure 1.4 Frontal or coronal plane

The **transverse plane** divides the body into upper (*superior*) and lower (*inferior*) sections (Figure 1.5).

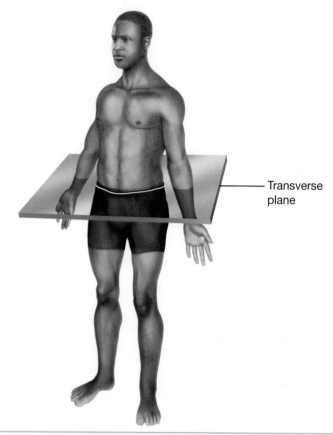
Transverse plane

Figure 1.5 Transverse plane

Anatomical Planes

Directions: Match the term with its correct definition.

Anatomical Plane

__C__	1. frontal plane
__F__	2. median plane
__D__	3. midsagittal plane
__E__	4. transverse plane
__A__	5. sagittal plane
__B__	6. coronal plane

Definition

A. divides the body into left and right sections

B. another term for *frontal plane*

C. divides the body into front (anterior/ventral) and back (posterior/dorsal) sections

D. divides the body into equal right and left halves

E. divides the body into upper (superior) and lower (inferior) sections

F. another term for *midsagittal plane*

SCORECARD: How Did You Do?

Number correct (_____), divided by 6 (_____), multiplied by 100 equals _____ (your score)

Terms of Position and Direction

In medical terminology, specific terms are used to describe the relative position of the body or of one body part in relation to another. Terms of position and direction are always based on anatomical position.

Just as road signs indicate the direction of a route (north, south, east, or west), directional terms in anatomy and physiology and in medical terminology often occur in pairs and generally have opposite meanings.

Common terms of position and direction are described in the table below and illustrated in Figures 1.6, 1.7, 1.8, and 1.9 on the pages that follow.

Term of Position or Direction	Definition
anterior	front of the body; ventral
anteroposterior	passing from the anterior (front) of the body to the posterior (rear)
caudal	toward the tailbone
cephalic	toward the head
distal	away from the point of origin
dorsal	back of the body; posterior
external	outer part of the body
inferior	body part located below another part or closer to the feet
internal	deep within the body
lateral	toward the side of the body
medial	toward the midline of the body
posterior	toward the back of the body
posteroanterior	passing from the posterior (rear) of the body to the anterior (front)
prone	lying face down with the palms facing downward
proximal	closer to the point of origin
superior	body part located above another part or closer to the head
supine	lying on the back with the palms facing upward
ventral	front of the body; anterior

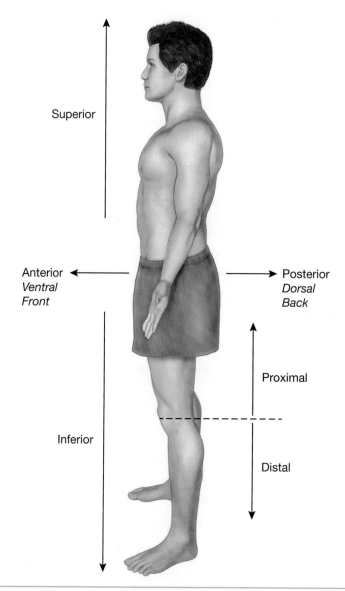

Figure 1.6 Superior/inferior, anterior/posterior, and proximal/distal views of human anatomy

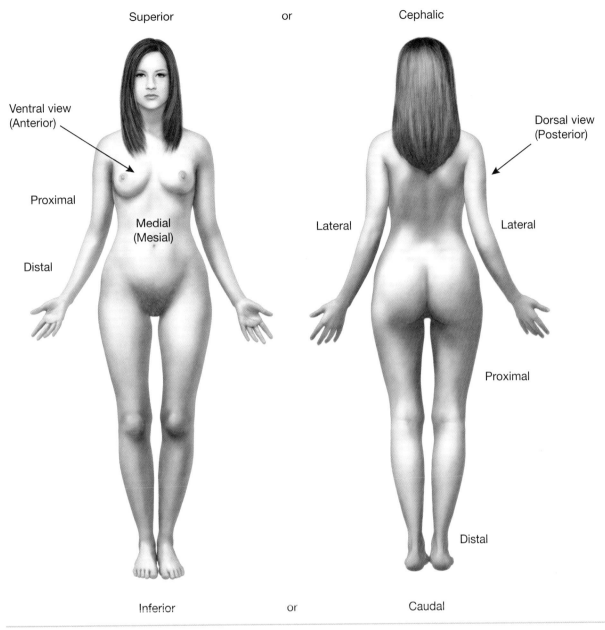

Figure 1.7 Major views of human anatomy

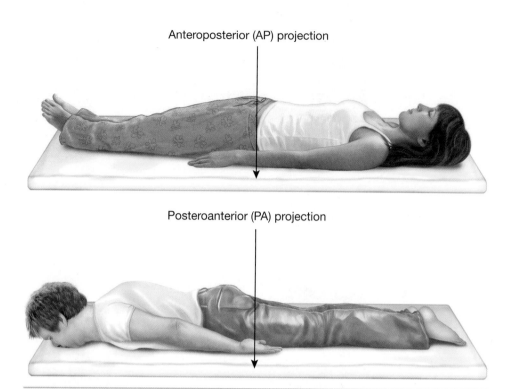

Anteroposterior (AP) projection

Posteroanterior (PA) projection

Figure 1.8 Superior/inferior, anterior/posterior, and proximal/distal views of human anatomy

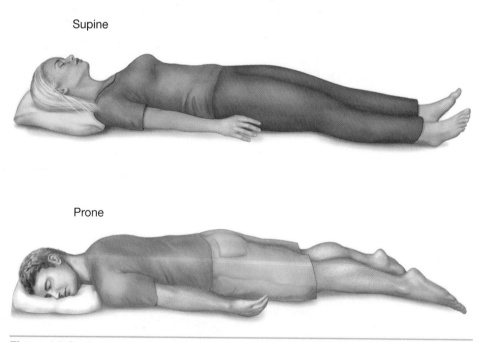

Supine

Prone

Figure 1.9 Supine and prone positions

Terms of Position and Direction

Directions: Match each term of position or direction with its definition.

Term of Position or Direction

__B__ 1. external
__I__ 2. prone
__Q__ 3. lateral
__K__ 4. superior
__D__ 5. anterior
__A__ 6. posteroanterior
__M__ 7. caudal
__L__ 8. ventral
__N__ 9. medial
__H__ 10. distal
__P__ 11. supine
__C__ 12. cephalic
__E__ 13. proximal
__J__ 14. dorsal
__R__ 15. anteroposterior
__G__ 16. internal
__O__ 17. posterior
__F__ 18. inferior

Definition

A. passing from the posterior (rear) of the body to the anterior (front)

B. outer part of the body

C. toward the head

D. front of the body; ventral

E. closer to the point of origin

F. body part located below another part or closer to the feet

G. deep within the body

H. away from the point of origin

I. lying face down with the palms facing downward

J. back of the body; posterior

K. body part located above another part or closer to the head

L. front of the body; anterior

M. toward the tailbone

N. toward the midline of the body

O. back of the body; dorsal

P. lying on the back with the palms facing upward

Q. toward the side of the body

R. passing from the anterior (front) of the body to the posterior (rear)

SCORECARD: How Did You Do?

Number correct (_____), divided by 18 (_____), multiplied by 100 equals _____ (your score)

Body Cavities

Body cavities protect and support internal organs (Figure 1.10). The human body contains two major cavities: the **dorsal cavity**, located posteriorly, and the **ventral cavity**, located anteriorly.

The dorsal cavity is subdivided into the **cranial cavity**, which contains the brain, and the **spinal cavity**, which contains the spinal cord. The spinal cavity is also called the *vertebral cavity*.

The ventral cavity is subdivided into the **thoracic** (chest) **cavity** and the **abdominopelvic cavity**. Because the abdominopelvic cavity is large, it is often subdivided into the **abdominal cavity** and the **pelvic cavity**.

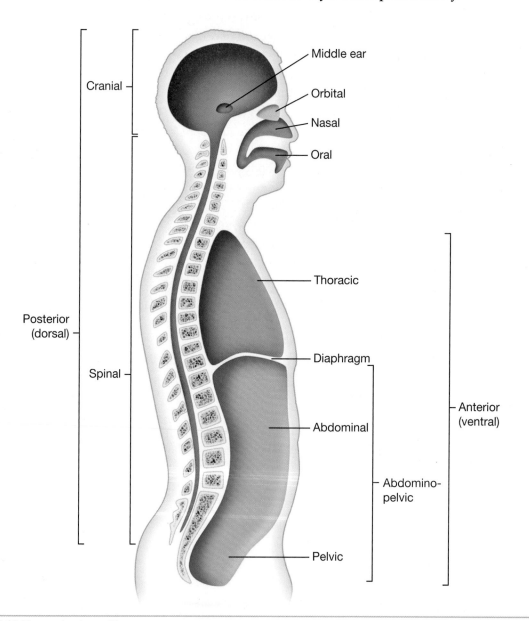

Figure 1.10 Human body cavities

Body Cavities

Directions: Match the term for each body cavity with its definition.

Body Cavity Term	*Definition*
_F_ 1. abdominopelvic cavity	A. the part of the dorsal cavity that contains the brain
_G_ 2. ventral cavity	
_E_ 3. thoracic cavity	B. one of the two major body cavities; located posteriorly
_B_ 4. dorsal cavity	C. the part of the dorsal cavity that contains the spine
_A_ 5. cranial cavity	
_C_ 6. spinal cavity	D. another term for the spinal cavity
_D_ 7. vertebral cavity	E. chest cavity; part of the ventral cavity
	F. the part of the ventral cavity that contains the abdominal and pelvic cavities
	G. one of the two major body cavities; located anteriorly

SCORECARD: How Did You Do?

Number correct (_____), divided by 7 (_____), multiplied by 100 equals _____ (your score)

Abdominopelvic Cavity: Quadrants

Because the abdominopelvic cavity is large, it is divided according to one of two systems: quadrants or regions. In the first system, the abdominopelvic cavity is divided into four quadrants (Figure 1.11). These four quadrants consist of the **left upper quadrant (LUQ)**, the **right upper quadrant (RUQ)**, the **left lower quadrant (LLQ)**, and the **right lower quadrant (RLQ)**. These directional terms refer to the left and right sides of the patient's body, not the perspective of the person viewing it. The quadrant system is used by healthcare professionals because the precise location of internal organs and structures varies from one patient to another.

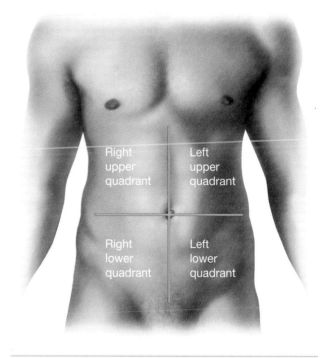

Figure 1.11 Four quadrants of the abdomen

Abdominopelvic Cavity: Regions

In the second, more detailed system of anatomical division, the abdominopelvic cavity is divided into nine regions that resemble the sections of a Tic-Tac-Toe grid (Figure 1.12). The nine regions include the **right and left hypochondriac regions**, the **epigastric region**, the **right and left lumbar regions**, the **umbilical region**, the **right and left inguinal** (or *iliac*) **regions**, and the **hypogastric region**. This method of dividing the abdominopelvic cavity is preferred by anatomists because of its more detailed precision.

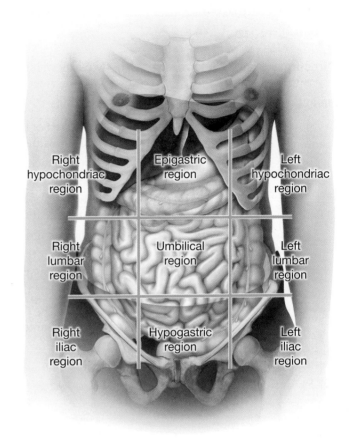

Right hypochondriac region

Epigastric region

Left hypochondriac region

Right lumbar region

Umbilical region

Left lumbar region

Right iliac region

Hypogastric region

Left iliac region

Figure 1.12 Nine regions of the abdomen

Common Medical Abbreviations for Anatomical Terms of Position, Direction, and Location

The following abbreviations are commonly used in place of medical terms that describe anatomical position, direction, and location.

Term	Abbreviation
anterior	Ant
anteroposterior	AP
inferior	Inf
lateral	Lat
left lower quadrant	LLQ
left upper quadrant	LUQ

(Continued)

Term	Abbreviation
medial	Med
posterior	Post
posteroanterior	PA
right lower quadrant	RLQ
right upper quadrant	RUQ
superior	Sup

Common Medical Abbreviations for Anatomical Terms of Position, Direction, and Location

Directions: Write the medical term that corresponds to each abbreviation.

1. Ant   anterior
2. LUQ   left upper quadrant
3. AP   anteroposterior
4. Inf   inferior
5. RUQ   right upper quadrant
6. Lat   lateral
7. Med   medial
8. LLQ   left lower quadrant
9. Post   posterior
10. PA   posteroanterior
11. RLQ   right lower quadrant
12. Sup   superior

Number correct (_____), divided by 12 (_____), multiplied by 100 equals _____ (your score)

Body Systems

From the most basic unit of matter—the microscopic atom—to the intricate architecture of the body systems, human anatomy is wondrously complex. There are eleven major organ systems in the body, each with its own specific function (Figure 1.13 on the next page). Some of these systems function complementarily to maintain homeostasis (a state of internal balance—a concept that will be discussed in a bit more detail later in this book).

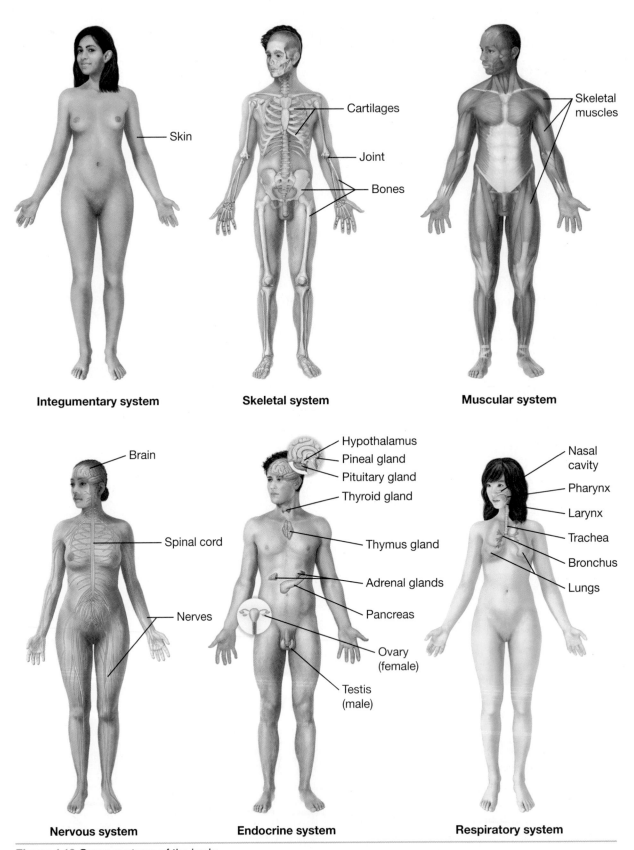

Integumentary system

Skeletal system

Muscular system

Nervous system

Endocrine system

Respiratory system

Skin

Cartilages

Joint

Bones

Skeletal muscles

Brain

Spinal cord

Nerves

Hypothalamus
Pineal gland
Pituitary gland
Thyroid gland
Thymus gland
Adrenal glands
Pancreas
Ovary
(female)
Testis
(male)

Nasal cavity
Pharynx
Larynx
Trachea
Bronchus
Lungs

Figure 1.13 Organ systems of the body

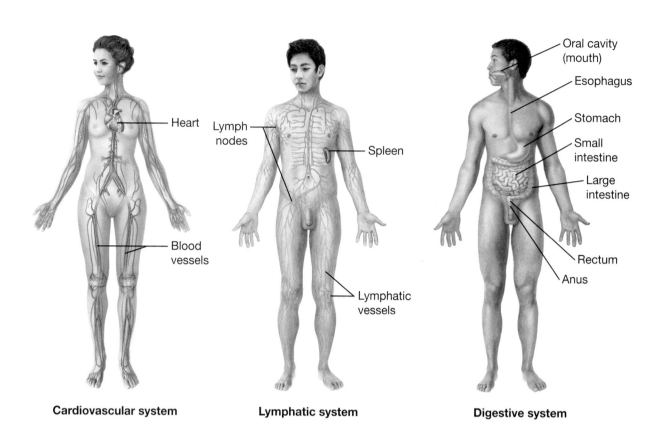

Cardiovascular system

Heart

Blood vessels

Lymphatic system

Lymph nodes

Spleen

Lymphatic vessels

Digestive system

Oral cavity (mouth)

Esophagus

Stomach

Small intestine

Large intestine

Rectum

Anus

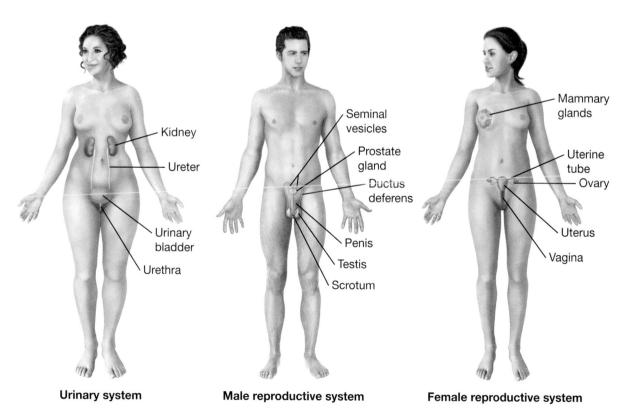

Urinary system

Kidney

Ureter

Urinary bladder

Urethra

Male reproductive system

Seminal vesicles

Prostate gland

Ductus deferens

Penis

Testis

Scrotum

Female reproductive system

Mammary glands

Uterine tube

Ovary

Uterus

Vagina

NOTE: In this textbook, medical terminology pertaining to the muscular and skeletal systems has been combined into one chapter titled *The Musculoskeletal System*. In addition, a separate chapter has been included on the special sensory organs of vision and hearing.

Mastering Medical Terminology

Congratulations! You have completed this chapter and are now ready to learn medical terms relating to the different body systems.

As you are aware, mastery of medical terminology requires memorization of word parts (prefixes, root words, and suffixes) and their meanings. Knowing the meanings of these word parts will enable you to break down and build medical terms that you do not know. You will find that as you gain mastery (which comes with practice, time, and patience), you will be able to rely less often on a dictionary to analyze medical terms and interpret their meanings.

Learning a lot of medical terms at once can be overwhelming. Following are some tips to help you study effectively, build mastery, and develop confidence in reading, writing, and speaking the language of medical terminology as you work your way through each chapter of this textbook.

1. Set aside time each day to review the key terms presented in the chapter. Listen to and practice the pronunciations of the terms. To hear the pronunciations of key terms, visit the Medical Terminology Companion Site (www.g-wlearning.com/healthsciences).

2. Don't wait until the last minute; spend time throughout the week studying the chapter material.

3. Practice with the e-Flash Card Activities at the companion website or mobile site. You can also make your own flash cards. Carry the flash cards with you wherever you go, and practice using them whenever you have a few free minutes.

4. Study regularly with a partner from your class, and take turns quizzing each other on the chapter material.

Chapter Review

More Practice: Activities and Games

The activities in this section will help you reinforce your skills and check your mastery of the material that you learned in this chapter. Visit the companion website for More Practice games and activities.

Identifying Anatomical Planes

Directions: Identify each anatomical plane below.

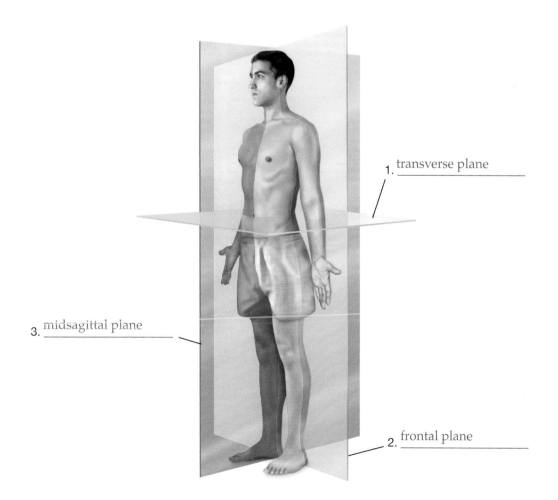

1. transverse plane

3. midsagittal plane

2. frontal plane

Major Views of Human Anatomy

Directions: Label each anatomical view in the diagram below.

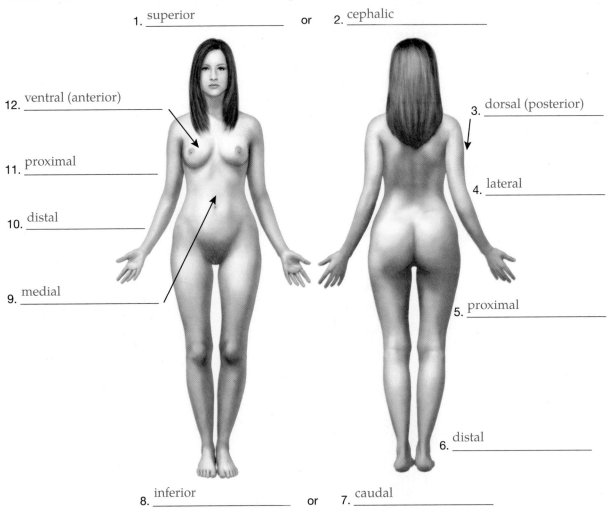

1. superior _____ or 2. cephalic _____

12. ventral (anterior) _____

11. proximal _____

10. distal _____

9. medial _____

3. dorsal (posterior) _____

4. lateral _____

5. proximal _____

6. distal _____

8. inferior _____ or 7. caudal _____

Identifying Prefixes

Directions: Match the prefix in column A with its correct meaning(s) in column B.

Column A

_E_	1.	para-
_C_	2.	epi-
_D_	3.	supra-
_F_	4.	brady-
_B_	5.	endo-
_A_	6.	tachy-

Column B

A. fast

B. within

C. upon

D. above

E. near; beside

F. slow

Identifying Suffixes

Directions: Read the definition of each medical term. For each term, choose the correct suffix from the Suffixes Chart on page 42 and write it on the blank line in the "Suffix" column. If a combining vowel is needed for a term, write it in the "Combining Vowel" space. Then build each medical term.

Definition	Root Word	Combining Vowel	Suffix	Build the Medical Term
1. pertaining to the esophagus	esophag		eal	esophageal
2. the study of the heart	cardi	o	logy	cardiology
3. rupture of a blood vessel	angi	o	rrhexis	angiorrhexis
4. cancerous tumor	carcin		oma	carcinoma
5. inflammation of the large intestine	col		itis	colitis
6. abnormal condition of the diverticulum	diverticul		osis	diverticulosis
7. pain in the stomach	gastr		algia	gastralgia
8. new surgical opening in the sigmoid colon	sigmoid		ostomy	sigmoidostomy
9. surgical removal of the thymus gland	thym		ectomy	thymectomy
10. specialist in the study and treatment of the skin	dermat	o	logist	dermatologist
11. instrument used to observe the joints	arthr	o	scope	arthroscope
12. weakness of the muscle	my		asthenia	myasthenia
13. disease of the bone	oste	o	pathy	osteopathy
14. record or image of the spinal cord	myel	o	gram	myelogram
15. new (surgical) opening in the trachea	trache	o	stomy	tracheostomy

Suffixes Chart

Suffix	Meaning
-al	pertaining to
-algia	pain
-asthenia	weakness
-eal	pertaining to
-ectomy	surgical removal; excision
-gram	record; image
-itis	inflammation
-logist	specialist in the study and treatment of
-logy	study of
-oma	tumor; mass
-osis	abnormal condition
-pathy	disease
-rrhexis	rupture
-scope	instrument used to observe
-scopy	process of observing
-stomy	new opening (created surgically)

Forming Plurals

Directions: For each medical term listed below, choose one of the endings to produce the correct plural form of each term. Write each plural form on the blanks provided.

a   ae   ata   ces   es   ges   i   ices   ies

1. diagnosis   diagnoses
2. vertebra   vertebrae
3. appendix   appendices
4. stigma   stigmata
5. spermatozoon   spermatozoa
6. sinus   sinuses
7. thorax   thoraces
8. bacterium   bacteria
9. adenoma   adenomata
10. ovum   ova
11. phalanx   phalanges
12. fungus   fungi
13. anomaly   anomalies

True or False

Directions: Indicate whether each statement below is true (T) or false (F).

True or False?

<u>T</u>   1. Many medical terms are formed from one or more word parts.

<u>T</u>   2. A suffix changes the meaning of a medical term.

<u>T</u>   3. Different suffixes may have the same meaning.

<u>F</u>   4. Every medical term must have a prefix.

<u>F</u>   5. If a suffix begins with a consonant, it must directly follow a root word; a combining vowel should not be inserted.

<u>T</u>   6. A prefix always appears at the beginning of a medical term.

<u>F</u>   7. All medical terms are formed from word parts such as prefixes, root words, combining forms, and suffixes.

<u>F</u>   8. Prefixes are used only in medical terms that pertain to body systems.

<u>F</u>   9. All medical terms contain at least two root words.

<u>F</u>   10. All medical terms contain a combining vowel.

<u>T</u>   11. A spelling error can change the meaning of a medical term.

<u>F</u>   12. Diacritical marks are placed above consonants to aid in pronouncing them.

<u>F</u>   13. When a patient lies flat on her back with her palms facing upward, she is in the prone position.

<u>F</u>   14. The human body can be divided into sections along four different planes.

<u>F</u>   15. The coronal plane divides the body into equal right and left halves.

<u>T</u>   16. Terms of body position and direction are always based on anatomical position.

<u>F</u>   17. For anatomical purposes, the human body can be divided into ten regions.

<u>F</u>   18. There are five major cavities in the human body.

<u>T</u>   19. When combined, the abdominal cavity and the pelvic cavity are referred to as the *abdominopelvic cavity*.

<u>T</u>   20. The integumentary system consists of the skin, hair follicles, nails, sweat glands, and sebaceous glands.

Chapter 2
The Integumentary System

dermat / o / logy: the study of the skin

Chapter Organization

- Intern Experience
- Overview of Integumentary System Anatomy and Physiology
- Word Elements
- Breaking Down and Building Integumentary System Terms
- Diseases and Disorders
- Tests, Procedures, and Treatments
- Analyzing the Intern Experience
- Working with Medical Records
- Chapter Review

Chapter Objectives

After completing this chapter, you will be able to

1. label an anatomical diagram of the integumentary system;
2. dissect and define common medical terminology related to the integumentary system;
3. build terms used to describe integumentary system diseases and disorders, diagnostic tests and procedures, and therapeutic treatments;
4. pronounce and spell common medical terminology related to the integumentary system;
5. understand that the processes of building and dissecting a medical term based on its prefix, word root, and suffix enable you to analyze an extremely large number of medical terms beyond those presented in this chapter;
6. interpret the meaning of abbreviations associated with the integumentary system; and
7. interpret medical records containing terminology and abbreviations related to the integumentary system.

You will see this icon [icon] at various points throughout this chapter. The icon indicates that you will find interactive activities and games on the Medical Terminology Companion Website. These activities and games will help you learn, practice, and expand your medical terminology knowledge and skills. Some of these activities are also available on the Medical Terminology Mobile Website.

Companion Website
www.g-wlearning.com/healthsciences

Mobile Site
www.m.g-wlearning.com/5800

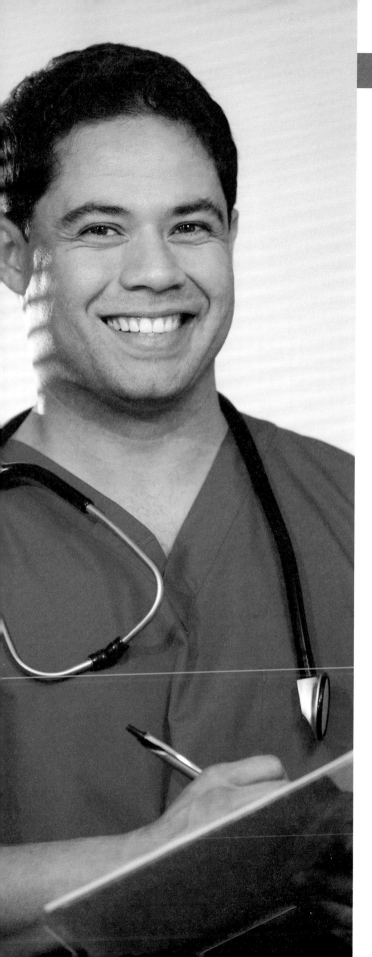

Intern Experience

Adrián Hernandez, an intern with Dr. Gaskins' office, meets Kate and one of her friends in examination room 1. Adrián learns that Kate and several of her friends, all members of the local high school lacrosse team, were watching a movie on TV, eating pizza, and painting their nails when Kate noticed redness and swelling in her right big toe, thickness and discoloration in the toenail, and pus around the nail. Her friends became nervous. With the prom only two weeks away, they persuaded Kate to go to the clinic.

Kate is experiencing a problem with her integumentary system, the body system that consists of the skin and related structures, including the nails, sweat and sebaceous glands, and hair. To help you understand what's happening to Kate, this chapter will present word elements (combining forms, prefixes, and suffixes) that make up medical terminology related to the integumentary system. As you continue to read, you will see many word parts that are also used in medical terms related to other body systems.

Before you begin this chapter, take some time to review the strategies presented in chapter 1 for analyzing medical terms. Reviewing these strategies will help you understand and recall the word elements and definitions of the terms that you are about to learn.

After you have learned the medical terminology presented in this chapter, you will practice analyzing medical records, commonly known as *patient chart notes*. Accurate interpretation of these chart notes will demonstrate that you have a solid understanding of medical terminology related to the integumentary system.

Let's begin our study with a brief overview of integumentary system anatomy and physiology.

Overview of Integumentary System Anatomy and Physiology

The **integumentary** (ĭn-TĔG-yū-MĔN-tă-rē) system is the body system made up of the skin, hair, nails, sweat glands, and oil-secreting glands. The word *integumentary* comes from the Latin *integumentum*, which means "covering." The skin covers the entire body and is the largest organ of the body. The skin and accessory structures of the integumentary system—the hair, nails, sweat glands, and oil-secreting glands—protect us from the external environment by preventing harmful substances from entering our bodies.

The sweat glands, called **sudoriferous** (sū-dō-RĬF-ĕr-ŭs) glands, cool the body by secreting perspiration, or sweat. The oil-secreting **sebaceous** (sĕ-BĀ-shŭs) glands produce an oily substance called **sebum** (SĒ-bŭm), which lubricates the skin, keeping it soft and supple.

The skin is our first line of defense against microorganisms that cause infection or disease, the ultraviolet (UV) rays of the sun, and harmful chemicals. The skin also protects internal body structures from injuries caused by blows, cuts, and burns. The terms **cutaneous** (kyŭ-TĀ-nē-ŭs) and **dermal** (DĔR-măl) are synonyms that both mean "pertaining to the skin." Although the integumentary system performs many different functions, its primary role is that of protection.

Main Functions of the Integumentary System

The primary functions of the integumentary system are to
1. protect the body by serving as a physical barrier between the internal organs and the external environment. The integumentary system protects us from pathogenic (disease-causing) microorganisms, harmful chemicals, the UV rays of the sun, and bodily harm due to physical trauma. It keeps harmful substances out of the body and helps prevents fluid loss by retaining water and electrolytes;
2. produce vitamin D, which is necessary for the absorption of calcium in the intestines;
3. regulate body temperature through blood vessels and sweat glands; and
4. provide sensory information to the brain about pain, pressure, touch, texture, and temperature through nerve receptors in the skin.

Major Structures of the Integumentary System

We mentioned that the skin—which includes the hair, nails, sweat and sebaceous glands, as well as specialized nerve receptors—is the most extensive organ system of the body. Figure 2.1 shows the two layers that make up the skin: the outer layer, or **epidermis** (ĕp-ĭ-DĔR-mĭs), and the inner layer, or dermis.

The epidermis is composed of epithelial (ĕp-ĭ-THĒ-lē-ăl) tissue, membranous tissue that covers the surface of the body, and does not contain blood vessels.

Within the epidermis are **melanocytes** (MĔL-ăn-ō-sīts), specialized cells responsible for the production of a pigment called **melanin** (MĔL-ă-nĭn). Melanin may be black, dark brown, or reddish-brown. Our skin color is determined primarily by the amount of melanin produced by melanocytes. The darker the skin, the greater the concentration of melanin.

Beneath the epidermis is the **dermis**, sometimes referred to as the "true skin" because most of the essential functions of the skin are performed within this layer. The dermis is thicker than the epidermis, is made of connective tissue, and contains blood vessels. Beneath the dermis is the **subcutaneous** (sŭb-kyū-TĀ-nē-ŭs) layer, which contains adipose (fat) tissue that provides insulation to the body (Figure 2.1).

Dermatology (dĕr-mă-TŎL-ō-jē) is the study of the skin and related structures. A **dermatologist** (dĕr-mă-TŎL-ō-jĭst) is a physician who specializes in the study and treatment of the skin and related structures.

Dermatologists commonly **biopsy** (BĪ-ŏp-sē) skin tissue (that is, remove the tissue for microscopic examination) and send the specimen to a **pathologist** (pă-THŎL-ō-jĭst). A pathologist is a physician who specializes in the study, diagnosis, and treatment of disease through the examination of cells, tissues, and bodily fluids. The pathologist examines the specimen to determine the **etiology** (ē-tē-ŎL-ō-jē), or cause, of a disease. The pathologist's report is correlated with the clinical findings of the dermatologist. Then a diagnosis, treatment plan, and **prognosis** (expected outcome) are determined.

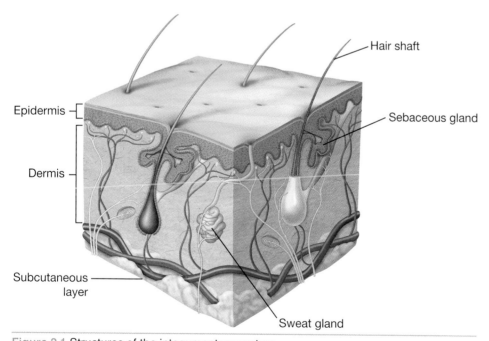

Figure 2.1 Structures of the integumentary system

Anatomy and Physiology Vocabulary

Now that you have been introduced to the basic structure and functions of the integumentary system, let's explore in more detail the key terms presented in the introduction.

Key Term	Definition
biopsy	removal of tissue for microscopic examination
cutaneous	pertaining to the skin
dermal	pertaining to the skin, especially the dermis
dermatologist	physician who specializes in the study and treatment of the skin and related structures
dermatology	study of the skin and related structures
dermis	the layer of skin beneath the epidermis; the "true skin"
epidermis	the outer layer of the skin
etiology	cause of a disease or disorder
integumentary	pertaining to the skin, which covers the body
melanin	black pigment that is primarily responsible for skin color
melanocytes	specialized cells in the epidermis that produce skin pigment
pathologist	physician who specializes in the study, diagnosis, and treatment of disease
prognosis	expected outcome
sebaceous	pertaining to oil
sebum	oily substance secreted by the sebaceous glands
subcutaneous	beneath the skin (pertaining to the layer of skin that lies below the dermis)
sudoriferous	pertaining to the sweat glands

E-Flash Card Activity: Anatomy and Physiology Vocabulary

Directions: After you have reviewed the anatomy and physiology vocabulary related to the integumentary system, practice with the e-flash cards until you are comfortable with the spelling and definition of each term.

Identifying Major Structures of the Integumentary System

Directions: Label the diagram of the integumentary system.

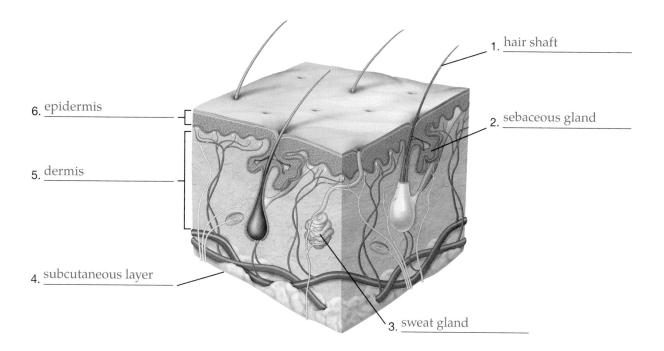

1. hair shaft

6. epidermis

2. sebaceous gland

5. dermis

4. subcutaneous layer

3. sweat gland

SCORECARD: How Did You Do?

Number correct (_____), divided by 6 (_____), multiplied by 100 equals _____ (your score)

Matching Anatomy and Physiology Vocabulary

Directions: Match the vocabulary term in Column A with its meaning in Column B. Some meanings may be used more than once.

Column A

- __N__ 1. dermatologist
- __I__ 2. melanin
- __E__ 3. dermis
- __G__ 4. prognosis
- __D__ 5. biopsy
- __H__ 6. etiology
- __J__ 7. sebum
- __C__ 8. epidermis
- __L__ 9. sudoriferous
- __A__ 10. cutaneous
- __A__ 11. dermal
- __K__ 12. sebaceous
- __M__ 13. subcutaneous
- __F__ 14. integumentary
- __B__ 15. dermatology
- __O__ 16. pathologist
- __P__ 17. melanocytes

Column B

A. pertaining to the skin

B. the study of the skin and related structures

C. the outer layer of the skin

D. removal of tissue for microscopic examination

E. the layer of skin beneath the epidermis; the "true skin"

F. pertaining to the skin, which covers the body

G. expected outcome

H. cause of a disease or disorder

I. black pigment primarily responsible for skin color

J. oily substance secreted by the sebaceous glands

K. pertaining to oil

L. pertaining to the sweat glands

M. beneath the skin (below the dermis)

N. physician who specializes in the study and treatment of the skin and related structures

O. physician who specializes in the study, diagnosis, and treatment of disease

P. specialized cells in the epidermis that produce skin pigment

SCORECARD: How Did You Do?

Number correct (_____), divided by 17 (_____), multiplied by 100 equals _____ (your score)

Word Elements

In this section you will learn word elements—prefixes, combining forms, and suffixes—that are common to the integumentary system. By learning these word parts and understanding how they are combined to build medical terms, you will be able to analyze Kate's skin problem (described in the Intern Experience at the beginning of this chapter) and identify a large number of terms associated with the integumentary system.

E-Flash Card Activity: Word Elements

Directions: Review the word elements in the tables that follow. Then, practice with the e-flash cards until you are able to quickly recognize the different word parts (prefixes, combining forms, and suffixes) and their meanings. The e-flash cards are grouped together by prefixes, combining forms, and suffixes, followed by a cumulative review of all the word elements that you learned in this chapter.

Prefixes

Let's start our study of integumentary system word elements by looking at the prefixes listed in the table below. These prefixes appear not only in medical terms related to the integumentary system but also in many terms pertaining to other body systems.

Prefix	Meaning
epi-	upon
hypo-	below; below normal
intra-	within
per-	through
sub-	beneath; below
trans-	across

Combining Forms

Listed below are common combining forms used in medical terms related to the integumentary system. As you will discover, some of these combining forms are used in medical terms related to other body systems as well.

Root Word/Combining Vowel	Meaning
carcin/o	cancer
cry/o	cold
contus/o	bruising
cutane/o	skin
cyan/o	blue
cyst/o	sac containing fluid
derm/a, derm/o, dermat/o	skin
ecchym/o	blood in the tissues
erythemat/o	redness
erythr/o	red
hemat/o	blood
lip/o	fat
malign/o	causing harm, cancer
melan/o	black

(Continued)

Root Word/Combining Vowel	Meaning
myc/o	fungus
necr/o	death
onych/o	nail
path/o	disease
prurit/o	itching
py/o	pus
schiz/o	split
seb/o	oil or sebum
squam/o	scale-like
topic/o	place
trich/o	hair
xer/o	dry

Suffixes

Listed below are suffixes used in medical terms pertaining to the integumentary system. You will also encounter these suffixes in your study of terms related to other body systems.

Suffix	Meaning
-al	pertaining to
-ancy	state of
-cyte	cell
-ectomy	surgical removal; excision
-gen	producing; originating; causing
-ia	condition
-ic	pertaining to
-ion	condition
-itis	inflammation
-logist	specialist in the study and treatment of
-logy	study of
-oid	like; resembling
-oma	tumor; mass
-osis	abnormal condition
-ous	pertaining to
-rrhea	flow; discharge
-tic	pertaining to
-tomy	incision; cut into

Matching Prefixes, Combining Forms, and Suffixes

Directions: In each exercise below, match the word element in Column A with its meaning in Column B. Some meanings may be used more than once.

Prefixes

Column A

F___ 1. per-
D___ 2. epi-
A___ 3. trans-
E___ 4. sub-
C___ 5. hypo-
B___ 6. intra-

Column B

A. across
B. within
C. below; below normal
D. upon
E. beneath; below
F. through

Combining Forms

Column A

C___ 1. schiz/o
J___ 2. melan/o
Q___ 3. cyan/o
A___ 4. malign/o
B___ 5. xer/o
S___ 6. carcin/o
N___ 7. myc/o
I___ 8. prurit/o
H___ 9. trich/o
L___ 10. topic/o
M___ 11. seb/o
K___ 12. cry/o
F___ 13. derm/a, derm/o, dermat/o
W___ 14. erythemat/o
F___ 15. cutane/o
P___ 16. py/o
D___ 17. lip/o
G___ 18. squam/o
X___ 19. ecchym/o
U___ 20. contus/o

Column B

A. causing harm, cancer
B. dry
C. split
D. fat
E. nail
F. skin
G. scale-like
H. hair
I. itching
J. black
K. cold
L. place
M. oil or sebum
N. fungus
P. pus
Q. blue
R. death
S. cancer
T. red
U. bruising

E	21. onych/o	V. blood
T	22. erythr/o	W. redness
R	23. necr/o	X. blood in the tissues
V	24. hemat/o	Y. sac containing fluid
Y	25. cyst/o	Z. disease
Z	26. path/o	

Suffixes

Column A

A	1. -al
K	2. -cyte
J	3. -rrhea
C	4. -ectomy
A	5. -tic
G	6. -ia
A	7. -ic
F	8. -itis
B	9. -logist
I	10. -logy
E	11. -oid
H	12. -oma
N	13. -tomy
D	14. -ancy
G	15. -ion
A	16. -ous
L	17. -gen
M	18. -osis

Column B

A. pertaining to

B. specialist in the study and treatment of

C. surgical removal; excision

D. state of

E. like; resembling

F. inflammation

G. condition

H. tumor; mass

I. study of

J. flow; discharge

K. cell

L. producing; originating; causing

M. abnormal condition

N. incision; cut into

SCORECARD: How Did You Do?

Number correct (_____), divided by 50 (_____), multiplied by 50 equals _____ (your score)

Breaking Down and Building Integumentary System Terms

You are now able to dissect and build medical terms pertaining to the integumentary system. Whether you merely want to understand TV shows with medical content, interpret what your doctor is saying to you, or prepare for a career in healthcare, the ability to recognize the prefixes, combining forms, and suffixes used in medical terms is essential. In fact, having a solid grasp of these medical word parts gives you the ability to figure out the definitions of an enormous number of medical terms. Simply by breaking down a word into its prefix, combining form(s), and suffix, you can determine the meaning of a medical term that you have never seen before.

Below are some common medical terms related to the integumentary system. For each term, a dissection has been provided, along with the meaning of each word part and the definition of the term as a whole.

Term	Dissection	Word Part/Meaning	Term Definition
Note: *For simplification, combining vowels have been omitted from the Word Part/Meaning column.*			
1. **contusion** (kŏn-TŪ-zhŭn)	contus/ion	**contus** = bruising **ion** = condition	condition of bruising
2. **cyanodermal** (SĪ-ă-nō-DĔR-măl)	cyan/o/derm/al	**cyan** = blue **derma** = skin **al** = pertaining to	pertaining to blue skin
3. **cyanosis** (sī-ă-NŌ-sĭs)	cyan/osis	**cyan** = blue **osis** = abnormal condition	abnormal condition of blue
4. **cystic** (SĬS-tĭk)	cyst/ic	**cyst** = sac containing fluid **ic** = pertaining to	pertaining to a sac containing fluid
5. **dermal** (DĔR-măl)	derm/al	**derm** = skin **al** = pertaining to	pertaining to the skin
6. **dermatitis** (DĔR-mă-TĪ-tĭs)	dermat/itis	**dermat** = skin **itis** = inflammation	inflammation of the skin
7. **dermatologist** (DĔR-mă-TŎL-ō-jĭst)	dermat/o/logist	**dermat** = skin **logist** = specialist in the study and treatment of	specialist in the study and treatment of the skin
8. **dermatology** (DĔR-mă-TŎL-ō-jē)	dermat/o/logy	**dermat** = skin **logy** = study of	study of the skin
9. **ecchymosis** (ĕk-ĭ-MŌ-sĭs)	ecchym/osis	**ecchym** = blood in the tissues **osis** = abnormal condition	abnormal condition of blood in the tissues
10. **epidermis*** (ĕp-ĭ-DĔR-mĭs)	epi/dermis	**epi** = upon **dermis** = skin	upon the skin
11. **epidermal** (ĕp-ĭ-DĔR-măl)	epi/derm/al	**epi** = upon **derm** = skin **al** = pertaining to	pertaining to upon the skin
12. **erythematous** (ĕr-ĭ-THĔM-ă-tŭs)	erythemat/ous	**erythemat** = redness **ous** = pertaining to	pertaining to redness of the skin
Prefixes = **Green** Root Words = **Red** Suffixes = **Blue**			

*The term *epidermis* is made up of the prefix *epi-* and an unusual blending of the Greek word *derma*, which means "skin," and the Latin word *cutis*, which means "surface layer of the skin."

Term	Dissection	Word Part/Meaning	Term Definition
13. **erythrodermal** (ĕ-RĬTH-rō-DĔR-măl)	erythr/o/derm/al	**erythr** = red **derm** = skin **al** = pertaining to	pertaining to red skin
14. **hematoma** (hēm-ă-TŌ-mă)	hemat/oma	**hemat** = blood **oma** = tumor; mass	tumor/mass of blood
15. **hypodermic** (hī-pō-DĔR-mĭk)	hypo/derm/ic	**hypo** = below **derm** = skin **ic** = pertaining to	pertaining to below the skin
16. **intradermal** (ĭn-tră-DĔR-măl)	intra/derm/al	**intra** = within **derm** = skin **al** = pertaining to	pertaining to within the skin
17. **lipocyte** (LĬP-ō-sīt)	lip/o/cyte	**lip** = fat **cyte** = cell	fat cell
18. **lipoid** (LĬP-oyd)	lip/oid	**lip** = fat **oid** = like; resembling	like or resembling fat
19. **lipoma** (lĭ-PŌ-mă)	lip/oma	**lip** = fat **oma** = tumor; mass	tumor/mass of fat
20. **malignancy** (mă-LĬG-năn-sē)	malign/ancy	**malign** = causing harm, cancer **ancy** = state of	state of cancer
21. **melanocyte** (MĔL-ăn-ō-sīt)	melan/o/cyte	**melan** = black **cyte** = cell	black cell
22. **melanoma** (mĕl-ă-NŌ-mă)	melan/oma	**melan** = black **oma** = tumor; mass	black tumor
23. **mycotic** (mī-KŎT-ĭk)	myc/o/tic	**myc** = fungus **tic** = pertaining to	pertaining to fungus
24. **necrotic** (nĕ-KRŎT-ĭk)	necr/o/tic	**necr** = death **tic** = pertaining to	pertaining to death
25. **onychectomy** (ŏn-ĭ-KĔK-tō-mē)	onych/ectomy	**onych** = nail **ectomy** = surgical removal; excision	excision of the nail (of a finger or toe)
26. **onychoma** (ŏn-ĭ-KŌ-mă)	onych/oma	**onych** = nail **oma** = tumor; mass	tumor of the nail
27. **onychomycosis** (ŎN-ĭ-kō-mī-KŌ-sĭs)	onych/o/myc/osis	**onych** = nail **myc** = fungus **osis** = abnormal condition	abnormal condition of nail fungus
28. **onychosis** (ŏn-ĭ-KŌ-sĭs)	onych/osis	**onych** = nail **osis** = abnormal condition	abnormal condition of the nail
29. **onychotomy** (ŏn-ĭ-KŎT-ō-mē)	onych/o/tomy	**onych** = nail **tomy** = incision; cut into	incision/cut into the nail

Prefixes = Green   Root Words = Red   Suffixes = Blue

Term	Dissection	Word Part/Meaning	Term Definition
30. **pathologist** (pă-THŎL-ō-jĭst)	path/o/logist	path = disease logist = specialist in the study, diagnosis, and treatment of	specialist in the study, diagnosis, and treatment of disease
31. **percutaneous** (pĕr-kyū-TĀ-nē-ŭs)	per/cutane/ous	per = through cutane = skin ous = pertaining to	pertaining to through the skin
32. **pruritic** (prū-RĬT-ĭk)	prurit/ic	prurit = itching ic = pertaining to	pertaining to itching
33. **pyogenic** (pī-ō-JĔN-ĭk)	py/o/gen/ic	py = pus gen = producing ic = pertaining to	pertaining to producing pus
34. **pyorrhea** (pī-ō-RĒ-ă)	py/o/rrhea	py = pus rrhea = flow; discharge	flow/discharge of pus
35. **schizotrichia** (skĭt-sō-TRĬK-ē-ă)	schiz/o/trich/ia	schiz = split trich = hair ia = condition	condition of split hair
36. **seborrhea** (sĕb-ō-RĒ-ă)	seb/o/rrhea	seb = sebum or oil rrhea = flow; discharge	flow/discharge of sebum or oil
37. **squamous** (SKWĀ-mŭs)	squam/ous	squam = scale-like ous = pertaining to	pertaining to scale-like
38. **subcutaneous** (sŭb-kyū-TĀ-nē-ŭs)	sub/cutane/ous	sub = beneath; below cutane = skin ous = pertaining to	pertaining to beneath the skin
39. **topical** (TŎP-ik-ăl)	topic/al	topic = place; location al = pertaining to	pertaining to location
40. **transdermal** (trans-DĔR-măl)	trans/derm/al	trans = across derm = skin al = pertaining to	pertaining to across the skin
41. **trichomycosis** (trĭk-ō-mī-KŌ-sĭs)	trich/o/myc/osis	trich = hair myc = fungus osis = abnormal condition	abnormal condition of fungus in the hair
42. **xeroderma** (zē-rō-DĔR-mă)	xer/o/derma	xer = dry derma = skin	dry skin

Prefixes = Green   Root Words = Red   Suffixes = Blue

Using the pronunciation guide in the Breaking Down and Building chart, practice saying each medical term aloud. To hear the pronunciation of each term, go to the Pronounce It activity at the G-W companion website.

Studying medical terminology is similar to learning a foreign language. At first, pronouncing new medical terms can be challenging. To develop fluency, it is necessary to practice pronouncing the terms until you are comfortable saying them aloud.

Audio Activity: Pronounce It

Directions: At the companion website, listen as each of the following medical terms is pronounced. Practice pronouncing the terms until you are comfortable saying them aloud.

contusion
(kŏn-TŪ-zhŭn)

cyanodermal
(SĪ-ă-nō-DĔR-măl)

cyanosis
(sī-ă-NŌ-sĭs)

cystic
(SĬS-tĭk)

dermal
(DĔR-măl)

dermatitis
(DĔR-mă-TĪ-tĭs)

dermatologist
(DĔR-mă-TŎL-ō-jĭst)

dermatology
(DĔR-mă-TŎL-ō-jē)

ecchymosis
(ĕk-ĭ-MŌ-sĭs)

epidermis
(ĕp-ĭ-DĔR-mĭs)

epidermal
(ĕp-ĭ-DĔR-măl)

erythematous
(ĕr-ĭ-THĔM-ă-tŭs)

erythrodermal
(ĕ-RĬTH-rō-DĔR-măl)

hematoma
(hēm-ă-TŌ-mă)

hypodermic
(hī-pō-DĔR-mĭk)

intradermal
(ĭn-tră-DĔR-măl)

lipocyte
(LĬP-ō-sīt)

lipoid
(LĬP-oyd)

lipoma
(lĭ-PŌ-mă)

malignancy
(mă-LĬG-năn-sē)

melanocyte
(MĔL-ăn-ō-sīt)

melanoma
(mĕl-ă-NŌ-mă)

mycotic
(mī-KŎT-ĭk)

necrotic
(nĕ-KRŎT-ĭk)

onychectomy
(ŏn-ĭ-KĔK-tō-mē)

onychoma
(ŏn-ĭ-KŌ-mă)

onychomycosis
(ŎN-ĭ-kō-mī-KŌ-sĭs)

onychosis
(ŏn-ĭ-KŌ-sĭs)

onychotomy
(ŏn-ĭ-KŎT-ō-mē)

pathologist
(pă-THŎL-ō-jĭst)

percutaneous
(pĕr-kyū-TĀ-nē-ŭs)

pruritic
(prū-RĬT-ĭk)

pyogenic
(pī-ō-JĔN-ĭk)

pyorrhea
(pī-ō-RĒ-ă)

schizotrichia
(skĭt-sō-TRĬK-ē-ă)

seborrhea
(sĕb-ō-RĒ-ă)

squamous
(SKWĀ-mŭs)

subcutaneous
(sŭb-kyū-TĀ-nē-ŭs)

topical
(TŎP-ik-ăl)

transdermal
(trans-DĔR-măl)

trichomycosis
(trĭk-ō-mī-KŌ-sĭs)

xeroderma
(zē-rō-DĔR-mă)

Audio Activity: Spell It

Directions: Cover the medical terms in the Pronounce It activity above with a sheet of paper. At the companion website, listen as the terms are read aloud. Correctly spell each term below.

1. contusion

2. cyanodermal

3. cyanosis

4. cystic

5. dermal

6. dermatitis

7. dermatologist

8. dermatology

9. ecchymosis _____
10. epidermis _____
11. epidermal _____
12. erythematous _____
13. erythrodermal _____
14. hematoma _____
15. hypodermic _____
16. intradermal _____
17. lipocyte _____
18. lipoid _____
19. lipoma _____
20. malignancy _____
21. melanocyte _____
22. melanoma _____
23. mycotic _____
24. necrotic _____
25. onychectomy _____

26. onychoma _____
27. onychomycosis _____
28. onychosis _____
29. onychotomy _____
30. pathologist _____
31. percutaneous _____
32. pruritic _____
33. pyogenic _____
34. pyorrhea _____
35. schizotrichia _____
36. seborrhea _____
37. squamous _____
38. subcutaneous _____
39. topical _____
40. transdermal _____
41. trichomycosis _____
42. xeroderma _____

Assessment

Break It Down

Directions: Dissect each medical term below into its word elements by placing a slash between each word part (prefix, root word, combining vowel, and suffix). Then define each term.

Example:

Medical Term: schizotrichia

Dissection: schiz/o/trich/ia

Definition: condition of split hair (ends)

Medical Term   **Dissection**

1. cyanodermal   c y a n/o/d e r m/a l

Definition: pertaining to blue skin _____

2. onychosis   o n y c h/o s i s

Definition: abnormal condition of the nail _____

Medical Term	Dissection

3. schizotrichia   s c h i z/o/t r i c h/i a

Definition: condition of split hair

4. ecchymosis   e c c h y m/o s i s

Definition: abnormal condition of blood in the tissues

5. lipocyte   l i p/o/c y t e

Definition: fat cell

6. contusion   c o n t u s/i o n

Definition: condition of bruising

7. erythematous   e r y t h e m a t/o u s

Definition: pertaining to redness of the skin

8. pyogenic   p y/o/g e n/i c

Definition: pertaining to producing pus

9. cyanosis   c y a n/o s i s

Definition: abnormal condition of blue

10. melanocyte   m e l a n/o/c y t e

Definition: black cell

Medical Term	Dissection
11. percutaneous	p e r / c u t a n e / o u s

Definition: pertaining to through the skin

| 12. onychectomy | o n y c h / e c t o m y |

Definition: excision of the nail

| 13. subcutaneous | s u b / c u t a n e / o u s |

Definition: pertaining to beneath the skin

| 14. cystic | c y s t / i c |

Definition: pertaining to a sac containing fluid

| 15. erythrodermal | e r y t h r / o / d e r m / a l |

Definition: pertaining to red skin

| 16. pathologist | p a t h / o / l o g i s t |

Definition: specialist in the study, diagnosis, and treatment of disease

| 17. lipoma | l i p / o m a |

Definition: tumor/mass of fat

| 18. onychomycosis | o n y c h / o / m y c / o s i s |

Definition: abnormal condition of nail fungus

Medical Term	Dissection

19. dermal

d e r m/a l

Definition: pertaining to the skin

---

20. xeroderma

x e r/o/d e r m a

Definition: dry skin

---

21. topical

t o p i c/a l

Definition: pertaining to location

---

22. dermatology

d e r m a t/o/l o g y

Definition: study of the skin

---

23. transdermal

t r a n s/d e r m/a l

Definition: pertaining to across the skin

---

24. hypodermic

h y p o/d e r m/i c

Definition: pertaining to below the skin

---

25. epidermis

e p i/d e r m i s

Definition: upon the skin

---

26. squamous

s q u a m/o u s

Definition: pertaining to scale-like

Medical Term	Dissection
27. malignancy	m a l i g n/a n c y

Definition: state of cancer

28. mycotic	m y c/o/t i c

Definition: pertaining to fungus

29. dermatitis	d e r m a t/i t i s

Definition: inflammation of the skin

30. onychotomy	o n y c h/o/t o m y

Definition: incision/cut into the nail

31. onychoma	o n y c h/o m a

Definition: tumor of the nail

32. pruritic	p r u r i t/i c

Definition: pertaining to itching

33. dermatologist	d e r m a t/o/l o g i s t

Definition: specialist in the study and treatment of the skin

34. intradermal	i n t r a/d e r m/a l

Definition: pertaining to within the skin

Medical Term	Dissection

35. necrotic n e c r / o / t i c

Definition: pertaining to death _____

_____

36. hematoma h e m a t / o m a

Definition: tumor/mass of blood _____

_____

37. epidermal e p i / d e r m / a l

Definition: pertaining to upon the skin _____

_____

38. melanoma m e l a n / o m a

Definition: black tumor _____

_____

39. seborrhea s e b / o / r r h e a

Definition: flow/discharge of sebum or oil _____

_____

40. lipoid l i p / o i d

Definition: like or resembling fat _____

_____

41. pyorrhea p y / o / r r h e a

Definition: flow/discharge of pus _____

_____

42. trichomycosis t r i c h / o / m y c / o s i s

Definition: abnormal condition of fungus in the hair _____

_____

SCORECARD: How Did You Do?

Number correct (_____), divided by 42 (_____), multiplied by 100 equals _____ (your score)

Build It

Directions: Build the medical terms that match the definitions provided below by supplying the correct word elements.

P (Prefixes) = Green
RW (Root Words) = Red
S (Suffixes) = Blue
CV (Combining Vowel) = Purple

1. pertaining to blue skin

cyan	o	derm	al
RW	CV	RW	S

2. specialist in the study, diagnosis, and treatment of disease

path	o	logist
RW	CV	S

3. fat cell

lip	o	cyte
RW	CV	S

4. pertaining to red skin

erythr	o	derm	al
RW	CV	RW	S

5. pertaining to through the skin

per	cutane	ous
P	RW	S

6. tumor of blood

hemat	oma
RW	S

7. pertaining to a sac containing fluid

cyst	ic
RW	S

8. condition of bruising

contus	ion
RW	S

9. pertaining to producing pus

py	o	gen	ic
RW	CV	S	S

10. condition of split hair

schiz	o	trich	ia
RW	CV	RW	S

11. inflammation of the skin

dermat	itis
RW	S

12. abnormal condition of nail fungus

onych	o	myc	osis
RW	CV	RW	S

13. pertaining to scale-like

squam	ous
RW	S

14. pertaining to below the skin (two possible answers)

hypo	derm	ic
P	RW	S

sub	cutane	ous
P	RW	S

15. flow or discharge of pus

py	o	rrhea
RW	CV	S

16. pertaining to the skin

derm	al
RW	S

17. black cell

melan	o	cyte
RW	CV	S

18. pertaining to upon the skin

epi	derm	al
P	RW	S

19. flow or discharge of sebum or oil

seb	o	rrhea
RW	CV	S

20. incision/cut into the nail

onych	o	tomy
RW	CV	S

21. specialist in the study and treatment of the skin

dermat	o	logist
RW	CV	S

22. pertaining to death

necr	o	tic
RW	CV	S

23. abnormal condition of blood in the tissues

ecchym	osis
RW	S

24. abnormal condition of fungus in the hair

trich	o	myc	osis
RW	CV	RW	S

25. upon the skin

epi	dermis
P	RW

26. tumor of fat

lip	oma
RW	S

27. pertaining to across the skin

trans	derm	al
P	RW	S

28. abnormal condition of blue

cyan	osis
RW	S

29. the study of the skin

dermat	o	logy
RW	CV	S

30. tumor of the nail

onych	oma
RW	S

31. pertaining to within the skin

intra	derm	al
P	RW	S

32. state of cancer

malign	ancy
RW	S

33. like or resembling fat

lip	oid
RW	S

34. pertaining to itching

prurit	ic
RW	S

35. pertaining to fungus

myc	o	tic
RW	CV	S

36. abnormal condition of the nail

onych	osis
RW	S

37. surgical removal/excision of the nail

onych	ectomy
RW	S

38. black tumor

melan	oma
RW	S

39. pertaining to place/location

topic	al
RW	S

40. dry skin

xer	o	derma
RW	CV	RW

Diseases and Disorders

Diseases and disorders of the integumentary system range from the mild to the severe, and they have a wide variety of causes. We will now take a look at some problems that commonly affect this body system.

Acne

Acne is a disorder that affects the sebaceous glands. It is most common during puberty when the sebaceous glands secrete large amounts of sebum, predominantly on the face, shoulders, and back.

Acne develops when excess sebum accumulates around the hair shaft and then hardens, blocking the hair follicle. Oily sebum traps dirt, enlarges the skin pore, and then turns black when exposed to air. The result is a *comedo*, or blackhead. A hardened white bump, or *whitehead*, appears when the pore becomes clogged with sebum that cannot reach the skin's surface. Bacteria may also invade the clogged pore, causing the formation of a small, infected skin elevation called a *pustule*. When the pustule becomes red and inflamed, it is called a *pimple* (Figure 2.3).

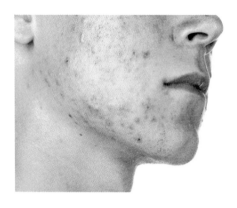

Suzanne Tucker/Shutterstock.com

Figure 2.3 Acne

Alopecia

Alopecia is an acute or chronic loss of scalp hair. Acute hair loss is usually a side effect of radiation or chemotherapy treatment in cancer patients. It can also be caused by a fungal infection or damage to the hair shaft or follicles.

There are two main forms of chronic hair loss. Chronic alopecia, also called *androgenetic alopecia,* is an inherited condition that typically begins during middle age and gradually worsens as a person gets older. Androgenetic alopecia is characterized by thinning of the hair on the top of the scalp; eventually, the hair disappears (Figure 2.4 on the next page). Hormonal changes in susceptible men and women may lead to alopecia, known as *male-pattern baldness* and *female-pattern baldness*. In some cases, a genetic predisposition may cause hair loss in men and women beginning in their twenties.

The second main form of chronic hair loss, *alopecia areata*, is caused by an autoimmune disorder. An autoimmune disorder is one in which the immune system of the body attacks its own tissues because it does not recognize and distinguish between that which is a normal part of the body (self) and a substance that is foreign to the body (non-self). In alopecia areata, the body's immune system attacks its own hair follicles, causing hair to fall out not only on the head but all over the body. (You will learn more about autoimmune disorders in Chapter 5: Lymphatic and Immune Systems.) Young children can be affected by alopecia areata.

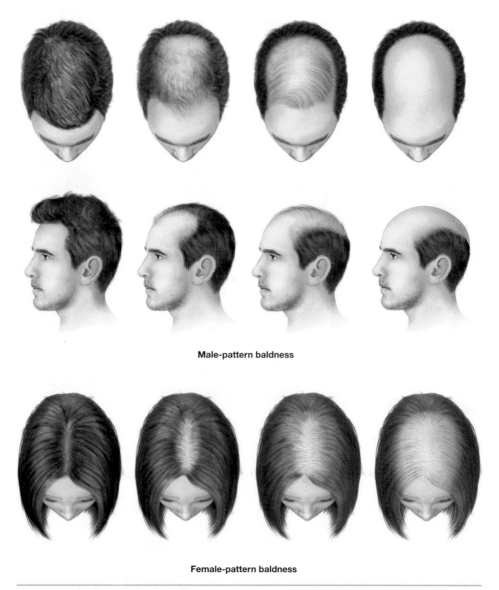

Male-pattern baldness

Female-pattern baldness

Figure 2.4 Androgenetic alopecia

Burns

Heat, electricity, chemicals, or radiation can cause burns to the skin. The severity of a burn is classified based on two factors: depth and extent of injury.

First-degree burns (Figure 2.5A) are mild burns that involve only the epidermis. They result in edema (swelling), pain, and **erythema** (ĕr-ĭ-THĒ-mă), or redness. Generally, however, first-degree burns do not produce scarring.

Second-degree burns (Figure 2.5B) extend through the epidermis and into the dermis, causing blisters, erythema, pain, edema, and sometimes scarring. A second-degree burn is also known as a *partial-thickness burn*.

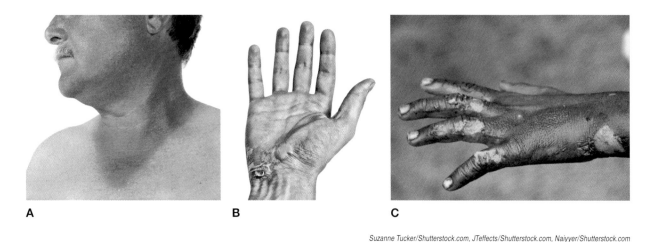

A   B   C

Figure 2.5 Different types of burns. A—First-degree burn. B—Second-degree burn. C—Third-degree burn.

Third-degree burns (Figure 2.5C) affect the epidermis, dermis, and sometimes the subcutaneous tissue and muscle. Third-degree burns, also called *full-thickness burns*, cause charred (black) skin and formation of a thick, crusty scar of necrotic tissue. Third-degree burns can become infected and delay healing, so they must be surgically removed.

Cancer of the Skin

Cancer is divided into two categories: **benign** (noncancerous) and **malignant** (causing cancer). **Malignant melanoma** is an aggressive form of skin cancer that originates in the melanocytes of the epidermis and quickly **metastasizes** (grows and spreads) to other parts of the body (Figure 2.6). Skin cancer can arise in areas that have been chronically exposed to the damaging ultraviolet light (UVA and UVB rays) of the sun.

People susceptible to UV damage include those with fair skin, which contains less melanin to absorb radiation, and the elderly, who have endured a lifetime of sunlight exposure. Regular self-examination of the skin, along with the use of sunscreen and avoidance of prolonged exposure to the sun, not only reduces damage to the skin but also helps prevent the development of skin cancer. Irregular changes in the color, shape, or size of skin moles or lesions should be examined by a dermatologist.

Contact Dermatitis

Contact dermatitis occurs when the skin comes in contact with an allergen or irritant, causing edema and pruritic (itchy) skin (Figure 2.7). Chemicals contained in deodorants,

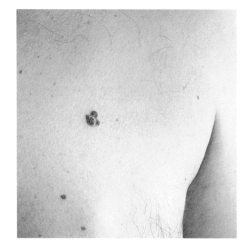

Figure 2.6 Skin cancer

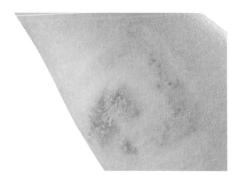

Figure 2.7 Contact dermatitis caused by exposure to poison ivy

soaps, perfumes, or makeup may cause the skin to become inflamed, red, and irritated. Small vesicles (fluid-filled sacs) may appear on the skin. Contact dermatitis may also be caused by exposure to animal dander, poison ivy, or synthetic products containing latex.

Edema

Edema comes from the Greek word *oidēma*, which means "swelling." This disorder is characterized by the buildup of excessive fluid in the body tissues, causing them to swell (Figure 2.8). Edema may result from large amounts of fluid moving from the blood into the dermis or subcutaneous tissues. Localized infections, allergic reactions, and some cardiovascular and urinary system diseases produce edema.

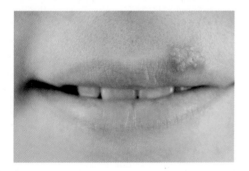

lekcej/Shutterstock.com

Figure 2.8 Edema

Herpes

Herpes comes from a Greek word meaning "to creep," an appropriate derivation given that this inflammatory disease is characterized by vesicles that appear to "creep" across the skin. Other symptoms include erythema, edema, and pain. Itching and soreness are usually present before the development of erythematous (ĕr-ĭ-THĔM-ă-tŭs) (red) patches. When the vesicles rupture, they release fluid that forms a crust.

The two most common types of herpes are herpes simplex and herpes zoster. **Herpes simplex** is caused by *herpes simplex virus 1* (HSV-1), which produces painful blisters on or around the lips (Figure 2.9). These blisters, commonly called *cold sores* or *fever blisters,* tend to recur during illness or stress. Topical or oral antiviral drugs are typically prescribed for herpes simplex.

Herpes zoster is an acute viral disease marked by inflammation of a nerve root, causing the appearance of painful blisters along the path of the nerve (Figure 2.10). Herpes zoster is more commonly called *shingles*. The herpes zoster virus is the same virus that causes chickenpox. The virus remains dormant in the nerves long after recovery from chickenpox, and it can become active due to stress or an immune system weakened with age.

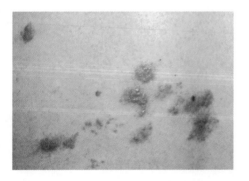

Levent Konuk/Shutterstock.com

Figure 2.9 Herpes simplex viral infection

Psoriasis

Psoriasis is a chronic skin disorder characterized by scaly, silvery-white patches and erythematous skin. The excessive production of epidermal cells associated with psoriasis is thought to be the result of an autoimmune disorder.

Stephen VanHorn/Shutterstock.com

Figure 2.10 Herpes zoster infection

The pruritic, erythematous, silvery scales and plaques (small, abnormal patches) caused by psoriasis usually appear on the scalp, elbows, hands, and knees (Figure 2.11). Psoriasis has a hereditary component, and the condition seems to worsen during physical, mental, or emotional stress. Because its etiology is unknown, there is no cure for psoriasis. Treatment consists of topical coal tar drugs, corticosteroid drugs, vitamin A and D supplements, and ultraviolet light therapy.

Procedures and Treatments

In this section, we will briefly describe some common diagnostic procedures used to help identify disorders and diseases of the integumentary system, as well as common therapeutic procedures used to treat certain conditions.

Biopsy

A **biopsy (Bx)** is a surgical procedure performed to remove all or part of a skin lesion for pathological evaluation (Figure 2.12). It may be performed using a knife, needle, brush, or punch (a sharp, round instrument). The biopsy specimen is sent to a laboratory, where a pathologist examines it under a microscope. The pathologist's findings are used to help make a diagnosis.

Figure 2.11 Psoriasis is characterized by pruritic, erythematous, silvery patches.

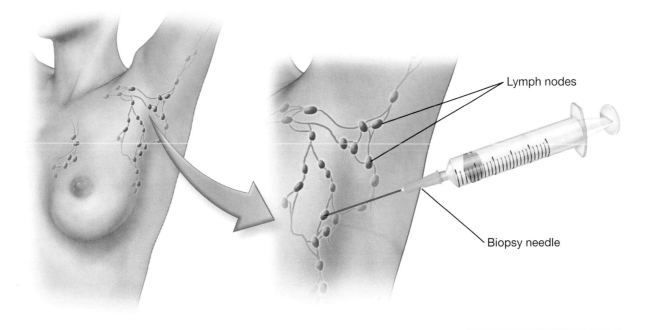

Lymph nodes

Biopsy needle

Figure 2.12 Needle biopsy

Cryosurgery

Cryosurgery is a technique in which liquid nitrogen, an extremely low-temperature fluid, is used to freeze and destroy abnormal skin cells or lesions (Figure 2.13). The nitrogen gas is applied directly to the tissue using an applicator, probe, or spray. This quick, simple, low-risk procedure can be performed in a doctor's office to freeze and destroy warts, moles, other benign lesions, or some small, malignant lesions.

Debridement

Debridement is a medical procedure in which damaged and necrotic tissue or foreign material is removed from a skin wound. Debridement of a wound prevents an infection from developing and helps the physician determine the depth and extent of the wound. Debridement is also used to remove thick, crusty, necrotic tissue that forms on a third-degree burn.

Incision and Drainage

Incision and drainage (I&D) is a dermatologic procedure commonly performed to treat a cyst or abscess. A scalpel or needle is used to puncture or cut the skin lesion above the cyst or abscess, which is then drained of fluid or pus.

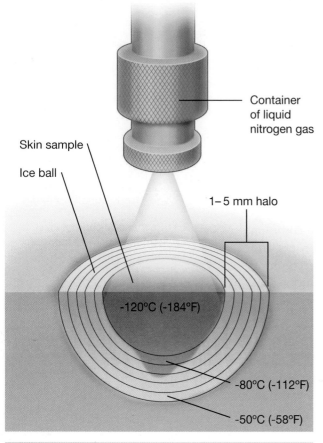

Container of liquid nitrogen gas

Skin sample

Ice ball

1– 5 mm halo

-120°C (-184°F)

-80°C (-112°F)

-50°C (-58°F)

Figure 2.13 Cryosurgery

Laser Surgery

A laser is a light beam that can be precisely focused on its target. It is used to treat diseased or damaged tissue by heating the targeted cells until they "burst."

Laser surgery is a medical procedure in which rapid pulses of light are used to remove diseased tissue or treat bleeding blood vessels. Laser surgery may also be used for cosmetic purposes, such as removing wrinkles, sunspots, birthmarks, tattoos, or enlarged blood vessels that are superficial (close to the skin's surface).

Onychectomy

An **onychectomy** is the surgical excision (removal) of a nail from a finger or toe. *Onychocryptosis* (ŎN-ĭ-kō-krĭp-TŌ-sĭs), more commonly known as an *ingrown toenail*, is a condition in which the nail grows into the soft flesh of the toe, causing pain, erythema, edema, and sometimes a fungal infection called *onychomycosis* (ŎN-ĭ-kō-mī-KŌ-sĭs). If the onychomycosis is unresponsive to treatment, the physician may recommend removing all or part of the nail plate.

Diseases, Disorders, Procedures, and Treatments

Directions: Define the disease, disorder, procedure, or treatment listed below.

1. biopsy a surgical procedure performed to remove all or part of a skin lesion for pathological evaluation

2. contact dermatitis a condition that occurs when the skin comes in contact with an allergen or irritant, causing edema and pruritic skin

3. malignant melanoma an aggressive form of skin cancer that originates in the melanocytes of the epidermis and quickly metastasizes to other parts of the body

4. cryosurgery a technique in which liquid nitrogen is used to freeze and destroy abnormal skin cells or lesions

5. edema a disorder characterized by the buildup of excessive fluid in the body tissues, causing them to swell

6. acne a disorder that affects the sebaceous glands

7. debridement a medical procedure in which damaged and necrotic tissue or foreign material is removed from a skin wound

8. onychectomy the surgical excision of a nail from a finger or toe

9. psoriasis a chronic skin disorder characterized by scaly, silvery-white patches and erythematous skin

10. alopecia an acute or chronic loss of scalp hair

11. laser surgery a medical procedure in which rapid pulses of light are used to remove diseased tissue or treat bleeding blood vessels

12. herpes an inflammatory disease characterized by vesicles that appear to "creep" across the skin

13. incision and drainage (I&D) <u>a dermatologic procedure commonly</u>
    <u>performed to treat a cyst or abscess</u>

14. first-degree burn <u>a mild burn that involves only the epidermis</u>

    _____

15. second-degree burn <u>a burn that extends through the epidermis into the</u>
    <u>dermis, causing blisters, erythema, pain, edema, and sometimes scarring</u>

    _____

16. third-degree burn <u>a burn that affects the epidermis, dermis, and</u>
    <u>sometimes the subcutaneous tissue and muscle</u>

    _____

SCORECARD: How Did You Do?

Number correct (_____), divided by 16 (_____), multiplied by 100 equals _____ (your score)

Identifying Abbreviations

Directions: Write the abbreviation for each medical term listed below.

Medical Term	Abbreviation
1. ultraviolet light	UVA and UVB
2. biopsy	Bx
3. herpes simplex virus 1	HSV-1
4. incision and drainage	I&D

SCORECARD: How Did You Do?

Number correct (_____), divided by 4 (_____), multiplied by 100 equals _____ (your score)

Analyzing the Intern Experience

As you know, all professionals in the healthcare field speak the same language—medical terminology. Patients come to the doctor's office with a variety of signs and symptoms that must be translated and communicated to other medical professionals using correct terminology. As a healthcare professional, you will be expected to pronounce, spell, write, and understand medical terms.

In the Intern Experience at the beginning of this chapter, Kate arrived at the doctor's office with specific signs and symptoms. Kate's doctor obtained a history of her health problems, performed a medical examination, and ordered a diagnostic test to help determine the cause of her condition. He analyzed all of this information, made a medical diagnosis, and formulated a treatment plan. The physician then made a dictated recording of Kate's health information, which was later transcribed into a medical record. In an outpatient setting, a medical record is commonly known as a *chart note*.

We will now analyze the Intern Experience scenario from a clinical perspective, interpreting the medical terms in Kate's chart note to gain an understanding of her health condition.

Audio Activity: Kate Stephano's Chart Note

Directions: At the companion website, listen and read along as the physician dictates Kate Stephano's chart note, shown below. Then do the exercise that appears after Kate's chart note.

CHART NOTE

Patient Name: Stephano, Kate
ID Number: 96453
Examination Date: January 23, 20xx

SUBJECTIVE
Kate was seen today for complaints of red and swollen, right great left toe. Patient denies injury. She is extremely anxious about the appearance of her toe.

OBJECTIVE
Examination reveals **erythematous** right great toe with purulent (pertaining to pus) drainage around the nail bed. The nail is thickened and appears to be **mycotic** in nature. It involves the entire nail plate.

ASSESSMENT
Onychomycosis

PLAN
Onychectomy. This is deferred due to patient anxiety and her desire to discuss this plan with her parents. Will follow up with phone call on how she wants to proceed.

Interpret Kate Stephano's Chart Note

Directions: After listening to the dictated recording and reading the chart note on Kate Stephano, provide the medical term that matches each definition below.

Example: condition of dry skin   *Answer:* xeroderma

1. pertaining to fungus
   mycotic

2. surgical removal/excision of the nail
   onychectomy

3. pertaining to redness of the skin
   erythematous

4. condition of nail fungus
   onychomycosis

SCORECARD: How Did You Do?

Number correct (_____), divided by 4 (_____), multiplied by 100 equals _____ (your score)

Working with Medical Records

In this activity, you will interpret the medical records (chart notes) of patients with health problems related to the integumentary system. These examples illustrate typical medical records prepared in a real-world healthcare environment. To interpret these chart notes, you will apply your knowledge of word elements (prefixes, combining forms, and suffixes), diseases and disorders, and procedures and treatments related to the integumentary system.

Audio Activity: Matthew Dixon's Chart Note

Directions: At the companion website, listen and read along as the physician dictates the following chart note on Matthew Dixon. Then do the exercise that appears after Matthew's chart note.

CHART NOTE

Patient Name: Dixon, Matthew
ID Number: 98651
Examination Date: February 16, 20xx

SUBJECTIVE
Patient presents with painful lump on right side of neck. Slight fever of 101°F, but denies any chills or sweating.

OBJECTIVE
There is an **erythematous** cystic lesion of the **epidermis** measuring 3×4 cm. The mass is fluctuant (movable and compressible) and slightly tender to the touch. No lymphadenomegaly (enlarged lymph glands) noted.

ASSESSMENT
Infected sebaceous cyst; right neck.

PLAN
Area was sterilely prepped and injected with 1% lidocaine (drug that numbs). A #11 scalpel blade was used to incise the **pyogenic** cyst. Copious amounts of purulent (pus-containing) material and sebum were extracted. Wound was irrigated with sterile saline solution and packed with ¼-inch gauze, and sterile dressing was applied. The **sebaceous** material was sent for culture. Prescribed cephalexin 250 mg q.i.d. × 10 days (take a 250 mg tablet of cephalexin, an antibiotic, 4 times per day for 10 days). Will return in 2 days for recheck.

Assessment

Interpret Matthew Dixon's Chart Note

Directions: After listening to the dictated recording and reading the chart note on Matthew Dixon, provide the medical term that matches each definition below.

Example: pertaining to within the skin   *Answer:* intradermal

1. pertaining to oil   sebaceous
2. upon the skin   epidermis
3. pertaining to redness of the skin   erythematous
4. pertaining to producing pus   pyogenic

SCORECARD: How Did You Do?

Number correct (_____), divided by 4 (_____), multiplied by 100 equals _____ (your score)

Audio Activity: Bennett Meira's Chart Note

Directions: Listen and read along as the physician dictates the following chart note on Bennett Meira. Then do the exercise that appears after Bennett's chart note.

CHART NOTE

Patient Name: Meira, Bennett
ID Number: 94421
Examination Date: February 20, 20xx

SUBJECTIVE
Patient is a 19-year-old male who was brought to FedDes Urgent Care by friends. He states that he was "knifed" due to a dispute over the outcome of a pool game. He has **contusions** to the abdomen and forehead and a stab wound of the right thigh. His tetanus is up to date. No other injuries. Denies any allergies and is not on any medications.

OBJECTIVE
Patient has a 2.5-cm vertical laceration of the lateral aspect of the right thigh that goes through the **epidermis**, **dermis**, and **subcutaneous** tissue down to the vascular layer of the thigh muscles. There does not appear to be any muscle injury, and there is no active bleeding, so no muscular tissue repair is necessary. **Ecchymosis** of the lower right anterior abdomen. Small **hematoma** of the forehead.

ASSESSMENT
Laceration, right lateral thigh.

PLAN
Suture repair and dressing applied. Wound care sheet given. Patient to return in 8 days for suture removal or earlier if signs of infection occur. He can use ibuprofen for pain. He was released in stable condition.

Assessment

Interpret Bennett Meira's Chart Note

Directions: After listening to the dictated recording and reading the chart note on Bennett Meira, provide the medical term that matches each definition below.

Example: pertaining to redness of the skin   *Answer:* erythematous

1. upon the skin   epidermis
2. beneath the skin   subcutaneous
3. "true skin"   dermis
4. tumor of blood   hematoma
5. condition of blood in tissue   ecchymosis
6. condition of bruising   contusion

SCORECARD: How Did You Do?

Number correct (_____), divided by 6 (_____), multiplied by 100 equals _____ (your score)

Chapter Review

Word Elements Summary

Prefixes

Prefix	Meaning
epi-	upon
hypo-	below; below normal
intra-	within
per-	through
sub-	beneath; below
trans-	across

Combining Forms

Root Word/Combining Vowel	Meaning
carcin/o	cancer
cry/o	cold
contus/o	bruising
cutane/o	skin
cyan/o	blue
cyst/o	sac containing fluid
derm/a, derm/o, dermat/o	skin
ecchym/o	blood in the tissues
erythemat/o	redness
erythr/o	red
hemat/o	blood
lip/o	fat
malign/o	causing harm, cancer
melan/o	black
myc/o	fungus
necr/o	death
onych/o	nail
path/o	disease

(Continued)

Root Word/Combining Vowel	Meaning
prurit/o	itching
py/o	pus
schiz/o	split
seb/o	oil or sebum
squam/o	scale-like
topic/o	place
trich/o	hair
xer/o	dry

Suffixes

Suffix	Meaning
-al	pertaining to
-ancy	state of
-cyte	cell
-ectomy	surgical removal; excision
-gen	producing; originating; causing
-ia	condition
-ic	pertaining to
-ion	condition
-itis	inflammation
-logist	specialist in the study and treatment of
-logy	study of
-oid	like; resembling
-oma	tumor; mass
-osis	abnormal condition
-ous	pertaining to
-rrhea	flow; discharge
-tic	pertaining to
-tomy	incision; cut into

More Practice: Activities and Games

The activities on the following pages will help you reinforce your skills and check your mastery of the medical terminology that you learned in this chapter. Visit the companion website for More Practice games and activities.

Multiple Choice: Diseases and Disorders

Directions: Write the letter of the disease or disorder that matches each numbered definition below.

__A__ 1. a disorder in which body tissues retain an excessive amount of fluid, causing them to swell
   a. edema   c. acne
   b. psoriasis   d. alopecia

__C__ 2. a disorder that is typically prominent during puberty, when the sebaceous glands secrete large amounts of sebum on the face, shoulders, and back
   a. edema   c. acne
   b. psoriasis   d. contact dermatitis

__C__ 3. a disorder associated with silvery-white, scaly patches and erythematous skin
   a. contact dermatitis   c. psoriasis
   b. edema   d. acne

__B__ 4. an acute loss of scalp hair
   a. contact dermatitis   c. herpes
   b. alopecia   d. psoriasis

__D__ 5. a condition produced by contact with an allergen or irritant, causing edema, pruritic skin, and, in many cases, small vesicles on the skin
   a. psoriasis   c. alopecia
   b. shingles   d. contact dermatitis

__C__ 6. an aggressive type of skin cancer that begins in the melanocytes of the epidermis and quickly metastasizes to other parts of the body; caused by chronic exposure to the sun's ultraviolet rays
   a. third-degree burn   c. malignant melanoma
   b. shingles   d. alopecia

Multiple Choice: Procedures and Treatments

Directions: Write the letter of the procedure or treatment that matches each numbered definition below.

__B__ 1. a surgical procedure in which liquid nitrogen is used to freeze and destroy abnormal cells
   a. biopsy   c. onychectomy
   b. cryosurgery   d. debridement

__C__ 2. excision, or surgical removal, of the nail from a finger or toe
   a. cryosurgery
   b. debridement
   c. onychectomy
   d. incision and drainage

__D__ 3. surgical removal of all or part of a skin lesion for pathological examination
   a. onychectomy   c. debridement
   b. cryosurgery   d. biopsy

__C__ 4. removal of foreign material or necrotic tissue from a skin wound
   a. laser surgery
   b. incision and drainage
   c. debridement
   d. biopsy

__A__ 5. a medical procedure performed to drain a cyst or abscess
   a. incision and drainage
   b. laser surgery
   c. debridement
   d. onychectomy

__B__ 6. the use of rapid pulses of light to remove wrinkles, sunspots, tattoos, birthmarks, or enlarged blood vessels that are close to the skin's surface
   a. incision and drainage
   b. laser surgery
   c. debridement
   d. onychectomy

True or False

Directions: Indicate whether each statement below is true or false.

True or False?

_F_   1. Sudoriferous glands produce an oily substance called *sebum.*

_T_   2. The skin is our first line of defense against microbes, harmful chemicals, and the sun's ultraviolet rays.

_F_   3. The skin is made up of five layers.

_T_   4. Skin color is determined by the amount of melanin produced by melanocytes.

_F_   5. A lipoma is a tumor of blood.

_F_   6. An onychoma is a fungus of the nail.

_T_   7. Vesicles are fluid-filled sacs.

_F_   8. First-degree burns involve only the dermis.

_F_   9. A benign melanoma is an aggressive form of skin cancer.

_F_   10. Fair-skinned individuals are less susceptible to UV damage from the sun.

_F_   11. *Psoriasis* is a Greek word meaning "creeping skin disease caused by a virus."

_T_   12. Laser surgery uses rapid pulses of light to remove diseased tissue.

_F_   13. Sebaceous glands cool the body by secreting perspiration, or sweat.

_F_   14. The outer layer of the skin is called the *dermis.*

_T_   15. Melanocytes are responsible for the production of melanin, a pigment in the skin.

_F_   16. The epidermis is sometimes referred to as the "true skin."

_T_   17. A dermatologist is a physician who specializes in the study and treatment of the skin.

_T_   18. A whitehead is a pustule that appears when a pore becomes clogged with sebum that cannot reach the skin's surface.

_T_   19. The medical terms *cutaneous* and *dermal* both mean "pertaining to the skin."

_F_   20. The term *intradermal* means "beneath the skin."

Break It Down

Directions: Separate each medical term below into its word elements by placing a slash between each word part (prefix, root word, combining vowel, and suffix). Then define each term.

Medical Term	Dissection
1. cystectomy	c y s t/e c t o m y

Definition: excision of a sac containing fluid

Medical Term	Dissection
2. dermatologic	d e r m a t / o / l o g / i c

Definition: pertaining to study of the skin
_____

| 3. transcutaneous | t r a n s / c u t a n e / o u s |

Definition: pertaining to across the skin
_____

| 4. carcinogen | c a r c i n / o / g e n |

Definition: producing cancer
_____

| 5. ecchymotic | e c c h y m / o / t i c |

Definition: pertaining to blood in the tissues
_____

| 6. subdermal | s u b / d e r m / a l |

Definition: pertaining to beneath the skin
_____

| 7. seborrheic | s e b / o / r r h e / i c |

Definition: pertaining to discharge of sebum
_____

| 8. intracystic | i n t r a / c y s t / i c |

Definition: pertaining to within a sac of fluid
_____

| 9. carcinogenic | c a r c i n / o / g e n / i c |

Definition: pertaining to producing cancer
_____

Medical Term	Dissection

10. cyanotic   c y a n/o/t i c

Definition: pertaining to blue

_____

11. dermatopathology   d e r m a t/o/p a t h/o/l o g y

Definition: study of disease of the skin

_____

12. hypotrichosis   h y p o/t r i c h/o s i s

Definition: abnormal condition of below-normal hair (little or no hair growth)

_____

13. necrogenic   n e c r o/g e n/i c

Definition: pertaining to producing death

_____

14. trichoid   t r i c h/o i d

Definition: like or resembling hair

_____

15. hypoliposis   h y p o/l i p/o s i s

Definition: abnormal condition of below-normal fat

_____

Working with Medical Records

Audio Activity: Gwenn Larson's Chart Note

Directions: At the companion website, listen and read along as the physician dictates the following chart note on Gwenn Larson. Then do the exercise that appears after Gwenn's chart note.

CHART NOTE

Patient Name: Larson, Gwenn
ID Number: 94671
Examination Date: February 24, 20xx

SUBJECTIVE
Patient returns with continued complaints of redness, swelling, and flaking of the skin around the elbow, **etiology** unknown. Patient wishes to discuss the results of her **biopsy.**

OBJECTIVE
Erythematous rash over left posterior elbow. Multiple trials of topical steroid applications have been unsuccessful.

ASSESSMENT
Biopsy report indicates chronic **psoriasis**.

PLAN
Prescribed new topical corticosteroid to be applied 3–4 times daily. **Prognosis** is favorable if the patient is compliant.

Assessment

Interpret Gwenn Larson's Chart Note

Directions: After listening to the dictated recording and reading the chart note on Gwenn Larson, provide the medical term that matches each definition below.

Example: condition of bruising   *Answer:* contusion

1. removal of tissue for microscopic examination   biopsy

2. pertaining to redness of the skin   erythematous

3. chronic skin disorder characterized by silvery-white, scaly patches   psoriasis

4. expected outcome   prognosis

5. cause of a disease or disorder   etiology

Chapter 3

The Digestive System

gastr / o / enter / o / logy: the study of the digestive system

Chapter Organization

- Intern Experience
- Overview of Digestive System Anatomy and Physiology
- Word Elements
- Breaking Down and Building Digestive System Terms
- Diseases and Disorders
- Procedures and Treatments
- Analyzing the Intern Experience
- Working with Medical Records
- Chapter Review

Chapter Objectives

After completing this chapter, you will be able to

1. label an anatomical diagram of the digestive system;
2. dissect and define common medical terminology related to the digestive system;
3. build terms used to describe digestive system diseases and disorders, diagnostic procedures, and therapeutic treatments;
4. pronounce and spell common medical terminology related to the digestive system;
5. understand that the processes of building and dissecting a medical term based on its prefix, word root, and suffix enable you to analyze an extremely large number of medical terms beyond those presented in this chapter;
6. interpret the meaning of abbreviations associated with the digestive system; and
7. interpret medical records containing terminology and abbreviations related to the digestive system.

You will see this icon ⬈ at various points throughout this chapter. The icon indicates that you will find interactive activities and games on the Medical Terminology Companion Website. These activities and games will help you learn, practice, and expand your medical terminology knowledge and skills. Some of these activities are also available on the Medical Terminology Mobile Website.

Companion Website
www.g-wlearning.com/healthsciences

Mobile Site
www.m.g-wlearning.com/5800

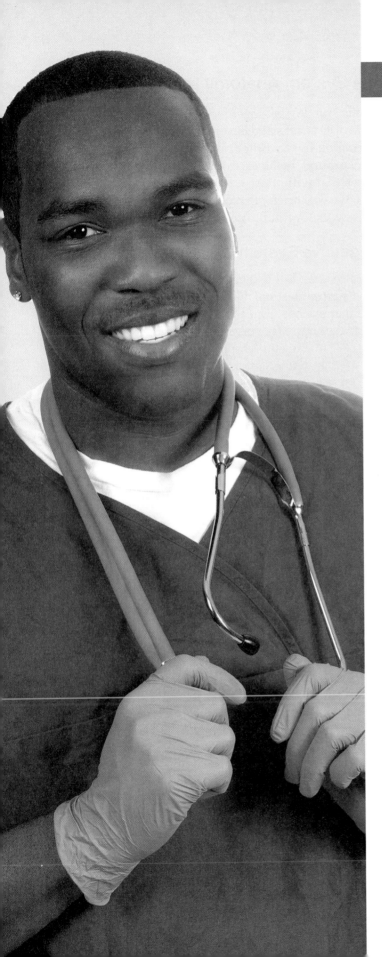

Evan Walker, an intern with Gratz Urgent Care Clinic, is working with Dr. Emily Stomack this week. Evan accompanies Dr. Stomack to exam room 3, where a nervous, young female patient is waiting with her mother.

Evan and Dr. Stomack learn that the patient, Sue, had the lead role in her high school play. Too nervous to eat before the performance, she skipped dinner. After the play, Sue was very hungry, so her mother took Sue and her friend to the Brickhouse, a new restaurant in town. All three gobbled down the deluxe burger special and turkey noodle soup.

When Sue arrived home, she took her dog for a walk. While walking the dog, Sue suddenly felt like something was caught in her throat. She had difficulty swallowing, and the sensation would not go away. A few hours later, the symptoms persisted, so Sue's mother suggested that she make an appointment with their family doctor first thing the next morning.

Sue is experiencing a problem with her digestive system, the body system that breaks down food and converts it into the "fuel" that the body needs for physical and cellular processes. To help you understand what is happening to Sue, this chapter will present word elements (combining forms, prefixes, and suffixes) that make up medical terminology related to the digestive system. As you progress through this book, you will see many word parts that are also used in medical terms related to other body systems.

Before you begin this chapter, take some time to review the strategies presented in chapter 1 for analyzing medical terms. Reviewing these strategies will help you understand and recall the word elements and definitions of medical terms that you are about to learn, as well as those you learned previously.

After you have learned the medical terms presented in this chapter, you will practice analyzing patient chart notes. Accurate interpretation of these chart notes will demonstrate that you have a solid understanding of medical terminology related to the digestive system.

Let's begin our study with a brief overview of the anatomy and physiology of the digestive system.

Overview of Digestive System Anatomy and Physiology

Super Bowl parties are great fun. We get together with friends, watch the game, and, of course, eat our favorite snacks and beverages. While we're caught up in the excitement of cheering on our favorite team, our digestive systems are quietly working in the background, breaking down those snacks into life-sustaining chemical substances that will nourish the cells in our bodies and give us energy. In this section, we will briefly explore the major organs of the digestive system and how they work together to accomplish these tasks.

Major Organs of the Digestive System

The **digestive system** is also called the **digestive tract**, the **alimentary** (ăl-ĭ-MĔN-tăr-ē) **canal**, and the **gastrointestinal (GI) tract**. The digestive tract consists of a long, hollow tube that extends from the **pharynx** (FĂR-inks), more commonly known as the *throat*, to the anus. Major organs of the GI tract include the mouth, esophagus, stomach, small intestine, large intestine (colon), rectum, and anus (Figure 3.1). The liver, gallbladder, pancreas, salivary glands, and teeth are accessory organs that aid in digestion.

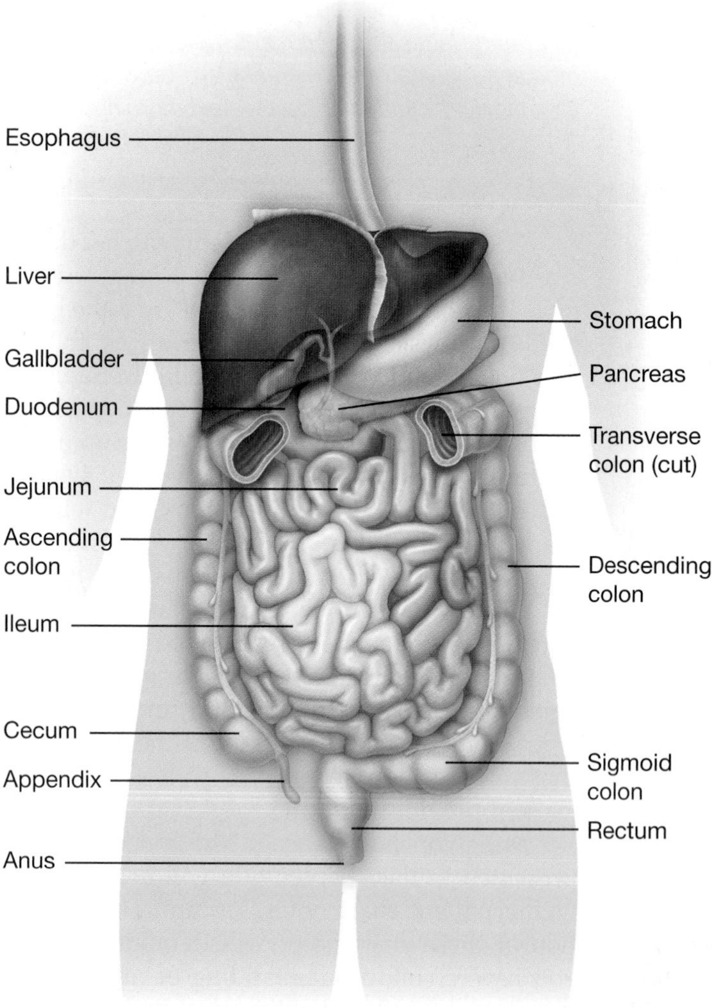

Main Functions of the Digestive System

The job of the digestive system is to ingest (take in), break down, and absorb nutrients from food and liquids and to eliminate waste products of the digestive process.

Digestion begins in the mouth, where the teeth and salivary glands work together to break down into smaller pieces the chicken wings, salsa, and chips consumed during the Super Bowl party. When the food is swallowed, it moves from the pharynx into the **esophagus** (ĕ-SŎF-ă-gŭs), a tubular structure that carries food into the stomach.

The **stomach** is an expandable organ, so it can accommodate a late-night pizza craving or a Super Bowl feeding frenzy. It acts like a blender by converting food into a paste-like mixture. Digestive juices and enzymes from the pancreas, liver, and gallbladder reduce the semi-digested

Figure 3.1 Organs of the digestive system

Esophagus

Liver

Gallbladder

Duodenum

Jejunum

Ascending colon

Ileum

Cecum

Appendix

Anus

Stomach

Pancreas

Transverse colon (cut)

Descending colon

Sigmoid colon

Rectum

food into smaller molecules, allowing nutrients to be absorbed into the small intestine and transported throughout the body by the blood.

The activities of chemical digestion and nutrient absorption both occur in the **small intestine**. The **duodenum** is the first segment of the small intestine, the **jejunum** is the middle part, and the **ileum** is the last—and the longest—segment of the small intestine.

The **large intestine** or **colon**, is the last section of the digestive system. It absorbs water and electrolytes and eliminates waste. The large intestine is so named because its diameter is wider than that of the small intestine. In comparison, the small intestine is much longer than the large intestine but smaller in diameter. The **rectum** receives waste products (feces) from the **sigmoid colon**, an S-shaped section of the large intestine, and stores it prior to elimination from the anus.

The study of the digestive system is called **gastroenterology** (GĂS-trō-ĕn-tĕr-ŎL-ō-jē). Even though the medical term *gastroenterology* literally means "the study of the stomach and intestines," the term is used to refer to the study of the entire digestive system. A **gastroenterologist** (GĂS-trō-ĕn-tĕr-ŎL-ō-jĭst) is a physician who specializes in the study and treatment of the digestive system.

Anatomy and Physiology Vocabulary

Now that you have been introduced to the basic structure and functions of the digestive system, let's explore in more detail the key terms presented in the introduction.

Key Term	Definition
digestive tract (also called **alimentary canal** or **gastrointestinal tract**)	long, hollow tube that starts at the pharynx and ends at the anus
duodenum	first part of the small intestine
esophagus	tubular structure that carries food from the pharynx (throat) to the stomach
gastroenterologist	physician who specializes in the study and treatment of the digestive system
gastroenterology	the study of the digestive system
ileum	final and longest part of the small intestine
jejunum	middle part of the small intestine
large intestine	last section of the digestive system, which absorbs water and electrolytes and eliminates waste; the colon
pharynx	the throat
rectum	last part of the large intestine leading to the anus
sigmoid	S-shaped section of the large intestine
small intestine	long, narrow, folded tube that extends from the stomach to the large intestine; the site where chemical digestion and absorption of food occur
stomach	an expandable organ that stores and breaks down food; located between the esophagus and small intestine

E-Flash Card Activity: Anatomy and Physiology Vocabulary

Directions: After you have reviewed the anatomy and physiology vocabulary related to the digestive system, practice with the e-flash cards until you are comfortable with the spelling and definition of each term.

Identifying Major Organs of the Digestive System

Directions: Label the diagram of the digestive tract.

16. esophagus

15. liver

14. gallbladder

13. duodenum

12. jejunum

11. ascending colon

10. ileum

9. cecum

8. appendix

7. anus

1. stomach

2. pancreas

3. transverse colon

4. descending colon

5. sigmoid colon

6. rectum

Matching Anatomy and Physiology Vocabulary

Directions: Match the vocabulary term in Column A with its meaning in Column B. Some meanings may be used more than once.

Column A

C	1. digestive tract
F	2. large intestine
B	3. esophagus
C	4. alimentary canal
K	5. small intestine
E	6. pharynx
D	7. gastroenterology
C	8. gastrointestinal (GI) tract
A	9. gastroenterologist
G	10. stomach
H	11. ileum
J	12. jejunum
I	13. duodenum
M	14. sigmoid
L	15. rectum

Column B

A. physician who specializes in the study and treatment of the digestive system

B. tubular structure that carries food from the pharynx (throat) to the stomach

C. long, hollow tube that starts at the pharynx and extends to the anus

D. the study of the digestive system

E. the throat

F. last section of the digestive system, which absorbs water and electrolytes and eliminates waste; also called the *colon*

G. expandable organ that stores and breaks down food; located between the esophagus and small intestine

H. last (and longest) part of the small intestine

I. first part of the small intestine

J. middle part of the small intestine

K. part of the digestive tract in which chemical digestion occurs

L. last part of the intestine leading to the anus

M. S-shaped section of the large intestine

SCORECARD: How Did You Do?

Number correct (_____), divided by 15 (_____), multiplied by 100 equals _____ (your score)

Word Elements

In this section you will learn word elements—prefixes, combining forms, and suffixes—that are common to the digestive system. By learning these word parts and understanding how they are combined to build medical terms, you will be able to analyze Sue's health problem (described in the Intern Experience at the beginning of this chapter) and identify a large number of terms associated with the digestive system.

E-Flash Card Activity: Word Elements

Directions: Review the word elements in the tables that follow. Then, practice with the e-flash cards until you are able to quickly recognize the different word parts (prefixes, combining forms, and suffixes) and their meanings. The e-flash cards are grouped together by prefixes, combining forms, and suffixes, followed by a cumulative review of all the word elements that you learned in this chapter.

Prefixes

Let's start our study of digestive system word elements by looking at the prefixes listed in the table below. These prefixes appear not only in medical terms related to the digestive system but also in many terms pertaining to other body systems.

Prefix	Meaning
a-	not; without
ad-	toward
anti-	against
brady-	slow
dia-	through
dys-	painful; difficult
epi-	upon; above
hyper-	above; above normal
pan-	all; everything
peri-	around
poly-	many
retro-	backward; behind

Combining Forms

Listed below are common combining forms used in medical terms related to the digestive system. As you progress through this book, you will discover that some of these combining forms are used in medical terms related to other body systems as well.

Root Word/Combining Vowel	Meaning
carcin/o	cancerous; cancer
celi/o	abdomen
chol/e	bile; gall
cholecyst/o	gallbladder
col/o, colon/o	colon; large intestine
dist/o	away from the point of origin
diverticul/o	diverticulum
duoden/o	duodenum
enter/o	intestines
esophag/o	esophagus
gastr/o	stomach
gingiv/o	gums
gloss/o	tongue
hemat/o	blood
hepat/o	liver
herni/o	hernia; rupture; protrusion
ile/o	ileum
jejun/o	jejunum
lapar/o	abdomen
lith/o	stone
or/o	mouth
organ/o	organ
pancreat/o	pancreas
peps/o	digestion
polyp/o	polyp; small growth
proct/o	anus and rectum
proxim/o	nearest the point of origin
rect/o	rectum
sial/o	saliva
sigmoid/o	sigmoid colon

Suffixes

Listed below are suffixes used in medical terms pertaining to the digestive system. You will also encounter these suffixes in your study of many terms related to other body systems.

Suffix	Meaning
-al	pertaining to
-algia	pain
-cele	hernia; swelling; protrusion
-dynia	pain
-eal	pertaining to
-ectomy	surgical removal; excision
-emesis	vomiting
-gram	record; image
-graphy	process of recording an image
-ia	condition
-iasis	abnormal condition
-ic	pertaining to
-itis	inflammation
-logist	specialist in the study and treatment of
-logy	study of
-megaly	enlargement
-oma	tumor; mass
-osis	abnormal condition
-phagia	condition of eating or swallowing
-pharynx	pharynx; throat
-plasty	surgical repair
-ptosis	drooping; downward displacement
-rrhea	flow; discharge
-scope	instrument used to observe
-scopy	process of observing
-stomy	new opening
-tomy	incision; cut into
-tripsy	crushing
-y	condition; process

Matching Prefixes, Combining Forms, and Suffixes

Directions: In each exercise below, match the word element in Column A with its meaning in Column B. Some meanings may be used more than once.

Prefixes

Column A

I	1.	peri-
G	2.	a-
H	3.	pan-
B	4.	brady-
D	5.	dys-
A	6.	ad-
L	7.	hyper-
E	8.	dia-
F	9.	poly-
C	10.	anti-
J	11.	retro-
K	12.	epi-

Column B

A. toward

B. slow

C. against

D. painful; difficult

E. through

F. many

G. not; without

H. all; everything

I. around

J. backward; behind

K. upon; above

L. above; above normal

Combining Forms

Column A

B	1.	sigmoid/o
I	2.	carcin/o
X	3.	hepat/o
AA	4.	chol/e
A	5.	gloss/o
P	6.	dist/o
W	7.	diverticul/o
V	8.	proxim/o
M	9.	pancreat/o
R	10.	duoden/o
E	11.	hemat/o

Column B

A. tongue

B. sigmoid colon

C. abdomen

D. saliva

E. blood

F. esophagus

G. jejunum

H. mouth

I. cancerous; cancer

J. hernia; rupture; protrusion

K. stomach

Column A

F	12. esophag/o
U	13. gingiv/o
S	14. lith/o
N	15. rect/o
G	16. jejun/o
Z	17. col/o
Z	18. colon/o
H	19. or/o
C	20. celi/o
CC	21. enter/o
K	22. gastr/o
Q	23. polyp/o
J	24. hern/o
D	25. sial/o
T	26. ile/o
L	27. proct/o
C	28. lapar/o
Y	29. cholecyst/o
BB	30. organ/o
DD	31. peps/o

Column B

L. anus and rectum

M. pancreas

N. rectum

P. away from the point of origin

Q. polyp; small growth

R. duodenum

S. stone

T. ileum

U. gums

V. nearest the point of origin

W. diverticulum

X. liver

Y. gallbladder

Z. colon; large intestine

AA. bile; gall

BB. organ

CC. intestines

DD. digestion

Suffixes

Column A

D	1. -dynia
B	2. -gram
F	3. -logist
L	4. -osis
S	5. -scope
E	6. -tripsy
A	7. -al

Column B

A. pertaining to

B. record; image

C. vomiting

D. pain

E. crushing

F. specialist in the study and treatment of

G. incision; cut into

Column A	Column B
_A_ 8. -eal	H. surgical removal; excision
_M_ 9. -graphy	I. surgical repair
_O_ 10. -logy	J. tumor; mass
_V_ 11. -megaly	K. condition
_Q_ 12. -scopy	L. abnormal condition
_D_ 13. -algia	M. process of recording an image
_H_ 14. -ectomy	N. inflammation
_K_ 15. -ia	O. study of
_R_ 16. -phagia	P. drooping; downward displacement
_G_ 17. -tomy	Q. process of observing
_Y_ 18. -cele	R. condition of eating or swallowing
_C_ 19. -emesis	S. instrument used to observe
_L_ 20. -iasis	T. new opening
_J_ 21. -oma	U. flow; discharge
_T_ 22. -stomy	V. enlargement
_A_ 23. -ic	W. throat
_I_ 24. -plasty	X. condition; process
_N_ 25. -itis	Y. hernia; swelling; protrusion
_W_ 26. -pharynx	
_P_ 27. -ptosis	
_U_ 28. -rrhea	
_X_ 29. -y	

SCORECARD: How Did You Do?

Number correct (_____), divided by 72 (_____), multiplied by 100 equals _____ (your score)

Breaking Down and Building Digestive System Terms

Now that you have mastered the prefixes, combining forms, and suffixes for digestive system terminology, you have the ability to dissect and build a large number of medical terms related to this system.

Below is a list of common medical terms related to the study, diagnosis, and treatment of the digestive system. For each term, a dissection has been provided, along with the meaning of each word element and the definition of the term as a whole.

Term	Dissection	Word Part/Meaning	Term Definition
Note: *For simplification, combining vowels have been omitted from the Word Part/Meaning column.*			
1. **aphagia** (ă-FĀ-jĕ-ă)	a/phagia	**a** = not; without **phagia** = condition of eating or swallowing	condition of without swallowing
2. **carcinoma** (kär-sĭ-NŌ-mă)	carcin/oma	**carcin** = cancerous; cancer **oma** = tumor; mass	cancerous tumor or mass
3. **celiectomy** (sē-lē-ĔK-tō-mē)	celi/ectomy	**celi** = abdomen **ectomy** = surgical removal; excision	excision of the abdomen
4. **cholecystitis** (KŌ-lĕ-sĭs-TĪ-tĭs)	cholecyst/itis	**cholecyst** = gallbladder **itis** = inflammation	inflammation of the gallbladder
5. **cholelithiasis** (KŌ-lĕ-lĭ-THĪ-ă-sĭs)	chol/e/lith/iasis	**chol** = bile; gall **lith** = stone **iasis** = abnormal condition	abnormal condition of gallstones
6. **colitis** (kō-LĪ-tĭs)	col/itis	**col** = colon **itis** = inflammation	inflammation of the colon
7. **colonoscopy** (kō-lŏn-ŎS-kō-pē)	colon/o/scopy	**colon** = colon **scopy** = process of observing	process of observing the colon
8. **colostomy** (kō-LŎS-tō-mē)	col/o/stomy	**col** = colon **stomy** = new opening	new opening in the colon
9. **diarrhea** (dī-ă-RĒ-ă)	dia/rrhea	**dia** = through **rrhea** = flow; discharge	flow through
10. **diverticulitis** (DĪ-vĕr-tĭk-ū-LĪ-tĭs)	diverticul/itis	**diverticul** = diverticulum **itis** = inflammation	inflammation of the diverticulum
11. **diverticulosis** (dī-vĕr-tĭk-ū-LŌ-sĭs)	diverticul/osis	**diverticul** = diverticulum **osis** = abnormal condition	abnormal condition of the diverticulum
Prefixes = Green Root Words = Red Suffixes = Blue			

Term	Dissection	Word Part/Meaning	Term Definition
12. **duodenal** (dū-ŏ-DĒ-năl) (dū-ŎD-ĕn-ăl)	duoden/al	**duoden** = duodenum **al** = pertaining to	pertaining to the duodenum
13. **dysentery** (DĬS-ĕn-tĕr-ē)	dys/enter/y	**dys** = painful; difficult **enter** = intestine **y** = condition; process	painful condition of the intestines
14. **dyspepsia** (dĭs-PĔP-sē-ă)	dys/peps/ia	**dys** = painful; difficult **peps** = digestion **ia** = condition	condition of painful or difficult digestion
15. **dysphagia** (dĭs-FĀ-jē-ă)	dys/phagia	**dys** = painful; difficult **phagia** = condition of eating or swallowing	condition of painful or difficult swallowing
16. **enteritis** (ĕn-tĕr-Ī-tĭs)	enter/itis	**enter** = intestine **itis** = inflammation	inflammation of the intestines
17. **epigastric** (ĕp-ĭ-GĂS-trĭk)	epi/gastr/ic	**epi** = upon; above **gastr** = stomach **ic** = pertaining to	pertaining to (the area) above the stomach
18. **esophageal** (ē-SŎF-ă-jē-ăl)	esophag/eal	**esophag** = esophagus **eal** = pertaining to	pertaining to the esophagus
19. **esophagogastro-duodenoscopy** (ē-SŎF-ă-gō-GĂS-trō-dū-ŏ-dĕ-NŎS-kō-pē)	esophag/o/gastr/o/duoden/o/scopy	**esophag** = esophagus **gastr** = stomach **duoden** = duodenum **scopy** = process of observing	process of observing the esophagus, stomach, and duodenum
20. **gastritis** (găs-TRĪ-tĭs)	gastr/itis	**gastr** = stomach **itis** = inflammation	inflammation of the stomach
21. **gastrodynia** (găs-trō-DĬN-ē-ă)	gastr/o/dynia	**gastr** = stomach **dynia** = pain	pain in the stomach
22. **gastroenterologist** (găs-trō-ĕn-tĕr-ŎL-ō-jĭst)	gastr/o/enter/o/logist	**gastr** = stomach **enter** = intestines **logist** = specialist in the study and treatment of	specialist in the study and treatment of the stomach and intestines
23. **gastroenterology** (găs-trō-ĕn-tĕr-ŎL-ō-jē)	gastr/o/enter/o/logy	**gastr** = stomach **enter** = intestines **logy** = study of	study of the stomach and intestines
24. **gastroesophageal** (găs-trō-ĕ-SŎF-ă-jē-ăl)	gastro/esophag/eal	**gastr** = stomach **esophag** = esophagus **eal** = pertaining to	pertaining to the stomach and esophagus
25. **gingivitis** (jĭn-jĭ-VĪ-tĭs)	gingiv/itis	**gingiv** = gums **itis** = inflammation	inflammation of the gums
26. **glossalgia** (glŏs-ĂL-jē-ă)	gloss/algia	**gloss** = tongue **algia** = pain	pain in the tongue

Prefixes = Green   Root Words = Red   Suffixes = Blue

Term	Dissection	Word Part/Meaning	Term Definition
27. **hematemesis** (HĒ-mă-TĔM-ĕ-sĭs)	hemat/emesis	**hemat** = blood **emesis** = vomiting	vomiting of blood
28. **hepatitis** (hĕp-ă-TĪ-tĭs)	hepat/itis	**hepat** = liver **itis** = inflammation	inflammation of the liver
29. **hepatomegaly** (HĔP-ă-tō-MĔG-ă-lē)	hepat/o/megaly	**hepat** = liver **megaly** = enlargement	enlargement of the liver
30. **laparoscope** (LĂP-ă-rō-skōp)	lapar/o/scope	**lapar** = abdomen **scope** = instrument used to observe	instrument used to observe the abdomen
31. **laparoscopy** (lăp-ă-RŎS-kō-pē)	lapar/o/scopy	**lapar** = abdomen **scopy** = process of observing	process of observing the abdomen
32. **organomegaly** (ŏr-gă-nō-MĔG-ă-lē)	organ/o/megaly	**organ** = organ **megaly** = enlargement	enlargement of an organ
33. **oropharynx** (or-ō-FĂR-inks)	or/o/pharynx	**or** = mouth **pharynx** = pharynx; throat	mouth and throat
34. **pancreatography** (păn-krē-ă-TŎG-ră-fē)	pancreat/o/graphy	**pancreat** = pancreas **graphy** = process of recording an image	process of recording an image of the pancreas
35. **polyposis** (pŏl-ĭ-PŌ-sĭs)	polyp/osis	**polyp** = polyp **osis** = abnormal condition	abnormal condition of polyps
36. **proctoplasty** (PRŎK-tō-plăs-tē)	proct/o/plasty	**proct** = anus and rectum **plasty** = surgical repair	surgical repair of the anus and rectum
37. **rectoscope** (RĔK-tō-skōp)	rect/o/scope	**rect** = rectum **scope** = instrument used to observe	instrument used to observe the rectum
38. **sialorrhea** (sī-ă-lō-RĒ-ă)	sial/o/rrhea	**sial** = saliva **rrhea** = flow; discharge	flow or discharge of saliva
39. **sigmoidoscopy** (sĭg-moy-DŎS-kō-pē)	sigmoid/o/scopy	**sigmoid** = sigmoid colon **scopy** = process of observing	process of observing the sigmoid colon

Prefixes = Green   Root Words = Red   Suffixes = Blue

Using the pronunciation guide in the Breaking Down and Building chart, practice saying each medical term aloud. To hear the pronunciation of each term, go to the Pronounce It activity at the G-W companion website.

Studying medical terminology is similar to learning a foreign language. At first, pronouncing new medical terms can be challenging. To develop fluency, it is necessary to practice pronouncing the terms until you are comfortable saying them aloud.

Audio Activity: Pronounce It

Directions: At the companion website, listen as each medical term shown below is pronounced. Practice pronouncing the terms until you are comfortable saying them aloud.

aphagia
(ă-FĀ-jĕ-ă)

carcinoma
(kär-sĭ-NŌ-mă)

celiectomy
(sē-lē-ĔK-tō-mē)

cholecystitis
(KŌ-lĕ-sĭs-TĪ-tĭs)

cholelithiasis
(KŌ-lĕ-lĭ-THĪ-ă-sĭs)

colitis
(kō-LĪ-tĭs)

colonoscopy
(kō-lŏn-ŎS-kō-pē)

colostomy
(kō-LŎS-tō-mē)

diarrhea
(dī-ă-RĒ-ă)

diverticulitis
(DĪ-vĕr-tĭk-ū-LĪ-tĭs)

diverticulosis
(dī-vĕr-tĭk-ū-LŌ-sĭs)

duodenal
(dū-ŏ-DĒ-năl)
(dū-ŎD-ĕn-ăl)

dysentery
(DĬS-ĕn-tĕr-ē)

dyspepsia
(dĭs-PĔP-sē-ă)

dysphagia
(dĭs-FĀ-jē-ă)

enteritis
(ĕn-tĕr-Ī-tĭs)

epigastric
(ĕp-ĭ-GĂS-trĭk)

esophageal
(ē-SŎF-ă-jē-ăl)

esophagogastro-
duodenoscopy
(ē-SŎF-ă-gō-GĂS-trō-
dū-ŏ-dĕ-NŎS-kō-pē)

gastritis
(găs-TRĪ-tĭs)

gastrodynia
(găs-trō-DĬN-ē-ă)

gastroenterologist
(găs-trō-ĕn-tĕr-ŎL-ō-jĭst)

gastroenterology
(găs-trō-ĕn-tĕr-ŎL-ō-jē)

gastroesophageal
(găs-trō-ĕ-SŎF-ă-jē-ăl)

gingivitis
(jĭn-jĭ-VĪ-tĭs)

glossalgia
(glŏs-ĂL-jē-ă)

hematemesis
(HĒ-mă-TĔM-ĕ-sĭs)

hepatitis
(hĕp-ă-TĪ-tĭs)

hepatomegaly
(HĔP-ă-tō-MĔG-ă-lē)

laparoscope
(LĂP-ă-rō-skōp)

laparoscopy
(lăp-ă-RŎS-kō-pē)

organomegaly
(ŏr-gă-nō-MĔG-ă-lē)

oropharynx
(or-ō-FĂR-inks)

pancreatography
(păn-krē-ă-TŎG-ră-fē)

polyposis
(pŏl-ĭ-PŌ-sĭs)

proctoplasty
(PRŎK-tō-plăs-tē)

rectoscope
(RĔK-tō-skōp)

sialorrhea
(sī-ă-lō-RĒ-ă)

sigmoidoscopy
(sĭg-moy-DŎS-kō-pē)

Audio Activity: Spell It

Directions: Cover the medical terms in the Pronounce It activity above with a sheet of paper. At the companion website, listen as the terms are read aloud. Correctly spell each term below.

1. aphagia
2. carcinoma
3. celiectomy
4. cholecystitis
5. cholelithiasis
6. colitis
7. colonoscopy
8. colostomy .

9. diarrhea _____

10. diverticulitis _____

11. diverticulosis _____

12. duodenal _____

13. dysentery _____

14. dyspepsia _____

15. dysphagia _____

16. enteritis _____

17. epigastric _____

18. esophageal _____

19. esophagogastroduodenoscopy _____

20. gastritis _____

21. gastrodynia _____

22. gastroenterologist _____

23. gastroenterology _____

24. gastroesophageal _____

25. gingivitis _____

26. glossalgia _____

27. hematemesis _____

28. hepatitis _____

29. hepatomegaly _____

30. laparoscope _____

31. laparoscopy _____

32. organomegaly _____

33. oropharynx _____

34. pancreatography _____

35. polyposis _____

36. proctoplasty _____

37. rectoscope _____

38. sialorrhea _____

39. sigmoidoscopy _____

Assessment

Break It Down

Directions: Dissect each medical term below into its word elements by placing a slash between each word part (prefix, root word, combining vowel, and suffix). Then define each term.

Example:

Medical Term: hepatomegaly

Dissection: hepat/o/megaly

Definition: enlargement of the liver

Medical Term

Dissection

1. dysphagia   d y s/p h a g i a

Definition: condition of painful or difficult swallowing _____

2. aphagia   a/p h a g i a

Definition: condition of without swallowing _____

Medical Term	Dissection

3. laparoscopy   l a p a r / o / s c o p y

Definition: process of observing the abdomen

_____

4. diverticulosis   d i v e r t i c u l / o s i s

Definition: abnormal condition of the diverticulum

_____

5. sialorrhea   s i a l / o / r r h e a

Definition: flow or discharge of saliva

_____

6. sigmoidoscopy   s i g m o i d / o / s c o p y

Definition: process of observing the sigmoid colon

_____

7. cholelithiasis   c h o l / e / l i t h / i a s i s

Definition: abnormal condition of gallstones

_____

8. hepatomegaly   h e p a t / o / m e g a l y

Definition: enlargement of the liver

_____

9. gastroesophageal   g a s t r o / e s o p h a g / e a l

Definition: pertaining to the stomach and esophagus

_____

10. gastrodynia   g a s t r / o / d y n i a

Definition: pain in the stomach

_____

Medical Term	Dissection

11. organomegaly organ/o/megaly

Definition: enlargement of an organ

12. dyspepsia dys/peps/ia

Definition: condition of painful or difficult digestion

13. oropharynx or/o/pharynx

Definition: mouth and throat

14. gastroenterology gastr/o/enter/o/logy

Definition: study of the stomach and intestines

15. colitis col/itis

Definition: inflammation of the colon

16. esophagogastroduodenoscopy esophag/o/gastr/o/duoden/o/scopy

Definition: process of observing the esophagus, stomach, and duodenum

17. enteritis enter/itis

Definition: inflammation of the intestines

Medical Term	Dissection
18. hematemesis	h e m a t/e m e s i s

Definition: vomiting of blood

19. epigastric	e p i/g a s t r/i c

Definition: pertaining to (the area) above the stomach

20. duodenal	d u o d e n/a l

Definition: pertaining to the duodenum

SCORECARD: How Did You Do?

Number correct (_____), divided by 20 (_____), multiplied by 100 equals _____ (your score)

Assessment

Build It

Directions: Build the medical term that matches each definition below by supplying the correct word elements.

P (Prefixes) = Green
RW (Root Words) = Red
S (Suffixes) = Blue
CV (Combining Vowel) = Purple

1. pertaining to the esophagus

esophag	eal
RW	S

2. cancerous tumor

carcin	oma
RW	S

3. new opening in the colon

col	o	stomy
RW	CV	S

4. process of observing the colon

colon	o	scopy
RW	CV	S

5. specialist in the study and treatment of the stomach and intestines

gastr	o	enter	o	logist
RW	CV	RW	CV	S

6. inflammation of the intestines

enter	itis
RW	S

7. pertaining to the duodenum

duoden	al
RW	S

8. inflammation of the gallbladder

chol	e	cyst	itis
RW	CV	RW	S

9. condition of painful or difficult swallowing

dys	phagia
P	S

10. process of observing the sigmoid colon

sigmoid	o	scopy
RW	CV	S

11. enlargement of the liver

hepat	o	megaly
RW	CV	S

12. inflammation of the colon

col	itis
RW	S

13. pertaining to the stomach and esophagus

gastr	o	esophag	eal
RW	CV	RW	S

14. painful digestion

dys	peps	ia
P	RW	S

15. process of observing the esophagus, stomach, and duodenum

esophag	o	gastr	o	duoden	o	scopy
RW	CV	RW	CV	RW	CV	S

16. pain in the stomach

gastr	o	dynia
RW	CV	S

17. vomiting of blood

hemat	emesis
RW	S

18. instrument used to observe the abdomen

lapar	o	scope
RW	CV	S

19. enlargement of an organ

organ	o	megaly
RW	CV	S

20. flow through

dia	rrhea
P	S

21. mouth and throat

or	o	pharynx
RW	CV	S

22. process of recording the pancreas

pancreat	o	graphy
RW	CV	S

23. inflammation of the liver

hepat	itis
RW	S

24. abnormal condition of polyps

polyp	osis
RW	S

SCORECARD: How Did You Do?

Number correct (_____), divided by 24 (_____), multiplied by 100 equals _____ (your score)

Diseases and Disorders

Diseases and disorders of the digestive system range from the mild to severe, and they have a wide variety of causes. We will now take a look at some problems that commonly affect the digestive system.

Crohn's Disease

Crohn's disease is a chronic **inflammatory bowel disease (IBD)** with clinical symptoms of bloody diarrhea, abdominal pain, weight loss, and fatigue. It is characterized by thickening and a gradual erosion of the inner lining of the intestinal wall (Figure 3.2). Ulcerations of the intestinal wall result in scar tissue formation, which can cause intestinal obstruction. Because the etiology (cause) is unknown, there is no cure for Crohn's disease.

Gastroesophageal Reflux Disease

Gastroesophageal reflux disease (GERD) is a chronic digestive disease that occurs when stomach acid flows back into the esophagus (Figure 3.3). The acidity of regurgitated food irritates the esophageal lining and may cause ulcerations in the lining. GERD produces heartburn after eating, dysphagia (condition of painful or difficult swallowing), and occasional hematemesis (vomiting of blood).

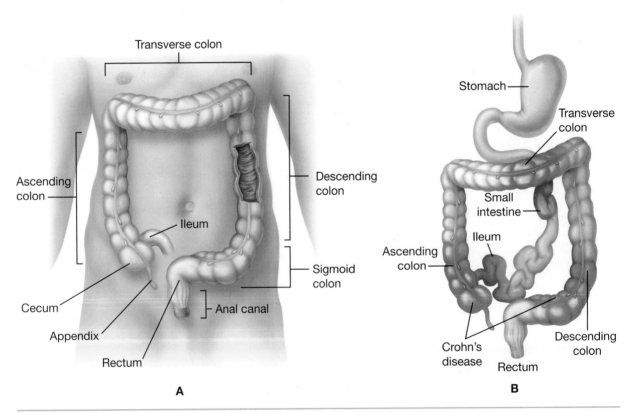

Figure 3.2 A—Normal large intestine. B—Intestinal inflammation of Crohn's disease.

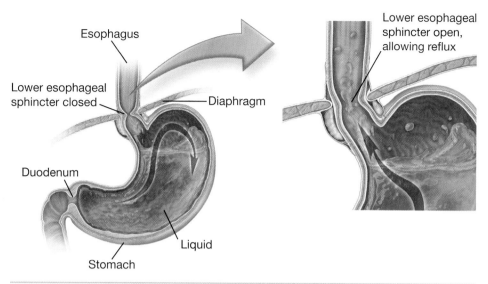

Figure 3.3 Gastroesophageal reflux disease (GERD) is characterized by backflow of stomach acids into the esophagus.

Hiatal Hernia

A **hiatal hernia** occurs when a portion of the stomach protrudes (bulges) through the diaphragm (Figure 3.4). The diaphragm, the major muscle involved in the breathing process, separates the thoracic (chest) cavity from the abdominal cavity.

The esophagus normally enters the abdominal cavity through an opening in the diaphragm. If the opening is weakened or enlarged, the stomach may herniate (bulge) upward through the diaphragm into the thoracic cavity. A large hiatal hernia causes heartburn, chest pain, belching, and nausea.

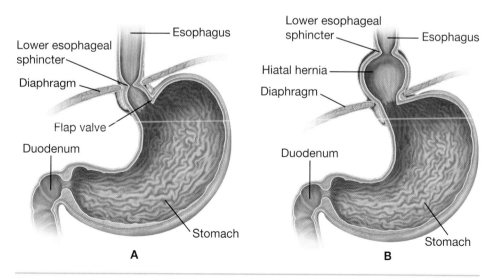

Figure 3.4 A—Normal muscle of the abdominal wall. B—In a hiatal hernia, a portion of the stomach bulges through the diaphragm.

Liver Disease

Hepatitis is an inflammation of the liver that causes abdominal pain, nausea, vomiting, and jaundice (yellowish discoloration of the skin and whites of the eyes). Most commonly, this inflammatory condition is caused by one of three viruses: hepatitis A, hepatitis B, or hepatitis C. Hepatitis can also result from chronic alcohol or drug abuse.

Cirrhosis is a chronic, irreversible liver disease in which normal liver cells are replaced with hard, fibrous scar tissue (Figure 3.5). Common symptoms include abdominal swelling, susceptibility to bruising, and renal failure. Cirrhosis is often associated with long-term alcoholism. There is no known cure.

Eating Disorders

Eating disorders are a group of serious conditions rooted in a negative or a distorted self-image. Those affected are so preoccupied with food and weight that they can focus on little else in their lives. Anorexia nervosa and bulimia nervosa are two common types of behavioral eating disorders. Both involve weight loss achieved by different methods.

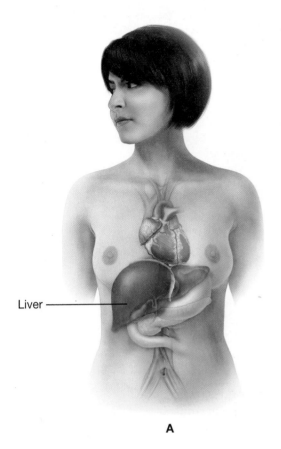

Liver

A

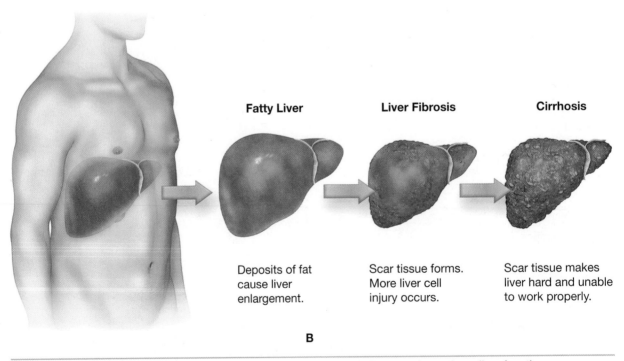

Fatty Liver

Deposits of fat cause liver enlargement.

Liver Fibrosis

Scar tissue forms. More liver cell injury occurs.

Cirrhosis

Scar tissue makes liver hard and unable to work properly.

B

Figure 3.5 A—Normal liver. B—The tissue scarring caused by cirrhosis severely weakens liver function.

Anorexia nervosa is characterized by an extreme aversion to food that results in weight loss and may lead to malnutrition (Figure 3.6). **Bulimia nervosa** involves repeated gorging of food followed by intentional vomiting and/or laxative abuse. Severe eating disorders can be life-threatening.

Ulcers

An **ulcer**, or *peptic ulcer*, is a breakdown in the mucosal lining of the esophagus, stomach, or duodenum caused by chronic irritation (Figure 3.7). This breakdown is caused by hydrochloric acid and pepsin, the acidic chemicals involved in the digestion of food. Esophageal, gastric, and duodenal ulcers are types of peptic ulcers.

Most ulcers are caused by *Helicobacter pylori* (*H. pylori*), a bacterium that attacks the weakened mucosa. Dyspepsia (epigastric pain with bloating and nausea) is a common symptom. Factors that may contribute to ulcer formation include stress, excessive caffeine consumption,

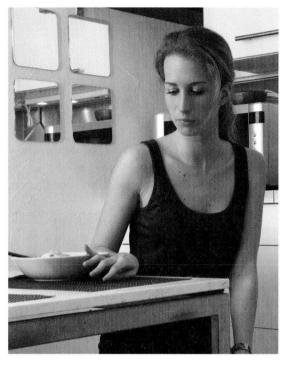

Hubert Raguet / Science Source

Figure 3.6 Distorted body image is a major symptom of anorexia nervosa.

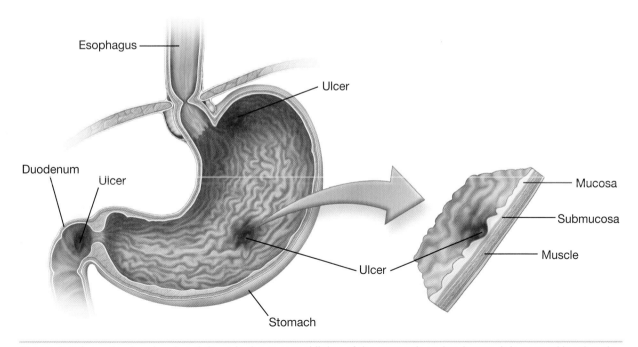

Figure 3.7 A peptic ulcer is a breakdown in the mucosal lining of the stomach or duodenum. It is caused by chronic irritation from highly acidic gastric chemicals.

smoking, and drugs such as aspirin and ibuprofen, which irritate the mucosal lining of the esophagus, stomach, and duodenum.

H. pylori infections are treated with antibiotic drugs and antacids. The patient is also instructed to avoid taking any drugs that contain aspirin.

Procedures and Treatments

In this section, we will briefly describe some common diagnostic procedures used to help identify diseases and disorders of the digestive system, as well as therapeutic procedures used to treat certain conditions.

Barium Enema

A **barium enema** is a diagnostic procedure in which barium is used as a contrast agent to enable radiographic visualization of the large intestine. A barium enema is also called a **lower gastrointestinal (LGI) series** (Figure 3.8).

Before a barium enema test, the patient cleanses the bowel by following a special diet and taking a laxative. The procedure involves infusing the barium through a catheter (tube) inserted through the anus and into the rectum, until the barium fills the large intestine. X-rays are then taken of the entire length of the colon (Figure 3.9).

A barium enema is used to define normal and abnormal anatomy of the colon. The procedure is performed to help diagnose disorders such as diverticulosis

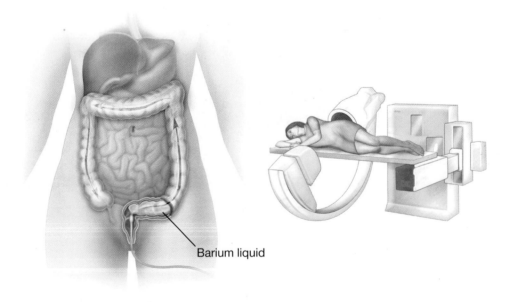

Barium liquid

Figure 3.8 During a barium enema, also called a *lower gastrointestinal* (LGI) *series*, a radioactive agent is introduced through a catheter inserted into the anus and rectum.

(the formation of pouches or sacs, called *diverticula*, in the colon wall), diverticulitis (inflammation of the diverticulum), polyps (small tissue masses that bulge or project outward or upward), intestinal blockages, abscesses, and cancer.

Colostomy

A **colostomy** is a surgical procedure in which one end of a healthy large intestine is brought out through the abdominal wall, and the edges of the bowel are stitched to the skin of the abdominal wall (Figure 3.10). The surgically created opening is called a *stoma*.

A colostomy drains stool (feces) from the colon into a colostomy bag attached to the abdomen. Most colostomy stool is softer and contains more liquid than stool that is passed normally. The procedure is usually performed after partial or complete intestinal obstruction (blockage of the large intestine), a severe infection, cancer, or trauma to the colon such as from a penetrating wound. Whether a colostomy is temporary or permanent depends on the extent of the disease or injury.

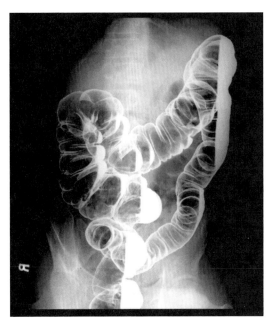

Living Art Enterprises, LLC / Science Source

Figure 3.9 X-ray from a contrast barium enema. This diagnostic procedure allows doctors to look for a variety of abnormalities, such as intestinal blockages, polyps, diverticulosis, and cancer.

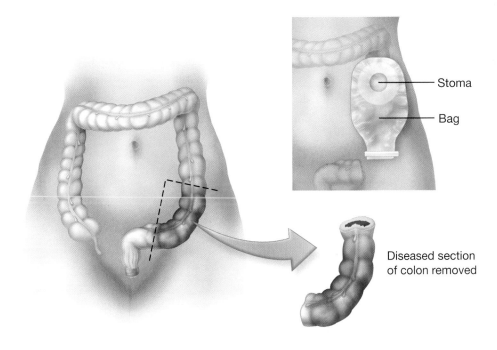

Stoma

Bag

Diseased section of colon removed

Figure 3.10 A colostomy drains stool from the large intestine into a colostomy bag. The surgically created opening is called a *stoma*.

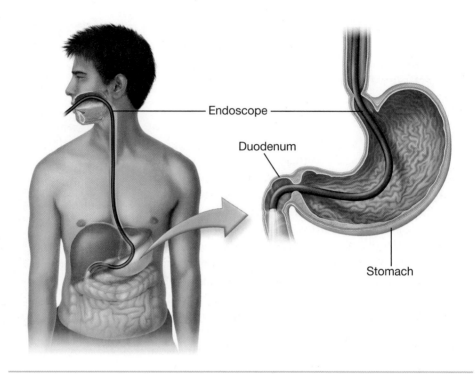

Figure 3.11 Endoscopy involves examination of internal body organs and structures with a flexible, fiber-optic instrument called an *endoscope*.

Endoscopy

An **endoscopy** (ĕn-DŎS-kō-pē) is a procedure in which an endoscope is used to examine internal body organs and structures (Figure 3.11). An *endoscope* is a flexible, fiber-optic instrument that contains a magnifying lens and a light source. It may also be equipped with a tool for removing tissue to be examined for signs of disease. The endoscope is inserted through an existing opening, such as the mouth or nose.

Esophagoscopy (ē-SŎF-a-GŎS-kō-pē) is examination of the esophagus with an *esophagoscope* (ē-SŎF-a-gō-skōp). If the endoscope passes farther into the stomach, the procedure is known as a **gastroscopy** (găs-TRŎS-kō-pē). If the endoscope is manipulated into the duodenum, the procedure is called an **esophagogastroduodenoscopy** (ē-SŎF-ă-gō-GĂS-trō-dū-ŏ-dĕ-NŎS-kō-pē), or **EDG**.

Endoscopic examination of the large intestine involves inserting the endoscope through the rectum. If the scope is passed through the rectum into the sigmoid colon, the procedure is called a **sigmoidoscopy** (sĭg-moy-DŎS-kō-pē). Endoscopic examination of the entire colon is called a **colonoscopy** (kō-lŏn-ŎS-kō-pē).

Upper Gastrointestinal Series

An **upper gastrointestinal (UGI) series** is a radiographic (X-ray) examination of the upper GI tract, which includes the esophagus, stomach, and duodenum (Figure 3.12). The patient drinks a milkshake-like mixture containing barium, a chemical element that serves as a contrast agent. The barium allows radiographic imaging of body organs and vessels that could not otherwise be seen on an X-ray. The barium mixture is flavored to make it more palatable to the patient.

During a UGI series, a radiologist views and records images as the barium flows through the esophagus and stomach. If the imaging procedure stops at the stomach, it is referred to as a **barium swallow**. If the entire small intestine also needs to be examined, the radiologist continues to record images of the duodenum, jejunum, and ileum until the barium reaches the beginning of the large intestine at the ileocecal valve. This valve prevents the backflow of waste from the large intestine into the small intestine. This diagnostic procedure is known as an **upper GI and small bowel series**.

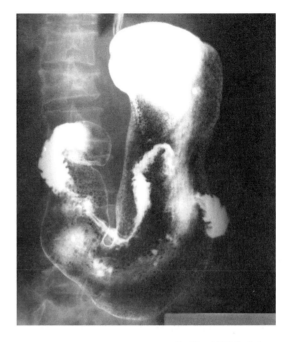

Figure 3.12 This upper gastrointestinal (UGI) study of an adult female shows a close-up of the stomach and duodenum.

Gastric Bypass Surgery

Gastric bypass surgery is a type of weight-loss surgery that limits food consumption by reducing the size of the stomach (Figure 3.13). In addition to limiting the amount of food that can be consumed in one sitting, this surgery reduces the absorption of nutrients from food. Gastric bypass and other weight-loss surgeries are performed when diet and exercise methods alone have been ineffective or when obesity causes serious health problems.

Typically, gastric bypass surgery is performed with a *laparoscope* (LĂP-ă-rō-skōp) inserted through small incisions made in the abdomen. The laparoscope is linked to a video monitor, which enables the surgeon to see and operate inside the abdomen without having to make large incisions. Compared to open surgery, laparoscopy (lăp-ă-RŎS-kō-pē) involves a shorter hospitalization period and faster recovery.

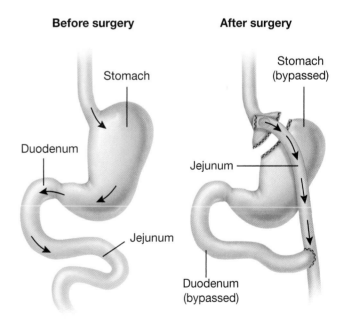

Figure 3.13 Gastric bypass surgery limits food consumption by reducing the size of the stomach.

Multiple Choice: Diseases and Disorders

Directions: Write the letter of the disease or disorder that matches each numbered definition below.

A   1. disorder in which a portion of the stomach protrudes through the diaphragm
   a. hiatal hernia
   b. gastroesophageal reflux disease
   c. Crohn's disease
   d. ulcer

B   2. chronic disease in which stomach acid backs up into the esophagus
   a. hiatal hernia
   b. gastroesophageal reflux disease
   c. Crohn's disease
   d. ulcer

D   3. disorder resulting from breakdown of the mucosal lining in the stomach or duodenum due to chronic irritation
   a. hiatal hernia
   b. gastroesophageal reflux disease
   c. Crohn's disease
   d. ulcer

C   4. chronic inflammatory bowel disease characterized by thickening and a gradual erosion of the inner lining of the intestinal wall
   a. hiatal hernia
   b. gastroesophageal reflux disease
   c. Crohn's disease
   d. ulcer

B   5. chronic, irreversible liver disease in which normal cells are replaced with hard, fibrous scar tissue; associated with long-term alcoholism
   a. hepatitis   c. Crohn's disease
   b. cirrhosis   d. peptic ulcer

C   6. inflammation of the liver that causes abdominal pain, nausea, vomiting, and jaundice
   a. bulimia nervosa   c. hepatitis
   b. cirrhosis   d. Crohn's disease

B   7. eating disorder characterized by repeated gorging of food followed by intentional vomiting and/or laxative abuse
   a. anorexia nervosa   c. reflux
   b. bulimia nervosa   d. hepatitis

SCORECARD: How Did You Do?

Number correct (_____), divided by 7 (_____), multiplied by 100 equals _____ (your score)

Multiple Choice: Procedures and Treatments

Directions: Write the letter of the diagnostic procedure or therapeutic treatment that matches each numbered definition below.

B   1. surgical procedure in which one end of a healthy large intestine is drawn through the abdominal wall, and the edges of the bowel are stitched to the skin of the abdominal wall
   a. gastric bypass surgery
   b. colostomy
   c. barium enema
   d. endoscopy

B   2. endoscopic examination of the esophagus
   a. upper gastrointestinal (UGI) series
   b. esophagoscopy
   c. barium swallow
   d. sigmoidoscopy

A   3. radiographic examination of the esophagus, stomach, and duodenum using barium as a contrast agent
   a. upper gastrointestinal (UGI) series
   b. endoscopy
   c. laparoscopy
   d. colostomy

D   4. procedure in which an endoscope is used to examine internal body structures
   a. barium enema
   b. sigmoidoscopy
   c. gastroscopy
   d. endoscopy

C   5. surgical procedure that reduces the size of the stomach to limit food consumption
  a. colostomy
  b. endoscopy
  c. gastric bypass surgery
  d. esophagogastroduodenoscopy

B   6. diagnostic procedure in which barium is used as a contrast agent to enable radiographic visualization of the large intestine
  a. upper GI and small bowel series
  b. barium enema
  c. gastroscopy
  d. colostomy

C   7. upper GI imaging procedure that stops at the stomach
  a. esophagoscopy   c. barium swallow
  b. barium enema   d. sigmoidoscopy

A   8. another term for *barium enema*
  a. lower gastrointestinal (LGI) series
  b. upper gastrointestinal (UGI) series
  c. barium swallow
  d. barium flow

B   9. radiographic examination of all three parts of the small intestine (duodenum, jejunum, and ileum)
  a. lower gastrointestinal (LGI) series
  b. upper GI and small bowel series
  c. sigmoidoscopy
  d. colonoscopy

C   10. endoscopic examination of the sigmoid colon
  a. colonoscopy
  b. colostomy
  c. sigmoidoscopy
  d. esophagogastroduodenoscopy

D   11. endoscopic examination of the entire colon
  a. barium swallow
  b. lower gastrointestinal (LGI) series
  c. colostomy
  d. colonoscopy

D   12. examination procedure that involves the use of an endoscope
  a. gastroscopy
  b. esophagogastroduodenoscopy
  c. colonoscopy
  d. all of the above

SCORECARD: How Did You Do?

Number correct (_____), divided by 12 (_____), multiplied by 100 equals _____ (your score)

Assessment

Identifying Abbreviations

Directions: Write the abbreviation for each medical term listed below.

Medical Term	Abbreviation
1. esophagogastroduodenoscopy	EGD
2. gastroesophageal reflux disease	GERD
3. lower gastrointestinal	LGI
4. upper gastrointestinal	UGI
5. inflammatory bowel disease	IBD

SCORECARD: How Did You Do?

Number correct (_____), divided by 5 (_____), multiplied by 100 equals _____ (your score)

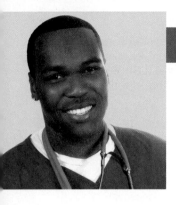

Analyzing the Intern Experience

In the Intern Experience described at the beginning of this chapter, Evan Walker encountered Sue, a young female patient who had difficulty swallowing. Sue was seen by Dr. Stomack, who obtained a history of her health problems and performed a physical examination. In addition, Dr. Stomack ordered a diagnostic test to help determine the cause of Sue's condition. When she received the test results, Dr. Stomack analyzed all the information that she had gathered, made a medical diagnosis, and developed a treatment plan. The physician then made a dictated recording of Sue's health information, which was later transcribed into a chart note.

We will now learn more about Sue's condition from a clinical perspective, interpreting the medical terms in her chart note as we analyze the scenario presented in the Intern Experience.

Audio Activity: Sue Resch's Chart Note

Directions: At the companion website, listen and read along as the physician dictates Sue Resch's chart note, shown below. Then do the exercise that appears after Sue's chart note.

CHART NOTE

Patient Name: Resch, Sue
ID Number: 76554
Examination Date: March 1, 20xx

SUBJECTIVE
Sue came into our office complaining of a feeling that something is caught in her throat. She thinks it might be a turkey bone from the soup she ate last night.

OBJECTIVE
Sensation of a foreign body in the **proximal** esophagus, near the **oropharynx**. Vital signs are normal. No known allergies. She states that this happened once before but denies any regular symptoms of **dysphagia** or **gastroesophageal reflux**.

ASSESSMENT
Sensation of foreign body.

PLAN
Recommend immediate **esophagogastroduodenoscopy** to exclude an **esophageal** foreign body.

Interpret Sue Resch's Chart Note

Directions: After listening to the dictated recording and reading the chart note on Sue Resch, provide the medical term that matches each definition below.

Example: inflammation of the intestine   *Answer:* enteritis

1. painful or difficult swallowing   dysphagia

2. mouth and throat   oropharynx

3. process of observing the esophagus, stomach, and duodenum   esophagogastroduodenoscopy

4. nearest the point of origin   proximal

5. backflow of stomach acid into the esophagus   gastroesophageal reflux

6. pertaining to the esophagus   esophageal

SCORECARD: How Did You Do?

Number correct (_____), divided by 6 (_____), multiplied by 100 equals _____ (your score)

Working with Medical Records

In this activity, you will interpret the medical records (chart notes) of patients with health problems related to the digestive system. These examples illustrate typical medical records prepared in a real-world healthcare environment. To interpret these chart notes, you will apply your knowledge of word elements (prefixes, combining forms, and suffixes), diseases and disorders, and procedures and treatments related to the digestive system.

Audio Activity: Ida Gundrum's Chart Note

Directions: At the companion website, listen and read along as the physician dictates the following chart note on Ida Gundrum. Then do the exercise that appears after Ida's chart note.

CHART NOTE

Patient Name: Gundrum, Ida
ID Number: 98774
Examination Date: October 11, 20xx

SUBJECTIVE
29-year-old female complains of **epigastric** discomfort, which she describes as a constant burning for several weeks. Initial treatment was successful with Tagamet® (drug that reduces gastric acid secretions), but discomfort has recurred several times over a 2-week period. She complains of nausea. No vomiting or **hematemesis**. Tagamet® partially relieves her symptoms. She has been under considerable stress at work due to job downsizing and outsourcing of personnel. Headache relief in the form of Tylenol® or Motrin® has been unsuccessful and seems to exacerbate (worsen) her condition.

OBJECTIVE
Abdomen is soft, flat, and nontender with normal bowel sounds. No masses or **organomegaly**.

ASSESSMENT
Gastritis, probably exacerbated by NSAIDs (nonsteroidal anti-inflammatory drugs), and stress.

PLAN
We discussed several methods of stress reduction, including support group websites. She will stop using Motrin® and Tylenol® for headaches. She was given a sample of Prilosec® 20 mg q.i.d. (4 times a day) to be taken for one month. The patient will return in 3–4 weeks for a follow-up visit.

Assessment

Interpret Ida Gundrum's Chart Note

Directions: After listening to the dictated recording and reading the chart note on Ida Gundrum, provide the medical term that matches each definition below.

Example: abnormal condition of gallstones   *Answer:* cholelithiasis

1. enlargement of an organ   organomegaly

2. vomiting blood   hematemesis

3. inflammation of the stomach   gastritis

4. pertaining to the area above the stomach   epigastric

SCORECARD: How Did You Do?

Number correct (_____), divided by 4 (_____), multiplied by 100 equals _____ (your score)

Audio Activity: Sally Nguyen's Chart Note

Directions: At the companion website, listen and read along as the physician dictates the following chart note on Sally Nguyen. Then do the exercise that appears after Sally's chart note.

CHART NOTE

Patient Name: Nguyen, Sally
ID Number: 22316
Examination Date: March 1, 20xx

PROCECURE
Flexible **sigmoidoscopy**

INDICATIONS
Patient is an 81-year-old female for routine screening flexible sigmoidoscopy. Patient has a maternal history of Crohn's disease and a paternal history of diabetes.

PROCEDURE REPORT
The 60 cm **sigmoidoscope** was introduced to 40 cm and was well tolerated. **Erythematous**, nonbleeding polyp, less than 1 cm, was found between 35 and 40 cm. Retroflex (backward) viewing is negative. Patient tolerated the procedure well.

DIAGNOSIS
Polyp at 35-40 cm on flexible sigmoidoscopy screening examination.

PLAN
She is referred to a **gastroenterologist** for **colonoscopy**. We discussed the risks of colonoscopy, its benefits, and the procedure. The patient was provided with a brochure describing the procedure and instructed to contact the office with any questions.

Assessment

Interpret Sally Nguyen's Chart Note

Directions: After listening to the dictated recording and reading the chart note on Sally Nguyen, provide the medical term that matches each definition below.

Example: inflammation of the stomach   *Answer:* gastritis

1. process of observing the colon   colonoscopy
2. specialist in the study of the stomach and intestine   gastroenterologist
3. instrument used to visualize the sigmoid colon   sigmoidoscope
4. process of observing the sigmoid colon   sigmoidoscopy

SCORECARD: How Did You Do?

Number correct (_____), divided by 4 (_____), multiplied by 100 equals _____ (your score)

Word Elements Summary

Prefixes

Prefix	Meaning
a-	not; without
ad-	toward
anti-	against
brady-	slow
dia-	through
dys-	painful; difficult
epi-	upon; above
hyper-	above; above normal
pan-	all; everything
peri-	around
poly-	many
retro-	backward; behind

Combining Forms

Root Word/Combining Vowel	Meaning
carcin/o	cancerous; cancer
celi/o	abdomen
chol/e	bile; gall
cholecyst/o	gallbladder
col/o, colon/o	colon; large intestine
dist/o	away from the point of origin
diverticul/o	diverticulum
duoden/o	duodenum
enter/o	intestines
esophag/o	esophagus

(Continued)

Root Word/Combining Vowel	Meaning
gastr/o	stomach
gingiv/o	gums
gloss/o	tongue
hemat/o	blood
hepat/o	liver
herni/o	hernia; rupture; protrusion
ile/o	ileum
jejun/o	jejunum
lapar/o	abdomen
lith/o	stone
or/o	mouth
organ/o	organ
pancreat/o	pancreas
peps/o	digestion
polyp/o	polyp; small growth
proct/o	anus and rectum
proxim/o	nearest the point of origin
rect/o	rectum
sial/o	saliva
sigmoid/o	sigmoid colon

Suffixes

Suffix	Meaning
-al	pertaining to
-algia	pain
-cele	hernia; swelling; protrusion
-dynia	pain
-eal	pertaining to
-ectomy	surgical removal; excision
-emesis	vomiting

(Continued)

Suffix	Meaning
-gram	record; image
-graphy	process of recording an image
-ia	condition
-iasis	abnormal condition
-ic	pertaining to
-itis	inflammation
-logist	specialist in the study and treatment of
-logy	study of
-megaly	enlargement
-oma	tumor
-osis	abnormal condition
-phagia	condition of eating or swallowing
-pharynx	pharynx; throat
-plasty	surgical repair
-ptosis	drooping; downward displacement
-rrhea	flow; discharge
-scope	instrument used to observe
-scopy	process of observing
-stomy	new opening
-tomy	incision; cut into
-tripsy	crushing
-y	condition; process

More Practice: Activities and Games

The activities on the following pages will help you reinforce your skills and check your mastery of the medical terminology that you learned in this chapter. Visit the companion website for More Practice games and activities.

True or False

Directions: Indicate whether each statement below is true or false.

True or False?

_T_   1. Major organs of the gastrointestinal (GI) tract include the mouth and stomach.

_T_   2. The liver, gallbladder, pancreas, salivary glands, and teeth are accessory organs that aid in digestion.

_F_   3. Chemical digestion and absorption of food occur in the stomach.

_F_   4. The small intestine is so named because its diameter is wider than that of the large intestine.

_F_   5. Crohn's disease is an acute inflammatory stomach disease.

_T_   6. A hiatal hernia occurs when a portion of the stomach protrudes through the diaphragm.

_T_   7. Hepatitis is an inflammation of the liver causing yellowish discoloration of the skin and eyes.

_T_   8. Ulcers can develop in the esophagus, stomach, or duodenum.

_T_   9. Gastric bypass is a type of weight-loss surgery.

_F_   10. Laparoscopic surgery involves a long, difficult recovery time.

_F_   11. The three parts of the small intestine are the duodenum, jejunum, and sigmoid.

_F_   12. The small intestine is known as the colon.

_T_   13. Anorexia nervosa and bulimia nervosa are two common types of behavioral eating disorders.

_T_   14. An endoscope is a flexible, fiber-optic instrument that has a magnifying lens and, in some cases, a tool for removing tissue to be checked for disease.

_F_   15. A colonoscopy drains stool from the colon into a colostomy bag attached to the abdomen.

_T_   16. A lower gastrointestinal (LGI) series can detect (for example) diverticulitis, polyps, abscesses, and cancer.

Dictionary Skills

Directions: Using a medical dictionary, such as *Taber's Cyclopedic Medical Dictionary*, look up the term **gastroparalysis**.

For each medical term shown below, indicate whether the term appears on the same page as **gastroparalysis**, before the page, or after the page. Use the following abbreviations in your answers:

O = on the same page   **B** = before the page   **A** = after the page

Write the definition of each term in the space provided.

Medical Term	O, B, A
	Answers in this column will vary.

1. gastropulmonary

Definition: pertaining to the lungs and the stomach

2. gastrology   _____

Definition: the study of the stomach

Medical Term	O, B, A
	Answers in this column will vary.

3. gastroptosis

Definition: downward displacement of the stomach

4. gastrulation

Definition: the process of becoming a gastrula

5. gastroscope

Definition: instrument used to observe the stomach

6. gastrolysis

Definition: the breaking up of adhesions around the stomach

7. gastrogastrostomy

Definition: surgical connection between two parts of the stomach

8. gastrojejunostomy

Definition: surgical connection between the stomach and the jejunum

9. gastrostenosis

Definition: narrowing or constriction of the stomach

10. gastromycosis

Definition: fungal infection of the stomach

Break It Down

Directions: Break down each medical term listed below by placing a slash between each word part (prefix, root word, combining vowel, and suffix). Then define each term.

Medical Term	Dissection
1. sigmoiditis	s i g m o i d / i t i s

Definition: inflammation of the sigmoid colon

| 2. rectocolitis | r e c t / o / c o l / i t i s |

Definition: inflammation of the rectum and large intestine

| 3. celioscopy | c e l i / o / s c o p y |

Definition: process of observing the abdomen

| 4. enterogram | e n t e r / o / g r a m |

Definition: record or image of the intestines

| 5. enterology | e n t e r / o / l o g y |

Definition: study of the intestines

| 6. gingival | g i n g i v / a l |

Definition: pertaining to the gums

| 7. enteroplasty | e n t e r / o / p l a s t y |

Definition: surgical repair of the intestines

Medical Term	Dissection

8. pancreatitis   p a n c r e a t/i t i s

Definition: inflammation of the pancreas
_____

9. gingivosis   g i n g i v/o s i s

Definition: abnormal condition of the gums
_____

10. glossoplasty   g l o s s o/p l a s t y

Definition: surgical repair of the tongue
_____

11. retrography   r e t r o/g r a p h y

Definition: process of recording an image behind
_____

12. glossalgia   g l o s s/a l g i a

Definition: pain in the tongue
_____

Audio Activity: Shana Laquisha's Chart Note

Directions: At the companion website, listen and read along as the physician dictates the following chart note on Shana Laquisha. Then do the exercise that appears after Shana's chart note.

RADIOLOGY REPORT

Patient Name: Laquisha, Shana
ID Number: 569801
Examination Date: March 1, 20xx

EXAMINATION
Upper GI

INDICATIONS
Patient has a history of **Crohn's disease** and uncontrolled diarrhea.

PROCEDURE
Swallowing mechanism appears normal. There is no evidence of aspiration (drawing of gastric contents into the throat). **Proximal esophagus** appears normal.
Fundus (base) of the **stomach** distends well. There is no suggestion of abnormal rugae (fold) pattern in the upper region of the stomach. The body and pyloris (passage at the lower end of the stomach that opens into the duodenum) of the stomach appear normal. There is a high-grade obstruction in the extreme distal end of the stomach. There is just a 2 to 3 mm passage of contrast agent beyond an "apple core" obstructing lesion. This certainly has to be considered a **carcinoma**; direct visualization is indicated. The **duodenal** bulb, loop, and proximal **jejunum** appear normal.

CONCLUSION
A 2 to 3 mm obstructing lesion in the distal end of the stomach, possibly carcinoma.

Assessment

Interpret Shana Laquisha's Chart Note

Directions: After listening to the dictated recording and reading the chart note on Shana Laquisha, provide the medical term that matches each definition below.

Example: inflammation of the diverticulum   *Answer:* diverticulitis

1. pertaining to the duodenum   duodenal

2. nearest the point of origin   proximal

3. cancerous tumor   carcinoma

4. an expandable organ that breaks food down for absorption by the body; located between the esophagus and small intestine   stomach

5. tubular structure that carries food from the pharynx to the stomach   esophagus

6. the section of the small intestine between the duodenum and the ileum   jejunum

7. chronic, inflammatory bowel disease characterized by thickening and gradual erosion of the inner lining of the intestinal wall   Crohn's disease

Chapter 4

The Musculoskeletal System

orth / o / ped / ics: the study of the musculoskeletal system

Chapter Organization

- Intern Experience
- Overview of Musculoskeletal System Anatomy and Physiology
- Word Elements
- Breaking Down and Building Musculoskeletal System Terms
- Diseases and Disorders
- Procedures and Treatments
- Analyzing the Intern Experience
- Working with Medical Records
- Chapter Review

Chapter Objectives

After completing this chapter, you will be able to

1. label an anatomical diagram of the musculoskeletal system;

2. dissect and define common medical terminology related to the musculoskeletal system;

3. build terms used to describe musculoskeletal system diseases and disorders, diagnostic procedures, and therapeutic treatments;

4. pronounce and spell common medical terminology related to the musculoskeletal system;

5. understand that the processes of building and dissecting a medical term based on its prefix, word root, and suffix enable you to analyze an extremely large number of medical terms beyond those presented in this chapter;

6. interpret the meaning of abbreviations associated with the musculoskeletal system; and

7. interpret medical records containing terminology and abbreviations related to the musculoskeletal system.

You will see this icon at various points throughout this chapter. The icon indicates that you will find interactive activities and games on the Medical Terminology Companion Website. These activities and games will help you learn, practice, and expand your medical terminology knowledge and skills. Some of these activities are also available on the Medical Terminology Mobile Website.

Companion Website
www.g-wlearning.com/healthsciences

Mobile Site
www.m.g-wlearning.com/5800

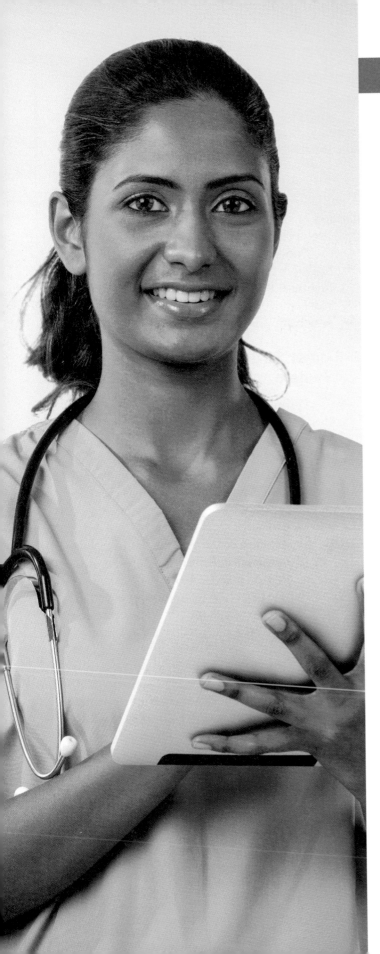

Aishandi Koshy is serving an internship at the DesFed Urgent Care Center, a facility that offers treatment to patients of all ages for illnesses and injuries such as the flu, asthma attacks, broken bones, cuts requiring stitches, and other health issues requiring time-sensitive care.

Aishandi's assignment this week is to observe and assist Dr. Geiger. Aishandi accompanies the doctor to exam room 5, where their next patient is waiting. Bill, a high school sophomore, recounts for Dr. Geiger the details of his injury.

It was Bill's first football game of the season. He was running the play pattern that the coach had drilled into the team. The quarterback hurled the ball in his direction, and as Bill was about to catch it, the harsh glare of the setting sun blocked his view. Out of nowhere his opponent tackled him, sliding sideways into his left knee. Dazed, Bill lay on the ground, clutching his knee in agony.

Bill is experiencing a problem with a part of his musculoskeletal system, the body system that provides a framework of support for muscles, ligaments, and tendons; protects delicate internal organs and tissues; and enables movement. To help you understand what is happening to Bill, this chapter will present word elements (combining forms, prefixes, and suffixes) that make up medical terminology related to the musculoskeletal system. As you progress through this book, you will see many word parts that are also used in medical terms related to other body systems.

We will begin our study of the musculoskeletal system with a brief overview of its anatomy and physiology. Major structures of both the muscular and skeletal systems will be covered, along with their main functions. Later in the chapter, you will learn about some common pathological conditions of the musculoskeletal system, tests and procedures used to diagnose these conditions, and common methods for treating them.

Overview of Musculoskeletal System Anatomy and Physiology

The primary functions of the musculoskeletal system are to
1. provide the framework and support for the body;
2. protect the internal organs;
3. allow bodily movement;
4. store calcium, phosphorus, and other vital minerals;
5. manufacture red blood cells; and
6. provide body heat through energy produced by the muscles.

The musculoskeletal system is a combination of two body systems that work together: the muscular system, which provides movement, and the skeletal system, which supports and protects the body.

Major Structures of the Muscular System

The **muscular system** is made up of muscles, tendons, and ligaments (Figure 4.1A). These structures are attached to bones, enabling us to move, bend, and manipulate objects. Muscular tissue is unique in its ability to contract, or shorten. In fact, as much as 70 percent of our body heat is generated by muscle contractions.

Muscles are categorized as either *voluntary* or *involuntary*. **Voluntary muscle**, also called *skeletal muscle*, is under conscious control. During voluntary muscular action, your brain sends neural (nerve) impulses to certain muscles, directing them to move. Examples of voluntary muscular action include sending a text message, closing a door, or walking up a flight of stairs.

By contrast, **involuntary muscle** is not under conscious control. Examples of involuntary muscle are the smooth muscle of the digestive tract, and cardiac muscle, which contracts to move blood into and out of the heart. Involuntary muscular movement happens unconsciously. Can you imagine if you had to think about contracting your heart to beat or your diaphragm muscle to breathe?

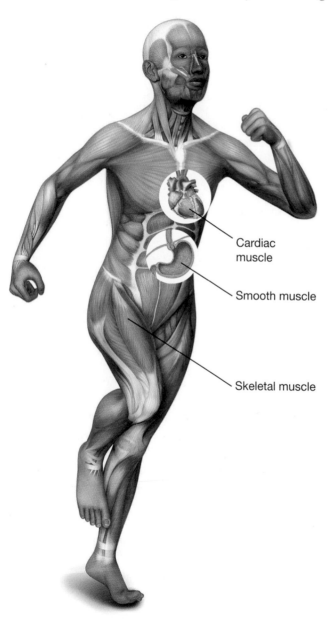

Cardiac muscle

Smooth muscle

Skeletal muscle

Figure 4.1A The muscular system.

Major Structures of the Skeletal System

The bones of the **skeletal system** provide a framework of support for the body and protect the internal organs (Figure 4.1B). Minerals such as calcium and phosphorus are stored in the bones, giving them their strength. The skeletal system also plays a crucial role in the production of red blood cells.

The adult skeletal system consists of 206 bones plus cartilage, ligaments, and tendons. **Cartilage** is connective tissue that acts as a shock absorber by cushioning bones that are linked together. This shock-absorbing function prevents friction between bones whenever we walk, run, or jump. The **meniscus** (mĕ-NĬS-kŭs) in the knee, for example, is a C-shaped disk of cartilage that cushions the knee joint. Actually, there are two *menisci* (mĕ-NĬS-ē) in each knee: one on the inner side of the knee and one on the outer side.

A **ligament** is a band of tissue that connects a bone to another bone. An example of a ligament is the **anterior cruciate** (KRŪ-shē-āt) **ligament** in the knee, which controls rotation and forward movement of the tibia (shin bone). A **tendon** is a cord of fibrous tissue that connects muscle to bone. Your Achilles tendon, for example, connects your heel bone to your calf (lower leg) muscles.

The point at which one bone meets another bone is called a **joint**. Joints make bodily motion possible. Without joints, your body movement would be limited and robotic.

Orthopedics is the study of the musculoskeletal system. The suffix **-ics** means "the organized knowledge, practice, or treatment" of a particular subject or field. An **orthopedist** is a physician who specializes in the study and treatment of the musculoskeletal system.

Anatomy and Physiology Vocabulary

Now that you have been introduced to the basic structure and functions of the musculoskeletal system, we will explore in more detail the key terms presented in the introduction.

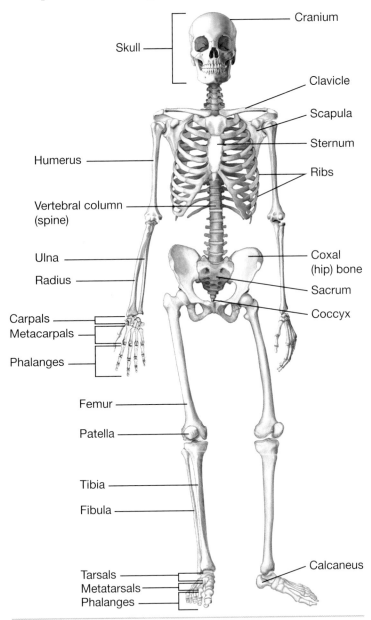

Figure 4.1B The skeletal system

Key Term	Definition
cartilage	connective tissue that acts as a shock absorber by cushioning bones that are linked together
involuntary muscle	muscle that is not under conscious control; smooth muscle and cardiac muscle
joint	the point at which one bone meets another bone
ligament	band of tissue that connects a bone to another bone
meniscus (plural *menisci*)	C-shaped disk of cartilage that cushions the knee joint
muscular system	the body system made up of muscles, tendons, and ligaments, all of which control movement
orthopedics	the study of the musculoskeletal system
orthopedist	physician who specializes in the study and treatment of the musculoskeletal system
skeletal system	the body system that provides a framework of support for organs and tissues, protects the internal organs, stores minerals such as calcium and phosphorus, and plays a crucial role in the production of erythrocytes (red blood cells)
tendon	band of fibrous tissue that attaches muscle to bone
voluntary muscle	muscle that is under conscious control; skeletal muscle

 ## E-Flash Card Activity: Anatomy and Physiology Vocabulary

Directions: After you have reviewed the anatomy and physiology vocabulary related to the musculoskeletal system, practice with the e-flash cards until you are comfortable with the spelling and definition of each term.

Identifying the Three Types of Muscle Tissue

Directions: Label the three types of muscular tissue in the diagram below.

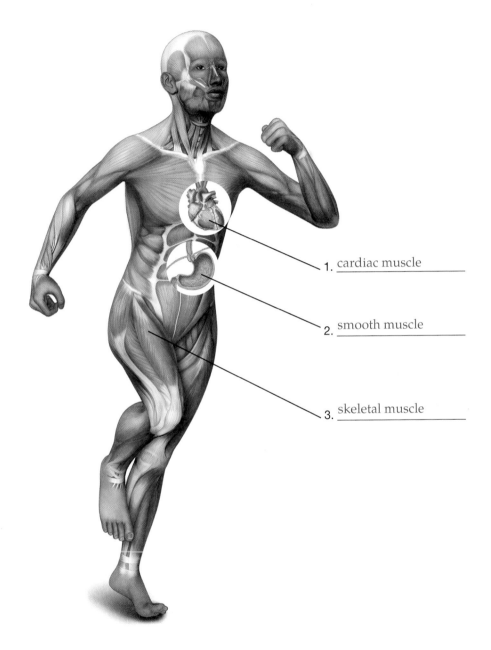

1. cardiac muscle _____

2. smooth muscle _____

3. skeletal muscle _____

Identifying Major Bones of the Skeletal System

Directions: Label the diagram of the skeletal system.

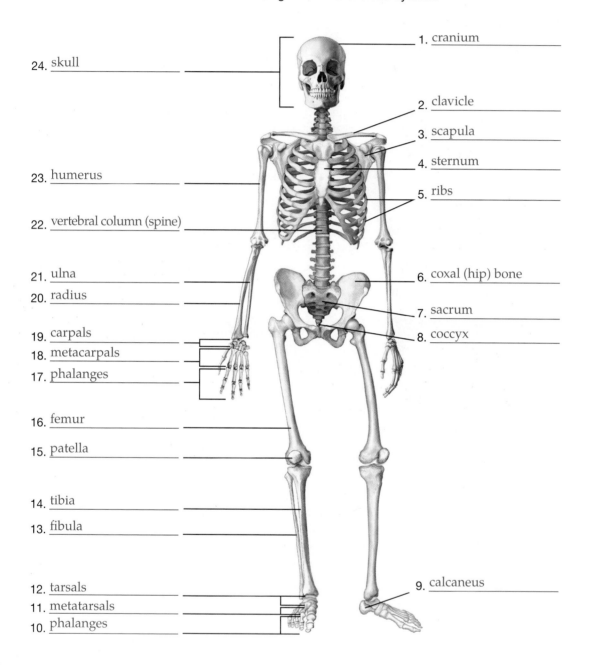

24. skull

23. humerus

22. vertebral column (spine)

21. ulna
20. radius

19. carpals
18. metacarpals
17. phalanges

16. femur

15. patella

14. tibia

13. fibula

12. tarsals
11. metatarsals
10. phalanges

1. cranium

2. clavicle

3. scapula

4. sternum

5. ribs

6. coxal (hip) bone

7. sacrum

8. coccyx

9. calcaneus

Matching Anatomy and Physiology Vocabulary

Directions: Match the vocabulary term in Column A with its meaning in Column B.

Column A

_J_	1.	cartilage
_F_	2.	involuntary muscle
_H_	3.	joint
_K_	4.	ligament
_A_	5.	meniscus
_C_	6.	orthopedics
_D_	7.	orthopedist
_B_	8.	skeletal system
_E_	9.	tendon
_G_	10.	voluntary muscle
_I_	11.	muscular system

Column B

A. C-shaped disk of cartilage that cushions the knee joint

B. the body system that provides a framework of support for organs and tissues, protects the internal organs, stores minerals such as calcium and phosphorus, and plays a crucial role in the production of red blood cells

C. the study of the musculoskeletal system

D. physician who specializes in the study and treatment of the musculoskeletal system

E. band of fibrous tissue that attaches muscle to bone

F. muscle that is not under conscious control; smooth muscle and cardiac muscle

G. muscle that is under conscious control; skeletal muscle

H. the point at which one bone meets another bone

I. the body system made up of muscles, tendons, and ligaments, all of which control movement

J. connective tissue that acts as a shock absorber by cushioning bones that are linked together

K. band of tissue that connects a bone to another bone

SCORECARD: How Did You Do?

Number correct (_____), divided by 11 (_____), multiplied by 100 equals _____ (your score)

Word Elements

In this section you will learn word elements—prefixes, combining forms, and suffixes—that are common to the musculoskeletal system. By learning these word elements and understanding how they are combined to build medical terms, you will be able to analyze Bill's musculoskeletal problem (described in the Intern Experience at the beginning of this chapter) and identify a large number of terms associated with the musculoskeletal system.

 ## E-Flash Card Activity: Word Elements

Directions: Review the word elements in the tables that follow. Then, practice with the e-flash cards until you are able to quickly recognize the different word parts (prefixes, combining forms, and suffixes) and their meanings. The e-flash cards are grouped together by prefixes, combining forms, and suffixes, followed by a cumulative review of all the word elements that you learned in this chapter.

Prefixes

Let's begin our study of musculoskeletal system word elements by looking at the prefixes listed in the table below.

Prefix	Meaning
a-	not; without
an-	not; without
brady-	slow
dys-	painful; difficult
endo-	within
epi-	upon; above
hyper-	above; above normal
inter-	between
intra-	within
meta-	change; beyond
per-	through
peri-	around
poly-	many
quadri-	four
sub-	beneath; below
supra-	above
sym-, syn-	together; with

Combining Forms

Listed below are common combining forms used in medical terms related to the musculoskeletal system.

Root Word/Combining Vowel	Meaning
anter/o	front
arthr/o	joint
articul/o	joint
burs/a, burs/o	bursa; sac
cardi/o	heart
carp/o	carpals (wrist bones)
chondr/o	cartilage
clavicul/o	clavicle (collar bone)
coccyg/o	coccyx (tailbone)
cost/o	rib
crani/o	skull
dist/o	away from the point of origin
dors/o	back (of the body)
ecchym/o	blood in the tissues
electr/o	electrical activity
erythemat/o	redness
erythr/o	red
femor/o	femur (thigh bone)
fibul/o	fibula
herni/o	hernia; rupture; protrusion
humer/o	humerus (upper arm bone)
ili/o	ilium
infer/o	below; beneath
ischi/o	ischium (part of hip bone)
kines/o, kinesi/o	movement
kyph/o	hump
later/o	side
lord/o	curve
medi/o	middle
metacarp/o	metacarpals (bones of the hand)
metatars/o	metatarsals (bones of the foot)
muscul/o	muscle

(Continued)

Root Word/Combining Vowel	Meaning
my/o	muscle
myel/o	bone marrow; spinal cord
necr/o	death
neur/o	nerve
orth/o	straight
oste/o	bone
patell/a, patell/o	patella (kneecap)
path/o	disease
phalang/o	phalanges (bones of fingers/toes)
por/o	pore; duct; small opening
poster/o	back (of the body)
proxim/o	nearest the point of origin
pub/o	pubis (part of the hip bone)
radi/o	radius (bone of the forearm); X-ray
sacr/o	sacrum (bone at base of the spine)
scapul/o	scapula (shoulder blade)
scoli/o	crooked; bent
spondyl/o	vertebra; spine
stern/o	sternum (breastbone)
tars/o	ankle bones
ten/o	tendon
tendin/o, tendon/o	tendon
tibi/o	tibia (shin bone)
uln/o	ulna (bone of the forearm)
vascul/o	blood vessel
vertebr/o	vertebra; spine

Suffixes

Listed below are suffixes used in medical terms pertaining to the musculoskeletal system. Many of these prefixes are used in medical terms related to other body systems as well.

Suffix	Meaning
-ac	pertaining to
-al	pertaining to
-algia	pain

(Continued)

Suffix	Meaning
-ar	pertaining to
-ary	pertaining to
-asthenia	weakness
-centesis	surgical puncture to remove fluid
-clasia	surgical breaking
-cyte	cell
-desis	to bind or tie together surgically
-dynia	pain
-eal	pertaining to
-ectomy	surgical removal; excision
-edema	swelling
-ema	condition
-gen	producing; originating; causing
-gram	record; image
-graphy	process of recording an image
-ia	condition
-ic	pertaining to
-ior	pertaining to
-itis	inflammation
-kinesia	movement
-kinesis	movement
-logist	specialist in the study and treatment of
-logy	study of
-lysis	breakdown; loosening; dissolving
-malacia	softening
-metry	process of measuring
-oma	tumor; mass
-osis	abnormal condition
-ous	pertaining to
-pathy	disease
-penia	deficiency; abnormal reduction
-plasty	surgical repair
-plegia	paralysis
-rrhaphy	suture

(Continued)

Suffix	Meaning
-rrhexis	rupture
-scope	instrument used to observe
-scopy	process of observing
-tome	instrument used to cut
-tomy	incision; cut into
-trophy	development

Matching Prefixes, Combining Forms, and Suffixes

Directions: In each exercise below, match the word element in Column A with its meaning in Column B. Some meanings may be used more than once.

Prefixes

Column A

- J 1. quadri-
- F 2. per-
- B 3. a-
- G 4. brady-
- A 5. dys-
- B 6. an-
- H 7. poly-
- L 8. hyper-
- O 9. meta-
- M 10. peri-
- C 11. epi-
- E 12. intra-
- N 13. sub-
- K 14. sym-
- I 15. supra-
- D 16. inter-
- K 17. syn-
- E 18. endo-

Column B

- A. painful; difficult
- B. not; without
- C. upon; above
- D. between
- E. within
- F. through
- G. slow
- H. many
- I. above
- J. four
- K. together; with
- L. above; above normal
- M. around
- N. beneath; below
- O. change; beyond

Combining Forms

Column A		Column B
C	1. orth/o	A. joint
A	2. arthr/o	B. carpals (wrist bones)
M	3. oste/o	C. straight
A	4. articul/o	D. skull
H	5. patell/a, patell/o	E. clavicle (collar bone)
L	6. phalang/o	F. rib
B	7. carp/o	G. radius (bone of the forearm); X-ray
K	8. femor/o	H. patella (kneecap)
I	9. chondr/o	I. cartilage
J	10. fibul/o	J. fibula
E	11. clavicul/o	K. femur; thigh bone
U	12. humer/o	L. phalanges (bones of the fingers and toes)
F	13. cost/o	M. bone
G	14. radi/o	N. vertebra; spine
D	15. crani/o	O. tendon
P	16. kines/o, kinesi/o	P. movement
Q	17. stern/o	Q. sternum (breastbone)
W	18. tibi/o	R. ankle bones
T	19. metatars/o	S. scapula (shoulder blade)
X	20. my/o	T. metatarsals (bones of the foot)
S	21. scapul/o	U. humerus (upper arm bone)
N	22. spondyl/o	V. metacarpals (bones of the hand)
R	23. tars/o	W. tibia (shin bone)
O	24. tendin/o, tendon/o	X. muscle
V	25. metacarp/o	

Suffixes

Column A		Column B
D	1. -ar	A. surgical puncture to remove fluid
A	2. -centesis	B. breakdown; loosening; dissolving
B	3. -lysis	C. instrument used to cut

M	4. -kinesis	D.	pertaining to
G	5. -metry	E.	condition
D	6. -ac	F.	pain
H	7. -gen	G.	process of measuring
D	8. -ior	H.	producing; originating; causing
M	9. -kinesia	I.	surgical breaking
L	10. -malacia	J.	weakness
N	11. -trophy	K.	paralysis
D	12. -ary	L.	softening
P	13. -osis	M.	movement
E	14. -ema	N.	development
F	15. -algia	O.	deficiency; abnormal reduction
D	16. -ic	P.	abnormal condition
K	17. -plegia	Q.	to bind or tie together surgically
J	18. -asthenia		
C	19. -tome		
I	20. -clasia		
Q	21. -desis		
D	22. -ous		
O	23. -penia		
E	24. -ia		
F	25. -dynia		

SCORECARD: How Did You Do?

Number correct (_____), divided by 68 (_____), multiplied by 100 equals _____ (your score)

Breaking Down and Building Musculoskeletal System Terms

Now that you have mastered the prefixes, combining forms, and suffixes for musculoskeletal system terminology, you have the ability to dissect and build a large number of medical terms related to this body system.

Below is a list of common medical terms related to the study and treatment of the musculoskeletal system. For each term, a dissection has been provided, along with the meaning of each word element and the definition of the term as a whole.

Term	Dissection	Word Part/Meaning	Term Definition
Note: *For simplification, combining vowels have been omitted from the Word Part/Meaning column.*			
1. **anterior** (ăn-TĒR-ē-or)	anter/ior	**anter** = front **ior** = pertaining to	pertaining to the front
2. **anteroinferior** (ĂN-tĕr-ō-ĭn-FĒR-ē-or)	anter/o/infer/ior	**anter** = front **infer** = below **ior** = pertaining to	pertaining to front and below
3. **arthralgia** (är-THRĂL-jē-ă)	arthr/algia	**arthr** = joint **algia** = pain	pain in the joint
4. **arthritis** (är-THRĪ-tĭs)	arthr/itis	**arthr** = joint **itis** = inflammation	inflammation of the joints
5. **arthrocentesis** (är-thrō-sĕn-TĒ-sĭs)	arthr/o/centesis	**arthr** = joint **centesis** = surgical puncture to remove fluid	surgical puncture to remove fluid from a joint
6. **arthrodesis** (är-thrō-DĒ-sĭs)	arthr/o/desis	**arthr** = joint **desis** = to bind or tie together surgically	to surgically bind/tie together joints
7. **arthroscope** (ÄR-thrō-skōp)	arthr/o/scope	**arthr** = joint **scope** = instrument used to observe	instrument used to observe the joints
8. **arthrochondritis** (är-thrō-kŏn-DRĪ-tĭs)	arthr/o/chondr/itis	**arthr** = joint **chondr** = cartilage **itis** = inflammation	inflammation of the joint and cartilage
9. **arthrogram** (ÄR-thrō-grăm)	arthr/o/gram	**arthr** = joint **gram** = record; image	image of the joint
10. **arthroscopy** (är-THRŎS-kō-pē)	arthr/o/scopy	**arthr** = joint **scopy** = process of observing	process of observing the joints
11. **arthrotome** (ÄR-thrō-tōm)	arthr/o/tome	**arthr** = joint **tome** = instrument used to cut	instrument used to cut joints
12. **atrophy** (ĂT-rō-fē)	a/trophy	**a** = not; without **trophy** = development	without development
13. **bradykinesia** (BRĂD-ē-kĭn-Ē-zē-ă)	brady/kinesia	**brady** = slow **kinesia** = movement	slow movement
14. **bursectomy** (bŭr-SĔK-tō-mē)	burs/ectomy	**burs** = bursa; sac **ectomy** = surgical removal; excision	excision of the bursa/sac
15. **bursotomy** (bŭr-SŎT-ō-mē)	burs/o/tomy	**burs** = bursa; sac **tomy** = incision; cut into	incision to the bursa/sac
16. **bursitis** (bŭr-SĪ-tĭs)	burs/itis	**burs** = bursa; sac **itis** = inflammation	inflammation of the bursa/sac

Prefixes = Green   Root Words = Red   Suffixes = Blue

Term	Dissection	Word Part/Meaning	Term Definition
17. **cardiorrhaphy** (kär-dē-OR-ă-fē)	cardi/o/rrhaphy	**cardi** = heart **rrhaphy** = suture	suture of the heart
18. **cardiorrhexis** (KÄR-dē-ō-RĔK-sĭs)	cardi/o/rrhexis	**cardi** = heart **rrhexis** = rupture	rupture of the heart
19. **carpal** (KÄR-păl)	carp/al	**carp** = carpals (wrist bones) **al** = pertaining to	pertaining to the carpals (wrist bones)
20. **chondrocostal** (kŏn-drō-KŎS-tăl)	chondr/o/cost/al	**chondr** = cartilage **cost** = rib **al** = pertaining to	pertaining to cartilage and ribs
21. **chondrogenic** (kŏn-drō-JĔN-ĭk)	chondr/o/gen/ic	**chondr** = cartilage **gen** = producing; originating; causing **ic** = pertaining to	pertaining to producing cartilage
22. **chondromalacia** (KŎN-drō-mă-LĀ-shē-ă)	chondr/o/malacia	**chondr** = cartilage **malacia** = softening	softening of the cartilage
23. **coccygeal** (kŏk-SĬJ-ē-ăl)	coccyg/eal	**coccyg** = coccyx (tailbone) **eal** = pertaining to	pertaining to the coccyx (tailbone)
24. **cranial** (KRĀ-nē-ăl)	crani/al	**crani** = skull **al** = pertaining to	pertaining to the skull
25. **craniotomy** (krā-nē-ŎT-ō-mē)	crani/o/tomy	**crani** = skull **tomy** = incision; cut into	incision to the skull
26. **dorsal** (DOR-săl)	dors/al	**dors** = back (of the body) **al** = pertaining to	pertaining to the back
27. **dyskinesia** (dĭs-kĭ-NĒ-zē-ă)	dys/kinesia	**dys** = painful; difficult **kinesia** = movement	painful or difficult movement
28. **dystrophy** (DĬS-trō-fē)	dys/trophy	**dys** = painful; difficult **trophy** = development	painful or difficult development
29. **ecchymosis** (ĕk-ĭ-MŌ-sĭs)	ecchym/osis	**ecchym** = blood in the tissues **osis** = abnormal condition	abnormal condition of blood in the tissues
30. **electromyogram** (ē-LĔK-trō-MĪ-ō-gram)	electr/o/my/o/gram	**electr** = electrical activity **my** = muscle **gram** = record; image	record/image of electrical activity in the muscle
31. **hypertrophy** (hī-PĔR-trō-fē)	hyper/trophy	**hyper** = above; above normal **trophy** = development	above-normal development
32. **intercostal** (ĭn-tĕr-KŎS-tăl)	inter/cost/al	**inter** = between **cost** = rib **al** = pertaining to	pertaining to between ribs
33. **intervertebral** (ĭn-tĕr-VĔR-tĕ-brăl)	inter/vertebr/al	**inter** = between **vertebr** = vertebra; spine **al** = pertaining to	pertaining to between vertebrae (plural form of *vertebra*)

Prefixes = Green   Root Words = Red   Suffixes = Blue

Term	Dissection	Word Part/Meaning	Term Definition
34. **kinesiology** (kĭ-nē-sē-ŎL-ō-jē)	kinesi/o/logy	**kinesi** = movement **logy** = study of	study of movement
35. **kyphosis** (kī-FŌ-sĭs)	kyph/osis	**kyph** = hump **osis** = abnormal condition	abnormal condition of a hump; humpback
36. **lateral** (LĂT-ĕr-ăl)	later/al	**later** = side **al** = pertaining to	pertaining to the side
37. **lordosis** (lor-DŌ-sĭs)	lord/osis	**lord** = curve **osis** = abnormal condition	abnormal condition of curve (of the spine)
38. **myitis** (mī-Ī-tĭs)	my/itis	**my** = muscle **itis** = inflammation	inflammation of the muscle
39. **myalgia** (mī-ĂL-jē-ă)	my/algia	**my** = muscle **algia** = pain	pain in the muscle
40. **myasthenia** (mī-ăs-THĒ-nē-ă)	my/asthenia	**my** = muscle **asthenia** = weakness	weakness of the muscle
41. **necrosis** (ně-KRŌ-sĭs)	necr/osis	**necr** = death **osis** = abnormal condition	abnormal condition of death
42. **osteomyelitis** (ŎS-tē-ō-mī-ě-LĪ-tĭs)	oste/o/myel/itis	**oste** = bone **myel** = bone marrow; spinal cord **itis** = inflammation	inflammation of the bone and bone marrow
43. **osteonecrosis** (ŎS-tē-ō-ně-KRŌ-sĭs)	oste/o/necr/osis	**oste** = bone **necr** = death **osis** = abnormal condition	abnormal condition of death of the bone
44. **osteopathy** (ŏs-tē-ŎP-ă-thē)	oste/o/pathy	**oste** = bone **pathy** = disease	disease of the bone
45. **osteoarthritis** (ŎS-tē-ō-är-THRĪ-tĭs)	oste/o/arthr/it is	**oste** = bone **arthr** = joint **itis** = inflammation	inflammation of the bone and joint
46. **osteochondritis** (ŎS-tē-ō-kŏn-DRĪ-tĭs)	oste/o/chondr/itis	**oste** = bone **chondr** = cartilage **itis** = inflammation	inflammation of the bone and cartilage
47. **osteomalacia** (ŎS-tē-ō-mă-LĀ-shē-ă)	oste/o/malacia	**oste** = bone **malacia** = softening	softening of the bone
48. **osteoporosis** (ŎS-tē-ō-por-Ō-sis)	oste/o/por/osis	**oste** = bone **por** = pore; duct; small opening **osis** = abnormal condition	abnormal condition of small openings in the bone
49. **osteopenia** (ŏs-tē-ō-PĒ-nē-ă)	oste/o/penia	**oste** = bone **penia** = deficiency; abnormal reduction	deficiency/abnormal reduction of bone

Prefixes = Green   Root Words = Red   Suffixes = Blue

Term	Dissection	Word Part/Meaning	Term Definition
50. **posterior** (pŏs-TĒR-ē-or)	poster/ior	**poster** = back (of the body) **ior** = pertaining to	pertaining to the back
51. **quadriplegia** (kwŏd-rĭ-PLĒ-jē-ă)	quadri/plegia	**quadri** = four **plegia** = paralysis	paralysis of four (extremities)
52. **scoliosis** (skō-lē-Ō-sĭs)	scoli/osis	**scoli** = crooked; bent **osis** = abnormal condition	abnormal condition of (being) crooked or bent
53. **spondylarthritis** (SPŎN-dĭl-är-THRĪ-tĭs)	spondyl/arthr/itis	**spondyl** = vertebra; spine **arthr** = joint **itis** = inflammation	inflammation of the vertebra and joint
54. **spondylodesis** (SPŎN-dĭ-lō-DĒ-sĭs)	spondyl/o/desis	**spondyl** = vertebra; spine **desis** = to bind or tie together surgically	to surgically bind/ tie together vertebrae (plural of *vertebra*)
55. **spondylosis** (spŏn-dĭ-LŌ-sĭs)	spondyl/osis	**spondyl** = vertebra; spine **osis** = abnormal condition	abnormal condition of the vertebra
56. **spondylolysis** (SPŎN-dĭ-lŏ-LĪ-sĭs)	spondyl/o/lysis	**spondyl** = vertebra; spine **lysis** = breakdown; loosening; dissolving	breakdown/ loosening/dissolving of the vertebra
57. **sternal** (STĔR-năl)	stern/al	**stern** = sternum (breastbone) **al** = pertaining to	pertaining to the sternum (breastbone)
58. **sternocostal** (stĕr-nō-KŎS-tăl)	stern/o/cost/al	**stern** = sternum (breastbone) **cost** = rib **al** = pertaining to	pertaining to the sternum (breastbone) and rib
59. **subcostal** (sŭb-KŎS-tăl)	sub/cost/al	**sub** = beneath; below **cost** = rib **al** = pertaining to	pertaining to below the rib
60. **synkinesis** (sĭn-kĭ-NĒ-sĭs)	syn/kinesis	**syn** = together; with **kinesis** = movement	movement together
61. **tendinitis** (tĕn-dĭ-NĪ-tĭs)	tendin/itis	**tendin** = tendon **itis** = inflammation	inflammation of the tendon
62. **vasculitis** (văs-kū-LĪ-tĭs)	vascul/itis	**vascul** = blood vessel **itis** = inflammation	inflammation of the blood vessel
63. **vertebral** (VĔR-tĕ-brăl)	vertebr/al	**vertebr** = vertebra; spine **al** = pertaining to	pertaining to the vertebra
64. **vertebrectomy** (vĕr-tĕ-BRĔK-tō-mē)	vertebr/ectomy	**vertebr** = vertebra **ectomy** = surgical removal; excision	excision of the vertebra

Prefixes = Green   Root Words = **Red**   Suffixes = Blue

Using the pronunciation guide in the Breaking Down and Building chart, practice saying each medical term aloud. To hear the pronunciation of each term, go to the Pronounce It activity at the G-W companion website.

Audio Activity: Pronounce It

Directions: At the companion website, listen as each medical term listed below is pronounced. Practice pronouncing the terms until you are comfortable saying them aloud.

anterior
(ăn-TĒR-ē-or)

anteroinferior
(ĂN-tĕr-ō-ĭn-FĒR-ē-or)

arthralgia
(är-THRĂL-jē-ă)

arthritis
(är-THRĪ-tĭs)

arthrocentesis
(är-thrō-sĕn-TĒ-sĭs)

arthrodesis
(är-thrō-DĒ-sĭs)

arthroscope
(ÄR-thrō-skōp)

arthrochondritis
(är-thrō-kŏn-DRĪ-tĭs)

arthrogram
(ÄR-thrō-grăm)

arthroscopy
(är-THRŎS-kō-pē)

arthrotome
(ÄR-thrō-tōm)

atrophy
(ĂT-rō-fē)

bradykinesia
(BRĂD-ē-kĭn-Ē-zē-ă)

bursectomy
(bŭr-SĔK-tō-mē)

bursotomy
(bŭr-SŎT-ō-mē)

bursitis
(bŭr-SĪ-tĭs)

cardiorrhaphy
(kär-dē-OR-ă-fē)

cardiorrhexis
(KÄR-dē-ō-RĔK-sĭs)

carpal
(KÄR-păl)

chondrocostal
(kŏn-drō-KŎS-tăl)

chondrogenic
(kŏn-drō-JĔN-ĭk)

chondromalacia
(KŎN-drō-mă-LĀ-shē-ă)

coccygeal
(kŏk-SĬJ-ē-ăl)

cranial
(KRĀ-nē-ăl)

craniotomy
(krā-nē-ŎT-ō-mē)

dorsal
(DOR-săl)

dyskinesia
(dĭs-kĭ-NĒ-zē-ă)

dystrophy
(DĬS-trō-fē)

ecchymosis
(ĕk-ĭ-MŌ-sĭs)

electromyogram
(ē-LĔK-trō-MĪ-ō-gram)

hypertrophy
(hī-PĔR-trō-fē)

intercostal
(ĭn-tĕr-KŎS-tăl)

intervertebral
(ĭn-tĕr-VĔR-tĕ-brăl)

kinesiology
(kĭ-nē-sē-ŎL-ō-jē)

kyphosis
(kī-FŌ-sĭs)

lateral
(LĂT-ĕr-ăl)

lordosis
(lor-DŌ-sĭs)

myitis
(mī-Ī-tĭs)

myalgia
(mī-ĂL-jē-ă)

myasthenia
(mī-ăs-THĒ-nē-ă)

necrosis
(nĕ-KRŌ-sĭs)

osteomyelitis
(ŎS-tē-ō-mī-ĕ-LĪ-tĭs)

osteonecrosis
(ŎS-tē-ō-nĕ-KRŌ-sĭs)

osteopathy
(ŏs-tē-ŎP-ă-thē)

osteoarthritis
(ŎS-tē-ō-är-THRĪ-tĭs)

osteochondritis
(ŎS-tē-ō-kŏn-DRĪ-tĭs)

osteomalacia
(ŎS-tē-ō-mă-LĀ-shē-ă)

osteoporosis
(ŎS-tē-ō-por-Ō-sis)

osteopenia
(ŏs-tē-ō-PĒ-nē-ă)

posterior
(pŏs-TĒR-ē-or)

quadriplegia
(kwŏd-rĭ-PLĒ-jē-ă)

scoliosis
(skō-lē-Ō-sĭs)

spondylarthritis
(SPŎN-dĭl-är-THRĪ-tĭs)

spondylodesis
(SPŎN-dĭ-lō-DĒ-sĭs)

spondylosis
(spŏn-dĭ-LŌ-sĭs)

spondylolysis
(SPŎN-dĭ-lŏ-LĪ-sĭs)

sternal
(STĔR-năl)

sternocostal
(stĕr-nō-KŎS-tăl)

subcostal
(sŭb-KŎS-tăl)

synkinesis
(sĭn-kĭ-NĒ-sĭs)

tendinitis
(tĕn-dĭ-NĪ-tĭs)

vasculitis
(văs-kū-LĪ-tĭs)

vertebral
(VĔR-tĕ-brăl)

vertebrectomy
(vĕr-tĕ-BRĔK-tō-mē)

Audio Activity: Spell It

Directions: Cover the medical terms in the Pronounce It activity on the preceding page with a sheet of paper. At the companion website, listen as the terms are read aloud. Correctly spell each term below.

1. anterior
2. anteroinferior
3. arthralgia
4. arthritis
5. arthrocentesis
6. arthrodesis
7. arthroscope
8. arthrochondritis
9. arthrogram
10. arthroscopy
11. arthrotome
12. atrophy
13. bradykinesia
14. bursectomy
15. bursotomy
16. bursitis
17. cardiorrhaphy
18. cardiorrhexis
19. carpal
20. chondrocostal
21. chondrogenic
22. chondromalacia
23. coccygeal
24. cranial
25. craniotomy
26. dorsal
27. dyskinesia
28. dystrophy
29. ecchymosis
30. electromyogram
31. hypertrophy
32. intercostal
33. intervertebral
34. kinesiology
35. kyphosis
36. lateral
37. lordosis
38. myitis
39. myalgia
40. myasthenia
41. necrosis
42. osteomyelitis
43. osteonecrosis
44. osteopathy
45. osteoarthritis
46. osteochondritis
47. osteomalacia
48. osteoporosis
49. osteopenia
50. posterior
51. quadriplegia
52. scoliosis
53. spondylarthritis
54. spondylodesis
55. spondylosis
56. spondylolysis
57. sternal
58. sternocostal
59. subcostal
60. synkinesis
61. tendinitis
62. vasculitis
63. vertebral
64. vertebrectomy

Break It Down

Directions: Dissect each medical term below into its word elements by placing a slash between each word part (prefix, root word, combining vowel, and suffix). Then define each term.

Example:
Medical Term: quadriplegia
Dissection: quadri / plegia
Definition: paralysis of four

Medical Term   **Dissection**

1. anterior   a n t e r / i o r

   Definition: pertaining to the front

2. arthritis   a r t h r / i t i s

   Definition: inflammation of the joints

3. bradykinesia   b r a d y / k i n e s i a

   Definition: slow movement

4. carpal   c a r p / a l

   Definition: pertaining to the carpals (wrist bones)

5. anteroinferior   a n t e r / o / i n f e r / i o r

   Definition: pertaining to front and below

Medical Term	Dissection

6. hypertrophy   h y p e r/t r o p h y

Definition: above-normal development

_____

7. arthralgia   a r t h r/a l g i a

Definition: pain in the joint

_____

8. dorsal   d o r s/a l

Definition: pertaining to the back

_____

9. arthroscope   a r t h r/o/s c o p e

Definition: instrument used to observe the joints

_____

10. myasthenia   m y/a s t h e n i a

Definition: weakness of the muscle

_____

11. osteoporosis   o s t e/o/p o r/o s i s

Definition: abnormal condition of small openings in the bone

_____

12. chondrogenic   c h o n d r/o/g e n/i c

Definition: pertaining to producing cartilage

_____

13. arthrogram   a r t h r/o/g r a m

Definition: image of the joint

_____

Medical Term	Dissection
14. atrophy	a/t r o p h y

Definition: without development

_____

| 15. kyphosis | k y p h/o s i s |

Definition: abnormal condition of a hump; humpback

_____

| 16. osteochondritis | o s t e/o/c h o n d r/i t i s |

Definition: inflammation of the bone and cartilage

_____

| 17. bursotomy | b u r s/o/t o m y |

Definition: incision to the bursa/sac

_____

| 18. dyskinesia | d y s/k i n e s i a |

Definition: painful or difficult movement

_____

| 19. spondylodesis | s p o n d y l/o/d e s i s |

Definition: to surgically bind/tie together vertebrae

_____

| 20. bursitis | b u r s/i t i s |

Definition: inflammation of the bursa/sac

_____

| 21. chondromalacia | c h o n d r/o/m a l a c i a |

Definition: softening of the cartilage

_____

Medical Term	Dissection

22. osteomyelitis   o s t e / o / m y e l / i t i s

Definition: inflammation of the bone and bone marrow

---

23. cranial   c r a n i / a l

Definition: pertaining to the skull

---

24. sternocostal   s t e r n / o / c o s t / a l

Definition: pertaining to the sternum (breastbone) and rib

---

25. arthrocentesis   a r t h r / o / c e n t e s i s

Definition: surgical puncture to remove fluid from a joint

---

26. coccygeal   c o c c y g / e a l

Definition: pertaining to the coccyx

---

27. lateral   l a t e r / a l

Definition: pertaining to the side

SCORECARD: How Did You Do?

Number correct (_____), divided by 27 (_____), multiplied by 100 equals _____ (your score)

Build It

Directions: Build the medical term that matches each definition below by supplying the correct word elements.

P (Prefixes) = Green
RW (Root Words) = Red
S (Suffixes) = Blue
CV (Combining Vowel) = Purple

1. to surgically bind/tie together the joint

arthr	o	desis
RW	CV	S

2. pertaining to front and below

anter	o	infer	ior
RW	CV	RW	S

3. abnormal condition of a hump; humpback

kyph	osis
RW	S

4. abnormal condition of small openings in the bone

oste	o	por	osis
RW	CV	RW	S

5. inflammation of the joints

arthr	itis
RW	S

6. incision to the skull

crani	o	tomy
RW	CV	S

7. surgical puncture to remove fluid from a joint

arthr	o	centesis
RW	CV	S

8. abnormal condition of death

necr	osis
RW	S

9. incision to the bursa

burs	o	tomy
RW	CV	S

10. instrument used to observe the joints

arthr	o	scope
RW	CV	S

11. pertaining to the side

later	al
RW	S

12. pertaining to the back (of the body) **(two possible answers)**

dors	al
RW	S

poster	ior
RW	S

13. inflammation of the joint and cartilage

arthr	o	chondr	itis
RW	CV	RW	S

14. study of movement

kinesi	o	logy
RW	CV	S

15. rupture of the heart

cardi	o	rrhexis
RW	CV	S

16. image of the joint

arthr	o	gram
RW	CV	S

17. pertaining to the carpals (wrist bones)

carp	al
RW	S

18. pertaining to the front

anter	ior
RW	S

19. abnormal condition of blood in the tissues

$$\frac{\text{ecchym}}{\text{RW}} \quad \frac{\text{osis}}{\text{S}}$$

20. process of observing the joints

$$\frac{\text{arthr}}{\text{RW}} \quad \frac{\text{o}}{\text{CV}} \quad \frac{\text{scopy}}{\text{S}}$$

21. record/image of electrical activity in the muscle

$$\frac{\text{electr}}{\text{RW}} \quad \frac{\text{o}}{\text{CV}} \quad \frac{\text{my}}{\text{RW}} \quad \frac{\text{o}}{\text{CV}} \quad \frac{\text{gram}}{\text{S}}$$

22. pertaining to the cartilage and rib

$$\frac{\text{chondr}}{\text{RW}} \quad \frac{\text{o}}{\text{CV}} \quad \frac{\text{cost}}{\text{RW}} \quad \frac{\text{al}}{\text{S}}$$

23. painful or difficult development

$$\frac{\text{dys}}{\text{P}} \quad \frac{\text{trophy}}{\text{S}}$$

24. slow movement

$$\frac{\text{brady}}{\text{P}} \quad \frac{\text{kinesia}}{\text{S}}$$

25. painful or difficult movement

$$\frac{\text{dys}}{\text{P}} \quad \frac{\text{kinesia}}{\text{S}}$$

26. without development

$$\frac{\text{a}}{\text{P}} \quad \frac{\text{trophy}}{\text{S}}$$

27. excision of the bursa/sac

$$\frac{\text{burs}}{\text{RW}} \quad \frac{\text{ectomy}}{\text{S}}$$

28. abnormal condition of curve (of the spine)

$$\frac{\text{lord}}{\text{RW}} \quad \frac{\text{osis}}{\text{S}}$$

29. pertaining to the coccyx (tailbone)

$$\frac{\text{coccyg}}{\text{RW}} \quad \frac{\text{eal}}{\text{S}}$$

30. inflammation of the bursa/sac

burs	itis
RW	S

31. above-normal development

hyper	trophy
P	S

32. suture of the heart

cardi	o	rrhaphy
RW	CV	S

33. pain in the joint

arthr	algia
RW	S

34. pertaining to producing cartilage

chondr	o	gen	ic
RW	CV	S	S

35. inflammation of the bone and cartilage

oste	o	chondr	itis
RW	CV	RW	S

36. weakness of the muscle

my	asthenia
RW	S

37. softening of the cartilage

chondr	o	malacia
RW	CV	S

38. disease of the bone

oste	o	pathy
RW	CV	S

39. abnormal condition of (being) crooked or bent

scoli	osis
RW	S

40. pertaining to the skull

crani	al
RW	S

41. inflammation of the vertebra and joint

spondyl	arthr	itis
RW	RW	S

42. pertaining to between ribs

inter	cost	al
P	RW	S

43. inflammation of the bone and bone marrow

oste	o	myel	itis
RW	CV	RW	S

44. to surgically bind/tie together vertebrae

spondyl	o	desis
RW	CV	S

45. softening of the bone

oste	o	malacia
RW	CV	S

46. breakdown/loosening/dissolving of the vertebra

spondyl	o	lysis
RW	CV	S

47. pertaining to below the rib

sub	cost	al
P	RW	S

48. inflammation of the bone and joint

oste	o	arthr	itis
RW	CV	RW	S

49. abnormal condition of death of the bone

oste	o	necr	osis
RW	CV	RW	S

SCORECARD: How Did You Do?

Number correct (_____), divided by 49 (_____), multiplied by 100 equals _____ (your score)

Diseases and Disorders

Diseases and disorders of the musculoskeletal system range from the mild to the severe, and they have a wide variety of causes. We will briefly examine some problems that commonly affect this system.

Bursitis

Bursitis is an inflammation of the bursa, a pad-like sac filled with lubricating fluid (Figure 4.2). *Bursae* (plural form of *bursa*) are found in connective tissue near joints. These fluid-filled sacs reduce friction between tendons, muscles, and bones.

Bursitis most commonly develops in the shoulder, elbow, or hip, but it can also occur in the knee, heel, or base of the great (big) toe. This condition is the result of frequent repetitive motion, a sudden impact injury, or lack of elasticity in aging tendons.

Fracture

A **fracture** is a break in a bone. There are two categories of bone fractures: simple and compound (Figure 4.3). A bone fracture that does not penetrate the skin is called a *simple* or *closed fracture*. If the broken bone protrudes through the skin, it is called a *compound* or *open fracture* (Figure 4.4).

Car accidents, falls, and athletic injuries are common causes of fractures. Low bone density from osteoporosis (discussed later in this section) may also result in bone fractures.

Herniated Disk

Spinal disks (also called *vertebral disks*) are rubbery cushions between the **vertebrae**, the individual bones that make up the spinal column. They have a soft interior surrounded by a tough exterior. Spinal disks cushion the bones of the spinal column and allow forward and side-to-side movement between the vertebrae.

With age, spinal disks become less flexible and more vulnerable to injury. Injury to a disk can cause

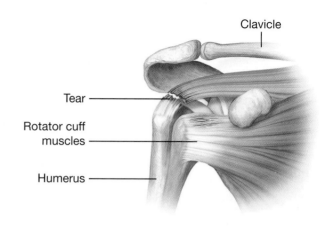

Figure 4.2 Bursitis is an inflammation of the bursa, a pad-like sac filled with lubricating fluid, which reduces friction between tendons, muscles, and bones.

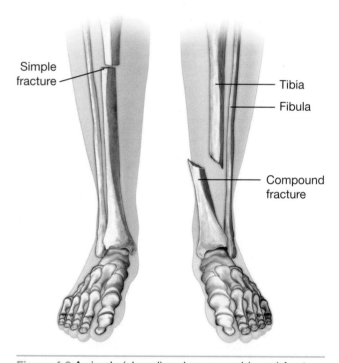

Figure 4.3 A simple (closed) and compound (open) fracture

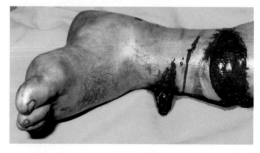

English / Custom Medical Stock Photo

Figure 4.4 A compound fracture of the ankle

it to slide out of place, resulting in what is commonly referred to as a *slipped disk*. As a spinal disk becomes less elastic, it may rupture. The result is a **herniated disk** (Figure 4.5). The rupture in the spinal disk causes a portion of the disk—the soft interior—to be forced through a weakened part of the tough, exterior part of the disk. When a herniated disk bulges out from between the vertebrae, it places pressure on nearby nerves. This can lead to pain, numbness, or weakness.

Joint Effusion

Joint effusion (ĕ-FYŪ-zhŭn) is an increase in the amount of fluid within the synovial (freely movable) compartment of a joint. Articular cartilage covers the ends of bones to prevent friction that would otherwise damage the bones during movement (Figure 4.6). A membrane encloses the joint in a capsule that contains synovial (lubricating) fluid. A small amount of synovial fluid exists in all freely movable joints.

When a joint has been affected by disease or trauma, synovial fluid buildup causes a freely movable joint to appear swollen. A doctor may drain the fluid to help relieve the pressure. If an infection is not suspected, a small amount of cortisone (anti-inflammatory medication) may be injected into the joint to provide pain relief and to help prevent the fluid from returning.

Knee Injuries

The knee joint contains four ligaments that provide stability and strength: the anterior and posterior cruciate ligaments (ACL and PCL, respectively) and the medial and lateral collateral ligaments (MCL and LCL, respectively). As you learned earlier in the chapter, the meniscus is a C-shaped cartilage pad that cushions the knee joint. Injury to the knee can affect any of the four stabilizing ligaments (Figure 4.7).

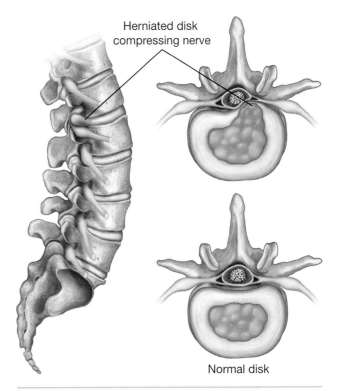

Figure 4.5 When a herniated disk bulges out between the vertebrae, it places pressure on nearby nerves, which can lead to pain, numbness, or weakness.

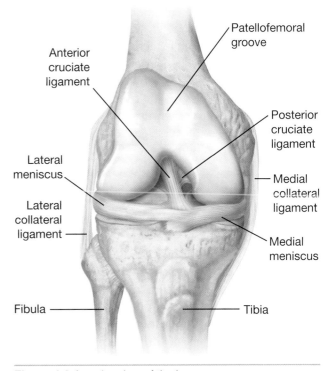

Figure 4.6 Anterior view of the knee

One of the most common knee injuries is a sprained or torn ACL, which can result from overextension of the knee joint, a severe blow to the side of the knee (a common occurrence during football games), or coming to a sudden stop and then quickly changing direction while running. Likewise, when the knee is struck from the outside, it may buckle, causing the MCL to stretch or tear. As with ACL injuries, MCL injuries are often the result of "clipping" during a football game, when a player is struck behind the knee. Both ACL and MCL injuries are characterized by swelling, pain, tenderness, and the sensation that the knee will "give way" when standing or moving.

Meniscus tears are typically caused by twisting or overextending the knee joint. A torn meniscus causes pain, swelling, and stiffness.

Lateral Epicondylitis

Lateral epicondylitis (ĔP-ĭ-kŏn-dĭ-LĪ-tĭs), the formal term for *tennis elbow*, is inflammation and pain on the lateral (outside) part of the upper arm near the elbow (Figure 4.8). This condition is caused by activity in which repetitive twisting of the wrist is frequent. Lateral epicondylitis is common in people who play a lot of tennis or other racquet sports—thus the name "tennis elbow."

As you learned earlier, tendons attach muscle to bone. When the tendons of the elbow are overworked, small tears can develop. Over time, this leads to irritation and pain where the tendons of the forearm muscles attach to the *lateral epicondyle* (ĕp-ĭ-KŎN-dīl), the bony prominence on the outside of the elbow. Rest and over-the-counter pain relievers often help alleviate discomfort from lateral epicondylitis. Surgery is recommended only when the pain is incapacitating (interferes significantly with activities of daily living) and has lasted six months or more.

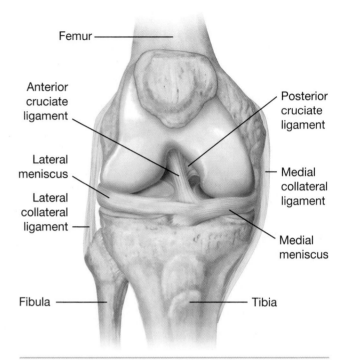

Figure 4.7 Major ligaments of the knee typically affected by injury

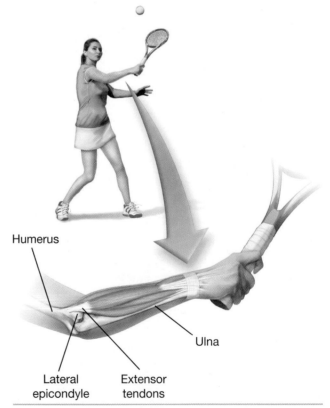

Figure 4.8 Lateral epicondylitis, more commonly known as *tennis elbow*

Muscular Dystrophy

Muscular dystrophy (DĬS-trō-fē) is a group of inherited muscular disorders characterized by progressive muscle degeneration, weakness, and atrophy (wasting away) without nerve involvement (Figure 4.9).

Duchenne (dū-SHĔN) *muscular dystrophy* (DMD), the most common form of the disease, occurs primarily in boys. DMD is characterized by mild muscle weakness in the legs and difficulty walking. The first signs of DMD are apparent by three years of age and become more severe with age. Death from respiratory or cardiac muscle weakness may occur in early adulthood.

Osteomyelitis

Osteomyelitis (ŎS-tē-ō-mī-ĕ-LĪ-tĭs) is an acute or chronic bone infection usually caused by bacteria (Figures 4.10, 4.11, and 4.12). It produces fever, chills, and pain in the area of the infection. The area may appear swollen, warm, and red. Sometimes, however, osteomyelitis does not cause any signs or symptoms, or those that are present may be difficult to distinguish from signs and symptoms of other health conditions.

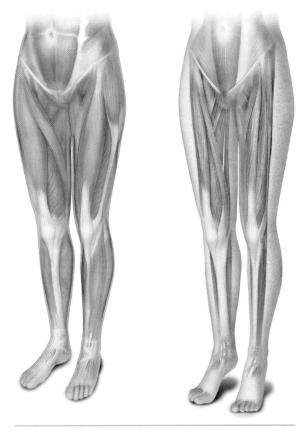

Figure 4.9 Muscular dystrophy is marked by degeneration and atrophy (wasting away) of the muscles.

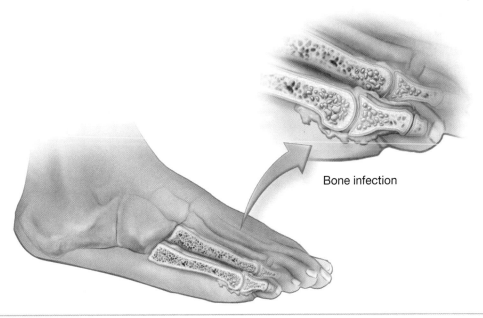

Bone infection

Figure 4.10 Osteomyelitis, an acute or chronic bone infection, is usually caused by bacteria.

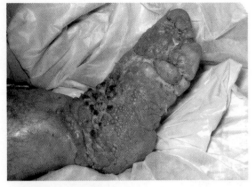

Mediscan/Visuals Unlimited, Inc.

Figure 4.11 Osteomyelitis

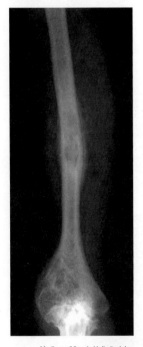

Mediscan/Visuals Unlimited, Inc.

Figure 4.12 Radiograph showing osteomyelitis in the leg

In osteomyelitis, bacteria may enter a bone via the bloodstream, from a nearby infection, or through direct contamination from an open fracture or surgery. Circulation problems can hinder leukocytes and lymphocytes (infection-fighting cells) from reaching the site of infection. (You will learn more about these infection-fighting microorganisms in Chapter 5: Lymphatic and Immune Systems.) Thus, what begins as a small infection may intensify, exposing bone and deep tissue to infection. Patients typically undergo extended intravenous antibiotic therapy (four to eight weeks).

Osteoporosis

Osteoporosis (ŎS-tē-ō-por-Ō-sis) is the thinning of bone tissue and the gradual loss of bone density (Figure 4.13). It is the most common type of bone disease. Usually, the loss of bone occurs gradually over a period of years.

Osteoporosis develops when the body fails to form enough new bone, when too much calcium moves from the bone into the blood, or both. Calcium and phosphate are two minerals essential for healthy bone formation. A diet deficient in calcium causes a decrease in bone production, which can result in brittle, fragile bones that are more prone to fracture, even without injury (Figure 4.14).

The leading cause of osteoporosis in women is reduced production of the hormone estrogen during menopause. In men, decreased production of the hormone testosterone heightens the risk of developing osteoporosis.

Normal bone　　　　　　　Osteoporosis

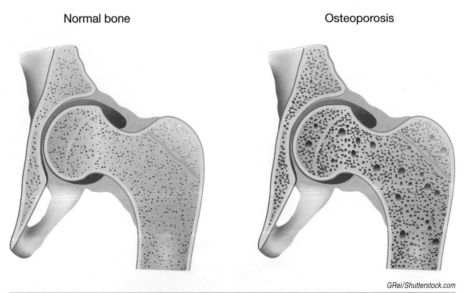

GRei/Shutterstock.com

Figure 4.13 In osteoporosis, the thinning of bone tissue and gradual loss of bone density makes bones more fragile and prone to fracture.

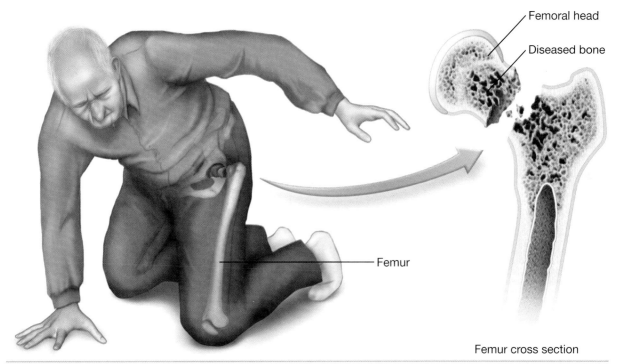

Femoral head

Diseased bone

Femur

Femur cross section

Figure 4.14 Osteoporosis causes the bones to thin and decreases their density, making them more fragile and susceptible to fracture.

Rotator Cuff Tear

The rotator cuff is a group of muscles and tendons that attach the humerus (upper arm) to the scapula (shoulder blade). It stabilizes the shoulder joint and allows broad range of motion. The rotator cuff holds the proximal humerus (the upper part of the arm, where the shoulder and elbow meet) within the joint socket of the scapula. This joint is called the *ball-and-socket joint* because it allows the shoulder to rotate.

Falling, lifting, and repetitive arm motions can irritate or damage the muscles or tendons of the rotator cuff, or cause a **rotator cuff tear** (Figure 4.15). Pain may occur when the shoulder is raised overhead. When a rotator cuff tear is suspected, a doctor may order a computerized tomography (CT) or magnetic resonance imaging (MRI) scan. (You will learn about these

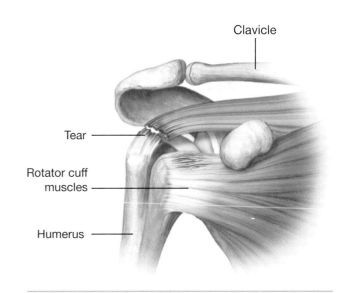

Clavicle

Tear

Rotator cuff muscles

Humerus

Figure 4.15 Rotator cuff tear

diagnostic procedures in the next section.) Arthroscopic (är-thrō-SKŎP-ik) surgery is often performed to repair the tendons in a torn rotator cuff.

Procedures and Treatments

We will now take a brief look at some common diagnostic tests and procedures used to help identify disorders and diseases of the musculoskeletal system, as well as some common therapeutic treatments.

Bone Scan

A **bone scan** is a type of nuclear medicine imaging (NMI) test. NMI involves the use of small amounts of radioactive materials called *radiopharmaceuticals* to generate images of bones, organs, soft tissues, and blood vessels. Bone scans are used to study body functions, analyze biological specimens, and help diagnose and treat a variety of musculoskeletal conditions. NMI technology aids doctors in determining the cause of a medical problem based on the *function* of a particular organ, tissue, or bone.

An NMI scan differs from a radiograph (X-ray), the latter of which helps doctors determine the presence of disease based on its *structural appearance* rather than on the function of a particular organ, tissue, or bone. By contrast, nuclear medicine is an extremely sensitive technology; it can detect abnormalities in the very early stages of disease, long before other diagnostic tests might reveal their presence. Early detection means that treatment can be initiated immediately and a better prognosis can be achieved.

In a nuclear medicine bone scan, a special camera is used to capture images of the bone (Figure 4.16). A radioactive substance is injected into a vein and traced as it travels through the bloodstream and into the bones. The radioactive substance is referred to as a *tracer*. It often takes several hours for the entire procedure to be completed.

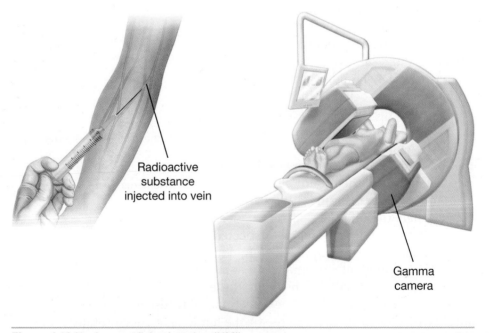

Radioactive substance injected into vein

Gamma camera

Figure 4.16 Nuclear medicine imaging (NMI) scanner

Bone scans are performed to help determine the cause of back pain, metastatic cancer (cancer that has spread, or moved to another site), or infection or trauma to the bones. An area of the body that absorbs little to no amount of the radioactive tracer appears as a dark area or "cold spot," indicating the presence of cancer or a decrease in blood supply to the bone. Conversely, an area of high bone activity, such as fast bone growth or repair, shows up as a bright area or "hot spot" on the scan. A hot spot on a bone scan can signify arthritis, a tumor, a fracture, or an infection. A bone scan can help identify certain health conditions days or even months earlier than a regular X-ray test.

Computerized Tomography

Computerized tomography (tō-MŎG-ră-fē), or CT, is a diagnostic procedure in which radiographs (X-rays) and a computer are used to display cross-sectional images of internal body structures (Figure 4.17). Computerized tomography is also called *computed tomography*. This cross-sectional imaging technique records details of human anatomy in the transverse (horizontal) or sagittal (right and left) planes. The CT scanner can be set to "image" (record images of) the body in different widths or sections. By contrast, plain-film radiographs or the more current digital radiography techniques can image anatomical structures in the anteroposterior (AP), lateral, and oblique planes. Computerized tomography is especially suited to imaging the bones, lungs, and chest and detecting cancerous growths.

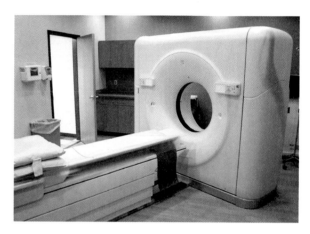

SNEHIT/Shutterstock.com

Figure 4.17 Computerized tomography (CT) scanner

CT scanning is similar to taking photographs of a friend or family member with a cell phone or digital camera. If a friend is facing you when you take a picture, she is in the anteroposterior position. If she is standing sideways, she is in the lateral position. With photography, we take photos in one dimension: from the front (AP) or the side (lateral). However, the human body is not one-dimensional. CT imaging is unique in its ability to view and record anatomy in the transverse and sagittal planes as well as in the anteroposterior and lateral planes.

If internal body structures were recorded only in one plane, then cancerous tumors, benign masses, and serious diseases could otherwise go undetected. Think of a sliced loaf of bread being photographed from the front and the side. We get the typical front and side views of the bread. Now remove a slice of bread, lay it down, and look at its internal structure. This view is what CT imaging allows us to see: internal "slices" of human anatomy.

A contrast agent, sometimes referred to as a *dye*, is often used during CT scanning to assist in visualizing body organs, blood vessels, and soft tissues (muscles, tendons, and ligaments). As you may recall from chapter 3, use of a contrast agent allows digital imaging of anatomical structures that are not dense enough to be viewed in an X-ray.

Electromyogram

An **electromyogram** (ē-lĕk-trō-MĪ-ō-gram), or **EMG**, is a test that records the electrical activity of muscles (Figure 4.18). It is used with patients who demonstrate impaired muscle strength. EMGs help detect various muscular diseases and conditions including pinched nerves, herniated disks, inflamed muscles, muscular dystrophy, and peripheral muscle damage (damage to specific muscles rather than to the muscles as a whole).

In an EMG, a needle is inserted into the muscle. The needle acts as an electrode, detecting electrical activity that is visually displayed on an *oscilloscope*, a laboratory instrument that graphically represents and analyzes the waveform of electrical signals. Functioning muscles produce an electrical current proportional to the level of muscular activity they generate. An EMG can help distinguish between muscle weakness caused by injury to a nerve that is attached to a muscle and muscle weakness resulting from a neurological disorder. EMG technology is also used to identify the degree of nerve irritation or injury.

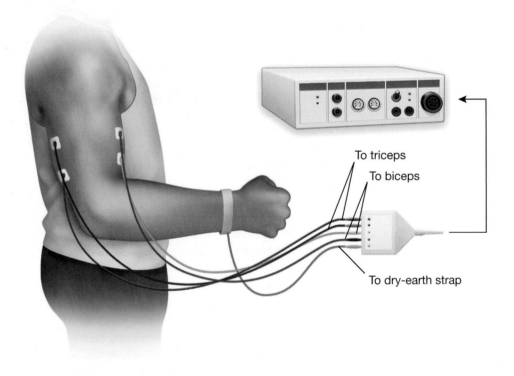

Figure 4.18 Electromyogram

Magnetic Resonance Imaging of the Bone

Magnetic resonance imaging, or **MRI**, is a diagnostic procedure in which a sophisticated magnet and a computer are used to generate cross-sectional images of blood vessels, bones, nerves, organs and other internal body structures (Figure 4.19). MR imaging is typically performed to evaluate soft tissues, major body joints, the spine for disk disease, and bones of the extremities. This procedure often shows more anatomical detail than plain radiographs or even CT scans. Imaging performed with a contrast agent enhances the diagnostic process.

Cross-sectional imaging modalities such as MRI and CT scanning are now considered standard in diagnosing osteomyelitis, and a combination of these techniques may be used to confirm the presence of the disease. These modalities reveal superior anatomic detail of the infected area and the surrounding soft tissues. MRI allows early detection of osteomyelitis and, in cases of chronic bone infection, assessment of the extent of osteomyelitic involvement and activity. MRI also assists the surgeon in planning optimal surgical management for the treatment of osteomyelitis.

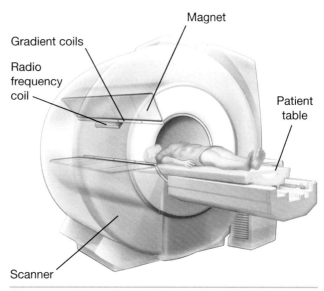

How MRI Technology Works

Figure 4.19 Magnetic resonance imaging (MRI) scanner

McMurray Test

The **McMurray test** is used to detect a meniscus tear in the knee (Figure 4.20). With the patient in the supine position (lying on the back with the face upward), the healthcare provider holds the heel of the injured leg with the knee flexed. The knee is gradually extended, and pressure is applied as the patient's lower leg is rotated both medially and laterally. The McMurray test is considered positive for meniscal injury if a clicking or cracking noise is heard.

Physical Therapy

Physical therapy (PT) is a form of rehabilitative treatment in which customized exercises and specially designed equipment are used to help patients regain or improve their mobility. Physical therapy benefits many different types of patients, from the infant born with a musculoskeletal defect

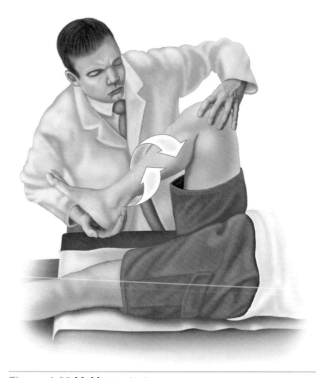

Figure 4.20 McMurray test

to the adult recovering from a stroke, injury, or surgery. PT is a conservative treatment method often used prior to, in conjunction with, or following more aggressive treatment options such as surgery or certain kinds of medication.

Rest, Ice, Compression, and Elevation

Often expressed as the acronym **RICE**, this first-aid regimen stands for **Rest, Ice, Compression, and Elevation**. RICE is a commonly recommended treatment for strains and sprains.

A *strain* is a stretched or torn muscle or tendon. The most common types of strains occur in the back and hamstring muscles (the muscles in the back of the upper leg). A *sprain*, by contrast, is a stretched or torn ligament. Sprains often occur in the ankle, knee, or wrist.

Spinal Fusion

Spinal fusion, also known as *spondylodesis* (SPŎN-dĭ-lō-DĒ-sĭs), is a surgical procedure in which two or more vertebrae are fused (joined together) (Figure 4.21). Trauma, degenerative disease, or a spinal deformity causes pain due to abnormal motion of the vertebrae. Bone tissue derived from either the patient or a donor is used to fuse the vertebrae, thus alleviating the pain.

Spinal fusion is often facilitated by a process called *fixation*, during which metallic screws or rods are used to stabilize the vertebrae. Following injury to the cervical or lumbar region (lower back), spinal fusion can help stabilize the area and prevent fractures of the spinal column, which could damage the spinal cord. Spinal fusion is also performed to remove or reduce pressure on nerves.

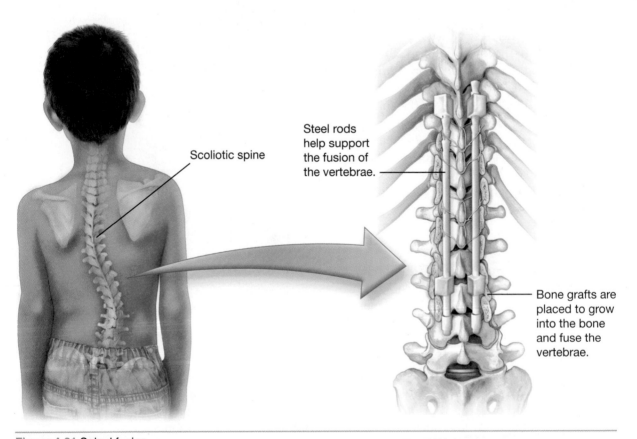

Scoliotic spine

Steel rods help support the fusion of the vertebrae.

Bone grafts are placed to grow into the bone and fuse the vertebrae.

Figure 4.21 Spinal fusion

Multiple Choice: Diseases and Disorders

Directions: Write the letter of the disease or disorder that matches each numbered definition below.

__A__ 1. the thinning of bone tissue and the gradual loss of bone density
   a. osteoporosis   c. joint effusion
   b. muscular dystrophy d. bursitis

__A__ 2. rupture of a vertebral disk that causes the soft interior of the disk to bulge between the vertebrae, creating pressure on nearby nerves
   a. herniated disk   c. muscular dystrophy
   b. bursitis   d. joint effusion

__D__ 3. acute or chronic bone infection often caused by bacteria
   a. muscular dystrophy c. osteoporosis
   b. bursitis   d. osteomyelitis

__D__ 4. the leading cause of osteoporosis is
   a. an increase in estrogen in women
   b. a reduction in estrogen in women
   c. a decrease in testosterone in men
   d. both b and c

__C__ 5. inflammation of a pad-like sac filled with lubricating fluid, found in connective tissue near joints
   a. muscular dystrophy c. bursitis
   b. osteoporosis   d. osteomyelitis

__D__ 6. a tear in one of the muscles or tendons that attach the humerus (upper arm) to the scapula (shoulder blade)
   a. meniscus tear   c. MCL tear
   b. ACL tear   d. rotator cuff tear

__C__ 7. an increase in the amount of fluid within the synovial compartment of a joint
   a. osteoporosis   c. joint effusion
   b. osteomyelitis   d. bursitis

__C__ 8. a group of inherited muscular disorders characterized by progressive muscle degeneration, weakness, and atrophy without nerve involvement
   a. joint effusion   c. muscular dystrophy
   b. osteomyelitis   d. bursitis

__B__ 9. a break in a bone
   a. osteoporosis   c. joint effusion
   b. fracture   d. bursitis

__A__ 10. an injury caused by twisting or overextending the knee joint
   a. ACL tear   c. lateral epicondylitis
   b. bursitis   d. rotator cuff tear

__C__ 11. inflammation of the lateral part of the upper arm due to repetitive twisting of the wrist
   a. rotator cuff tear   c. lateral epicondylitis
   b. bursitis   d. osteomyelitis

SCORECARD: How Did You Do?

Number correct (_____), divided by 11 (_____), multiplied by 100 equals _____ (your score)

Multiple Choice: Procedures and Treatments

Directions: Write the letter of the diagnostic procedure or therapeutic treatment that matches each numbered definition below.

__D__ 1. procedure involving the use of radiographs and a computer to display cross-sectional images of internal body structures
   a. magnetic resonance imaging (MRI)
   b. bone scan
   c. electromyogram (EMG)
   d. computerized tomography (CT)

__D__ 2. procedure in which a sophisticated magnet and a computer are used to generate cross-sectional images of bones, organs, nerves, blood vessels, and other structures; often shows more anatomical detail than other imaging tests
   a. McMurray test
   b. electromyogram (EMG)
   c. computerized tomography (CT)
   d. magnetic resonance imaging (MRI)

<u>A</u> 3. test that involves the use of a radioactive substance and a special camera to image the bone
   a. bone scan
   b. McMurray Test
   c. electromyogram (EMG)
   d. spondylodesis

<u>B</u> 4. surgical procedure in which two or more vertebrae are fused
   a. electromyogram (EMG)
   b. spinal fusion
   c. spondylodesis
   d. both b and c

<u>D</u> 5. test that records the electrical activity of muscles
   a. electromusculogram
   b. electromusculography
   c. McMurray Test
   d. electromyogram (EMG)

<u>B</u> 6. manual test used to detect a meniscus tear in the knee
   a. meniscal laceration test
   b. McMurray Test
   c. electromyogram
   d. magnetic resonance imaging (MRI)

SCORECARD: How Did You Do?

Number correct (_____), divided by 6 (_____), multiplied by 100 equals _____ (your score)

Assessment

Identifying Abbreviations

Directions: Write the abbreviation for each medical term listed below.

Medical Term	Abbreviation
1. computerized tomography	CT
2. magnetic resonance imaging	MRI
3. Duchenne muscular dystrophy	DMD
4. medial collateral ligament	MCL
5. anterior cruciate ligament	ACL
6. lateral collateral ligament	LCL
7. rest, ice, compression, and elevation	RICE
8. anteroposterior	AP
9. nuclear medicine imaging	NMI
10. physical therapy	PT
11. electromyogram	EMG

SCORECARD: How Did You Do?

Number correct (_____), divided by 11 (_____), multiplied by 100 equals _____ (your score)

Analyzing the Intern Experience

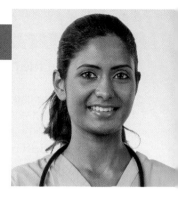

In the Intern Experience described at the beginning of this chapter, we met Aishandi, an intern with the DesFed Urgent Care Center. Aishandi "shadowed" (that is, followed and observed) Dr. Geiger as he interacted with Bill, a teenage patient who had suffered a knee injury during a football game. Dr. Geiger examined Bill and obtained his personal and family health history. He then made a medical diagnosis and provided Bill with a treatment plan. He also referred the teenager to an orthopedic specialist for further examination. Later, Dr. Geiger made a dictated recording of Bill's health information, which was subsequently transcribed into a chart note.

We will now learn more about Bill's injury from a clinical perspective, interpreting the medical terms in his chart note as we analyze the scenario presented in the Intern Experience.

Audio Activity: Bill Jesmann's Chart Note

Directions: At the companion website, listen and read along as the physician dictates Bill Jesmann's chart note, shown below. Then do the exercise that appears after Bill's chart note.

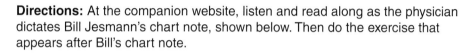

CHART NOTE

Patient Name: Jesmann, William
ID Number: 42645
Date of Service: October 26, 20xx

SUBJECTIVE
This 16-year-old male was tackled during a football game, twisting his left knee. The pain is worse on the lateral and inferior aspect of the left knee. It's worse if he pivots. He states that he has sometimes noticed a "catch" in his knee after practice. It has responded well to ice and ibuprofen.

OBJECTIVE
There is slight tenderness with active and passive ROM (range of motion) of the knee. The knee is not **erythematous** or warm. There is no crepitus (crackling or grating sound) or **edema**. There is tenderness with palpation of the left medial collateral **ligament**. There is lateral collateral ligament laxity (looseness, slackness, or displacement) but no medial collateral laxity. **McMurray test** is negative.

ASSESSMENT
Left lateral collateral ligament **sprain**.

PLAN
He will be sent to an **orthopedist** for consultation and possible **MRI** and/or **arthroscopy**. Follow-up **PT** is recommended.

Interpret William Jesmann's Chart Note

Directions: After listening to the dictated recording and reading the chart note on Bill Jesmann, provide the medical term that matches each definition below.

Example: inflammation of the muscle   *Answer:* myitis

1. band of tissue that connects bone to bone
ligament

2. specialist in the study and treatment of the musculoskeletal system
orthopedist

3. test manually performed to detect a meniscus tear in the knee
McMurray test

4. red
erythematous

5. diagnostic procedure in which a sophisticated magnet and a computer are used to generate cross-sectional images of body structures
MRI

6. process of observing the joint
arthroscopy

7. swelling
edema

8. rehabilitative treatment in which customized exercises and specially designed equipment are used to help patients regain or improve their mobility
PT

9. stretched or torn ligament
sprain

SCORECARD: How Did You Do?

Number correct (_____), divided by 9 (_____), multiplied by 100 equals _____ (your score)

Working with Medical Records

In this activity, you will interpret the medical records (chart notes) of patients with musculoskeletal conditions. These examples illustrate typical medical records prepared in a real-world healthcare environment. To interpret these chart notes, you will apply your knowledge of word elements (prefixes, combining forms, and suffixes), diseases and disorders, and procedures and treatments related to the musculoskeletal system.

Audio Activity: Ezilary Morales' Chart Note

Directions: At the companion website, listen and read along as the physician dictates the following chart note on Ezilary Morales. Then do the exercise that appears after Ezilary's chart note.

CHART NOTE

Patient Name: Morales, Ezilary
ID Number: 93668
Date of Service: March 14, 20xx

SUBJECTIVE
This 15-year-old female suffered an injury to her left hand during a gymnastics tournament. She was splinted and sent to the office for evaluation.

OBJECTIVE
She has diffuse (spread out; scattered) **edema** and **ecchymosis** over the **dorsal** aspect of her left hand in the 3rd and 4th **metacarpal** region. She has full range of motion of her fingers. Neurological and sensory exam is normal. Peripheral circulation (blood flow to the upper and lower extremities) is normal. X-ray imaging shows evidence of a nondisplaced oblique (slanted) shaft **fracture** of the **metacarpals** without involvement of the joints.

ASSESSMENT
Right 3rd and 4th metacarpal fractures, nondisplaced.

PLAN
Her fingers were taped for immobilization and placed in a short-arm splint. She will keep it elevated and use Advil® for pain relief. She is scheduled for a follow-up visit with Orthopedic Specialists, Inc. in the next 3 to 7 weeks.

Assessment

Interpret Ezilary Morales' Chart Note

Directions: After listening to the dictated recording and reading the chart note on Ezilary Morales, provide the medical term that matches each definition below.

Example: inflammation of the bone and cartilage   *Answer:* osteochondritis

1. break in a bone

   fracture

2. pertaining to the back (of the body)

   dorsal

3. bones of the hand

   metacarpals

4. swelling

   edema

5. abnormal condition of blood in the tissues

   ecchymosis

6. pertaining to the bones of the hand

   metacarpal

SCORECARD: How Did You Do?

Number correct (_____), divided by 6 (_____), multiplied by 100 equals _____ (your score)

Audio Activity: Amos Stoudt's Chart Note

Directions: At the companion website, listen and read along as the physician dictates the following chart note on Amos Stoudt. Then do the exercise that appears after Amos's chart note.

CHART NOTE

Patient Name: Stoudt, Amos
ID Number: 12114
Date of Service: May 19, 20xx

SUBJECTIVE
This 23-year-old male presents with lower right arm pain. Two days ago he was helping his father cut up tree branches from last week's violent storm when he was struck by a falling limb. When he uses his right hand, he has swelling and pain with **pronation** (turning of the hand and forearm so the palm faces downward), **supination** (turning of the hand and forearm so the palm faces upward), and gripping.

OBJECTIVE
He has mild **edema** over the **distal radius** (outer lateral bone of the forearm), approximately 8 cm **proximal** to the radial styloid process (small protrusion of bone). Neurovascularly intact. He has full range of motion of his hand and **phalanges**. X-rays confirm a nondisplaced **fracture** of the distal forearm.

ASSESSMENT
Right radial shaft fracture in good alignment.

PLAN
Fiberglass cast applied. Patient provided with arm sling and told to keep the arm elevated. Advised use of Advil®, aspirin, or Tylenol® for pain. Follow follow-up appointment in 10 days.

Assessment

Interpret Amos Stoudt's Chart Note

Directions: After listening to the dictated recording and reading the chart note on Amos Stoudt, provide the medical term that matches each definition below.

Example: painful or difficult movement   *Answer:* dyskinesia

1. nearest the point of origin   proximal
2. turning of the palm downward   pronation
3. swelling   edema
4. fingers   phalanges
5. break in a bone   fracture
6. outer lateral bone of the forearm   distal radius
7. turning of the palm upward   supination

SCORECARD: How Did You Do?

Number correct (_____), divided by 7 (_____), multiplied by 100 equals _____ (your score)

Chapter Review

Word Elements Summary

Prefixes

Prefix	Meaning
a-	not; without
an-	not; without
brady-	slow
dys-	painful; difficult
endo-	within
epi-	upon; above
hyper-	above; above normal
inter-	between
intra-	within
meta-	change; beyond
per-	through
peri-	around
poly-	many
quadri-	four
sub-	beneath; below
supra-	above
sym-, syn-	together; with

Combining Forms

Root Word/Combining Vowel	Meaning
anter/o	front
arthr/o	joint
articul/o	joint
burs/a, burs/o	bursa; sac
cardi/o	heart
carp/o	carpals (wrist bones)
chondr/o	cartilage
clavicul/o	clavicle (collar bone)

(Continued)

Root Word/Combining Vowel	Meaning
coccyg/o	coccyx (tailbone)
cost/o	rib
crani/o	skull
dist/o	away from the point of origin
dors/o	back (of the body)
ecchym/o	blood in the tissues
electr/o	electrical activity
erythemat/o	redness
erythr/o	red
femor/o	femur (thigh bone)
fibul/o	fibula
herni/o	hernia; rupture; protrusion
humer/o	humerus (upper arm bone)
ili/o	ilium
infer/o	below; beneath
ischi/o	ischium (part of hip bone)
kines/o, kinesi/o	movement
kyph/o	hump
later/o	side
lord/o	curve
medi/o	middle
metacarp/o	metacarpals (bones of the hand)
metatars/o	metatarsals (bones of the foot)
muscul/o	muscle
my/o	muscle
myel/o	bone marrow; spinal cord
necr/o	death
neur/o	nerve
orth/o	straight
oste/o	bone
patell/a, patell/o	patella (kneecap)
path/o	disease
phalang/o	phalanges (bones of the fingers and toes)

(Continued)

Root Word/Combining Vowel	Meaning
por/o	pore; duct; small opening
poster/o	back (of the body)
proxim/o	nearest the point of origin
pub/o	pubis (part of the hip bone)
radi/o	radius (bone of the forearm); X-ray
sacr/o	sacrum (bone at base of the spine)
scapul/o	scapula (shoulder blade)
scoli/o	crooked; bent
spondyl/o	vertebra; spine
stern/o	sternum (breastbone)
tars/o	ankle bones
ten/o	tendon
tendin/o, tendon/o	tendon
tibi/o	tibia (shin bone)
uln/o	ulna (bone of the forearm)
vascul/o	blood vessel
vertebr/o	vertebra; spine

Suffixes

Suffix	Meaning
-ac	pertaining to
-al	pertaining to
-algia	pain
-ar	pertaining to
-ary	pertaining to
-asthenia	weakness
-centesis	surgical puncture to remove fluid
-clasia	surgical breaking
-cyte	cell
-desis	to bind or tie together surgically
-dynia	pain
-eal	pertaining to
-ectomy	surgical removal; excision

(Continued)

Suffix	Meaning
-edema	swelling
-ema	condition
-gen	producing; originating; causing
-gram	record; image
-graphy	process of recording an image
-ia	condition
-ic	pertaining to
-ior	pertaining to
-itis	inflammation
-kinesia	movement
-kinesis	movement
-logist	specialist in the study and treatment of
-logy	study of
-lysis	breakdown; loosening; dissolving
-malacia	softening
-metry	process of measuring
-oma	tumor; mass
-osis	abnormal condition
-ous	pertaining to
-pathy	disease
-penia	deficiency; abnormal reduction
-plasty	surgical repair
-plegia	paralysis
-rrhaphy	suture
-rrhexis	rupture
-scope	instrument used to observe
-scopy	process of observing
-tome	instrument used to cut
-tomy	incision; cut into
-trophy	development

More Practice: Activities and Games

The activities on the following pages will help you reinforce your skills and check your mastery of the medical terminology that you learned in this chapter. Visit the companion website for More Practice games and activities.

Break It Down

Directions: Dissect each medical term below into its word elements by placing a slash between each word part (prefix, root word, combining vowel, and suffix). Then define each term.

Example:
Medical Term: arthritis
Dissection: arthr / itis
Definition: inflammation of the joint

Medical Term	Dissection

1. arthroscopy   a r t h r / o / s c o p y

   Definition: process of observing the joints
   _____

2. arthrotomy   a r t h r / o / t o m y

   Definition: incision to the joint
   _____

3. costochondral   c o s t / o / c h o n d r / a l

   Definition: pertaining to the rib and cartilage
   _____

4. craniectomy   c r a n i / e c t o m y

   Definition: excision of the skull
   _____

5. metacarpal   m e t a / c a r p / a l

   Definition: pertaining to beyond the carpals (wrist bones)
   _____

6. myelography   m y e l / o / g r a p h y

   Definition: process of recording an image of the spinal cord
   _____

Medical Term	Dissection

7. myocarditis   m y o / c a r d / i t i s

Definition: inflammation of the muscle of the heart

8. neuralgia   n e u r / a l g i a

Definition: pain in the nerve

9. craniology   c r a n i / o / l o g y

Definition: study of the skull

10. polyneural   p o l y / n e u r / a l

Definition: pertaining to many nerves

11. supracostal   s u p r a / c o s t / a l

Definition: pertaining to above the rib

12. posterolateral   p o s t e r / o / l a t e r / a l

Definition: pertaining to the back and side

13. iliocostal   i l i / o / c o s t / a l

Definition: pertaining to the ilium and rib

14. musculovascular   m u s c u l / o / v a s c u l / a r

Definition: pertaining to the muscles and blood vessels

Medical Term	Dissection
15. ischiofemoral	i s c h i / o / f e m o r / a l

Definition: pertaining to the ischium and femur

| 16. costectomy | c o s t / e c t o m y |

Definition: excision of the rib

| 17. supraclavicular | s u p r a / c l a v i c u l / a r |

Definition: pertaining to above the clavicle

| 18. costotome | c o s t / o / t o m e |

Definition: instrument used to cut the rib

| 19. subscapular | s u b / s c a p u l / a r |

Definition: pertaining to below the scapula

| 20. dorsalgia | d o r s / a l g i a |

Definition: pain in the back (of the body)

| 21. neuromuscular | n e u r / o / m u s c u l / a r |

Definition: pertaining to nerves and muscles

| 22. humeral | h u m e r / a l |

Definition: pertaining to the humerus

Medical Term	Dissection
23. ecchymoma	e c c h y m/o m a

Definition: tumor of blood in the tissues

| 24. femoral | f e m o r/a l |

Definition: pertaining to the femur

| 25. iliococcygeal | i l i/o/c o c c y g/e a l |

Definition: pertaining to the ilium and coccyx

Spelling

Directions: Circle the correctly spelled term in each item below.

1. bradikinesia | bradikynesia | (bradykinesia) | bradykynesia
2. artheralgia | (arthralgia) | arthralgea | artherelgia
3. echymosis | ecchimosis | eccymosis | (ecchymosis)
4. miasthenia | (myasthenia) | myaesthenia | miaesthenia
5. condromalacia | (chondromalacia) | chondromalaysia | khondromalacia
6. (kyphosis) | kyfosis | kifosis | kyphoses
7. diskinesia | (dyskinesia) | dyskenesia | dyskenasia
8. (osteomyelitis) | ostomyelitis | osteomielitis | osteomyalitis
9. laterel | (lateral) | latteral | laterral
10. epichondylitis | epicondilytis | epicondilitis | (epicondylitis)
11. intevertebral | intervertebrel | (intervertebral) | intervertabral
12. (scoliosis) | skoliosis | scholiosis | schoeliosis

True or False

Directions: Indicate whether each statement below is true or false.

True or False?

   F   1. The muscular system is made up of muscles and bones.

   T   2. Voluntary muscles are under conscious control.

   T   3. The skeletal system consists of bones plus cartilage, ligaments, and tendons.

   F   4. The suffix **-gram** means "process of recording an image."

   F   5. The prefix **inter-** means "within."

   F   6. The prefix **per-** means "around."

   T   7. The root word **articul** means "joint."

   T   8. The term *dystrophy* contains a prefix and a suffix.

   F   9. Skeletal muscle is an example of involuntary muscle.

   T   10. The root word **clavicul** means "collar bone."

   F   11. The rotator cuff is a group of muscles and ligaments that attach the humerus to the scapula.

   T   12. The term *bradykinesia* contains a prefix, root word, and suffix.

   F   13. The McMurray test is used to detect a meniscus tear in the elbow.

   T   14. The root words **spondyl** and **vertebr** mean "vertebra" or "spine."

   T   15. The suffixes **-ac**, **-al**, **-ar**, and **-ary** mean "pertaining to."

   T   16. A small amount of synovial fluid exists in all freely movable joints.

   F   17. The suffix **-oma** means "abnormal condition."

   F   18. The root word **oste** means "muscle."

   F   19. The suffix **-rrhexis** means "suture."

   T   20. The term *intervertebral* contains a prefix, root word, and suffix.

   T   21. The term *anteroinferior* contains two root words and a suffix.

   F   22. The acronym **RICE** stands for *rest, ice, contraction, and elevation.*

   F   23. The term *spondylarthritis* contains a prefix, root word, and suffix.

   T   24. Spinal disks cushion the bones of the spinal column.

   T   25. The prefix **brady-** means "slow."

   F   26. The root word **metacarp** means "bones of the feet."

   T   27. Lateral epicondylitis is commonly known as "tennis elbow."

   F   28. The suffixes **-ic** and **-ior** mean "posterior."

   T   29. Duchenne muscular dystrophy is the most common form of muscular dystrophy.

   T   30. The term *arthrocentesis* contains a root word and a suffix.

   T   31. Cardiac muscle is an example of involuntary muscle.

   F   32. There are three major ligaments that provide stability and strength to the knee joint.

Audio Activity: Emma Almondo's Chart Note

Directions: At the companion website, listen and read along as the physician dictates the following chart note on Emma Almondo. Then do the exercise that appears after Emma's chart note.

CHART NOTE

Patient Name: Almondo, Emma
ID Number: 14288
Date of Service: January 8, 20xx

SUBJECTIVE
Emma was babysitting her neighbor's 7-year-old son when he threw his spaghetti onto the floor. As she was cleaning the spaghetti off the floor, Emma slipped and fell to the floor, injuring her left wrist and left knee.

OBJECTIVE
The left wrist is swollen with obvious deformity. There is normal sensation of the fingers with normal motion of the fingers. Patient has pain with movement of the wrist. Left **patella** is tender to palpation (examination with the hands). There is **joint effusion** of the knee. Sensation and movement **distal** to the knee are both normal. X-rays of the left wrist reveal a **fracture** of the **distal radius** with approximately a 20-degree **dorsal** angulation, which is displaced about 30 percent from its normal position. There is no **ulna** (inner medial bone of the forearm) fracture. X-ray of the left patella shows a fracture with no displacement of the fragments.

ASSESSMENT
1. Fracture, left wrist
2. Patellar fracture, left knee

PLAN
Knee immobilizer was placed. She should bear as little weight as possible on the left knee. **Posterior** splint with elastic bandage was placed on the forearm. Patient was given acetaminophen with codeine for pain. An appointment with Orthopedic Specialists was made for Wednesday. Possible open reduction internal fixation (surgical realignment of bones with implants to guide the healing process).

Interpret Emma Almondo's Chart Note

Directions: After listening to the dictated recording and reading the chart note on Emma Almondo, provide the medical term that matches each definition below.

Example: weakness in the muscle   *Answer:* myasthenia

1. increase in the amount of fluid in the synovial compartment of a joint

   joint effusion

2. pertaining to the back (of the body) **(two possible answers)**

   dorsal

   posterior

3. break in a bone

   fracture

4. outer lateral bone of the forearm

   radius

5. kneecap

   patella

6. inner medial bone of the forearm

   ulna

7. pertaining to away from the point of origin

   distal

Cumulative Review

Chapters 2–4: Integumentary, Digestive, and Musculoskeletal Systems

Directions: Check your mastery of common word elements used in medical terminology related to the integumentary, digestive, and musculoskeletal systems. Write the definition(s) of each prefix, combining form, and suffix listed below. For more cumulative review practice, visit the companion website.

Prefixes

ad-	toward
an-	not; without
anti-	against
brady-	slow
dia-	through
dys-	painful; difficult
end-, end/o-	within
epi-	upon; above
hyper-	above; above normal
hypo-	below; below normal
inter-	between
intra-	within
meta-	change; beyond
pan-	all; everything
per-	through
peri-	around
poly-	many
quadri-	four
retro-	backward; behind
sub-	beneath; below
supra-	above

sym-, syn-	together; with
trans-	across

Combining Forms

arthr/o	joint
articul/o	joint
cardi/o	heart
celi/o	abdomen
chol/e	bile; gall
cholecyst/o	gallbladder
col/o, colon/o	colon; large intestine
contus/o	bruising
crani/o	skull
cyst/o	sac containing fluid
derm/a, derm/o, dermat/o	skin
dist/o	away from the point of origin
duoden/o	duodenum
ecchym/o	blood in the tissues
electr/o	electrical activity
enter/o	intestines
esophag/o	esophagus
femor/o	femur
fibul/o	fibula
gastr/o	stomach
gingiv/o	gums
gloss/o	tongue
hepat/o	liver
herni/o	hernia; rupture; protrusion
humer/o	humerus

ile/o	ileum
ili/o	ilium
infer/o	below; beneath
ischi/o	ischium
lapar/o	abdomen
melan/o	black
metacarp/o	metacarpals
myel/o	bone marrow; spinal cord
necr/o	death
onych/o	nail
orth/o	straight
pancreat/o	pancreas
phalang/o	phalanges
por/o	pore; duct; small opening
poster/o	back (of the body)
proct/o	anus and rectum
proxim/o	nearest the point of origin
prurit/o	itching
sacr/o	sacrum
scapul/o	scapula
schiz/o	split
scoli/o	crooked; bent
squam/o	scale-like
stern/o	sternum
tars/o	ankle bones
topic/o	place
uln/o	ulna
vertebr/o	vertebra; spine
xer/o	dry

Suffixes

-algia	pain
-ar	pertaining to
-ary	pertaining to
-cele	hernia; swelling; protrusion
-centesis	surgical puncture to remove fluid
-clasia	surgical breaking
-cyte	cell
-edema	swelling
-ema	condition
-gen	producing; originating; causing
-graphy	process of recording an image
-ia	condition
-iasis	abnormal condition
-ic	pertaining to
-ior	pertaining to
-itis	inflammation
-kinesia	movement
-kinesis	movement
-lysis	breakdown; loosening; dissolving
-malacia	softening
-metry	process of measuring
-penia	deficiency; abnormal reduction
-phagia	condition of eating or swallowing
-pharynx	pharynx; throat
-plasty	surgical repair
-ptosis	drooping; downward displacement
-rrhea	flow; discharge
-scopy	process of observing
-stomy	new opening

Chapter 5

The Lymphatic and Immune Systems

immun / o / logy: the study of the immune system

Chapter Organization

- Intern Experience
- Overview of Lymphatic and Immune System Anatomy and Physiology
- Word Elements
- Breaking Down and Building Terms Related to the Lymphatic and Immune Systems
- Diseases and Disorders
- Procedures and Treatments
- Analyzing the Intern Experience
- Working with Medical Records
- Chapter Review

Chapter Objectives

After completing this chapter, you will be able to

1. label an anatomical diagram of the lymphatic system;
2. dissect and define common medical terminology related to the lymphatic and immune systems;
3. build terms used to describe lymphatic and immune system diseases and disorders, diagnostic procedures, and therapeutic treatments;
4. pronounce and spell common medical terminology related to the lymphatic and immune systems;
5. understand that the processes of building and dissecting a medical term based on its prefix, word root, and suffix enable you to analyze an extremely large number of medical terms beyond those presented in this chapter;
6. interpret the meaning of abbreviations associated with the lymphatic and immune systems; and
7. interpret medical records containing terminology and abbreviations related to the lymphatic and immune systems.

You will see this icon [↗] at various points throughout this chapter. The icon indicates that you will find interactive activities and games on the Medical Terminology Companion Website. These activities and games will help you learn, practice, and expand your medical terminology knowledge and skills. Some of these activities are also available on the Medical Terminology Mobile Website.

Companion Website
www.g-wlearning.com/healthsciences

Mobile Site
www.m.g-wlearning.com/5800

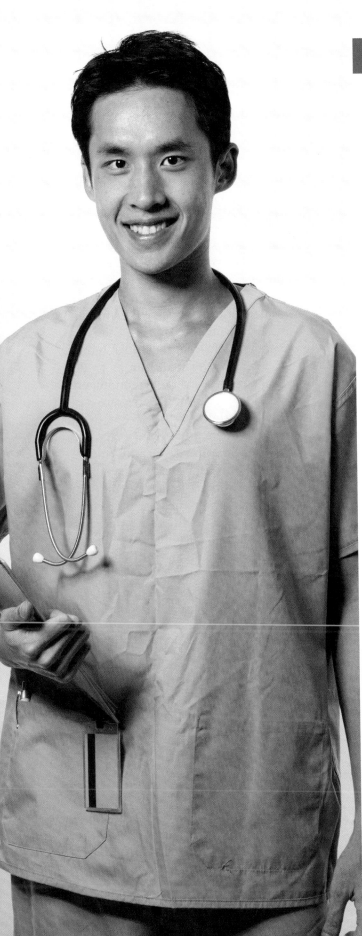

Sean, an intern with the Cassel County Clinic, is asked by the nurse manager to assist Dr. Rymus in exam room 2. His patient is William Shumaker, a 57-year-old accountant. Mr. Shumaker tells Sean that lately he has been feeling excessively fatigued, which he attributes to working long hours during the tax season. About a week ago, he noticed a small lump on the right side of his neck. Mr. Shumaker is also concerned about two other symptoms: persistent night sweats and weight loss.

Mr. Shumaker is experiencing a problem with his lymphatic system, which plays a vital role in protecting the body from infection. To help you understand what is happening to him, this chapter will present medical terms consisting of word elements (combining forms, prefixes, and suffixes) related to the lymphatic and immune systems.

By now, you recognize that many of the same medical word elements appear in terms used to describe different body systems. This systematic use of combining forms, prefixes, and suffixes helps make the study of medical terminology logical, consistent, and predictable.

We will begin our study of the lymphatic and immune systems with a brief overview of their anatomy and physiology. Later in the chapter, you will learn about some common pathological conditions of the lymphatic and immune systems, tests and procedures used to diagnose these conditions, and common methods for treating them.

Overview of Lymphatic and Immune System Anatomy and Physiology

The lymphatic and immune systems are covered together in this chapter because these two body systems are interdependent and complementary in structure and function.

The Lymphatic System

The **lymphatic** (lĭm-FĂT-ĭk) **system** is a sophisticated network of organs, glands, vessels, and cells that aid the immune system in filtering and destroying dead blood cells, particulate waste, and pathogens. A **pathogen** (PĂTH-ō-jĕn) is a disease-causing microorganism such as a bacterium, virus, fungus, toxin, parasite, or cancer cell. The fight against pathogens is a complex, coordinated effort between the immune and lymphatic systems. The lymphatic system manufactures **lymph**, or *lymphatic fluid*, a clear or milky-white fluid that contains **lymphocytes** (LĬM-fō-sīts). Lymphocytes are specialized **leukocytes** (LŪ-kō-sīts), white blood cells that protect the body from infection and disease by attacking foreign substances in the blood.

In addition to supporting the immune system, the lymphatic system supplements the functions of the cardiovascular system, also called the *circulatory system*. (You will learn more about the cardiovascular system in chapter 10.) Besides seeking out and destroying foreign "invaders" in the body, the lymphatic system works to maintain proper fluid balance and blood volume in the body.

The organs that make up the lymphatic system are the tonsils, adenoids, thymus gland, and spleen (Figure 5.1). The **tonsils** are two small, oval-shaped masses of lymphoid tissue in the back of the pharynx (throat). The tonsils protect the body from infection by trapping pathogens that enter through the mouth or nose. The **adenoids** (ĂD-ĕ-noyds) are small masses of lymphoid tissue located posterior to

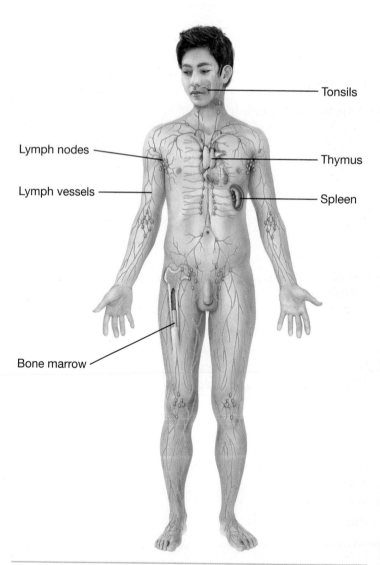

Tonsils

Lymph nodes

Lymph vessels

Thymus

Spleen

Bone marrow

Figure 5.1 Major organs and structures of the lymphatic system

the nasal cavity. The difference between tonsils and adenoids is that you can see your tonsils when you stand before a mirror and open your mouth very wide. Because your adenoids are situated in your nasopharynx (where the throat meets the nasal cavity), you cannot easily see them. Adenoids perform the same function as tonsils: they trap bacteria and viruses that enter through the nose or mouth. When infected, adenoids can enlarge and interfere with breathing.

The **thymus** (THĪ-mŭs) **gland**, or **thymus**, is a butterfly-shaped gland in the upper chest beneath the sternum (breastbone). The thymus receives from the bone marrow a specialized type of leukocyte called *T lymphocytes*, which are critical to a properly functioning immune system. T lymphocytes, or *T cells*, originate in the bone marrow and mature in the thymus. After they have matured, T cells reproduce and then differentiate into *helper T cells*, which control immune responses.

The **spleen** is a fist-sized organ that lies above the stomach and beneath the ribs on the left side of the body. The spleen contains infection-fighting leukocytes. The spleen also performs two other important functions: It controls the amount of blood in the body, and it destroys old or damaged red blood cells.

Immunology is the study of the immune system. An **immunologist** is a physician who specializes in the study and treatment of diseases and disorders of the immune system.

The Immune System

The **immune system** is a network of organs, tissues, and cells that work in tandem with those of the lymphatic system to protect the body from pathogenic invasion. For the immune system to function properly, it must distinguish between those cells that are part of the body ("self" cells) from cells that are foreign to the body ("non-self" cells). Once this distinction has been made, the immune system takes steps to attack the foreign cells.

When the immune system fails to differentiate between "self" and "non-self" cells, the body attacks its own cells and tissues. This is known as an **autoimmune disorder**. Examples of autoimmune disorders include allergies, rheumatoid arthritis, type I diabetes, and thyroid disease. You were introduced to some common autoimmune disorders in chapter 2, and you will learn about others as you continue to read this text.

The defense mechanisms of the immune system are classified as *nonspecific* or *specific* based on the way in which they respond to pathogenic invasion. **Nonspecific immunity** confers general protection against many different types of pathogens, such as viruses, bacteria, and fungi. A nonspecific immune response is one in which the body does not target a specific foreign substance. **Phagocytes** are an example of a nonspecific protective mechanism. These specialized cells (literally, "eating or swallowing cells") engulf and destroy pathogens in the body.

The first line of defense in nonspecific immunity is the skin. Intact skin serves as a barrier that keeps harmful microorganisms and other foreign substances from entering the body. Other nonspecific defense systems include the coughing and sneezing reflexes, which help dislodge irritants from the respiratory tract; mucous membranes, which trap bacteria and tiny particles; enzymes in our tears; and the lubricating oils in our skin.

By contrast, **specific immunity** affords protection against an **antigen**, a specific substance that, when introduced into the body, stimulates the production of an antibody. An **antibody** is a special kind of protein that the body produces to destroy or inactivate an antigen. The antibody confers protection against one specific substance and no others. Specific immunity involves "cell memory," the ability of cells in the body to recognize and respond to a specific harmful substance.

Anatomy and Physiology Vocabulary

Now that you have been introduced to the basic structure and functions of the lymphatic and immune systems, we will explore in more detail the key terms presented in the overview.

Key Term	Definition
adenoids	small masses of lymphoid tissue located posterior to the nasal cavity; when infected, can become enlarged and interfere with breathing
antibody	a special kind of protein that the body produces to destroy or inactivate an antigen
antigen	a specific substance that, when introduced into the body, stimulates the production of an antibody
autoimmune disorder	a disorder that arises when the immune system fails to differentiate between "self" and "non-self" cells, causing the body to attack its own cells and tissues
immune system	network of organs, tissues, and cells that work together to protect the body from disease-causing pathogens such as bacteria, viruses, toxins, and cancer cells
immunologist	physician who specializes in the study and treatment of diseases and disorders of the immune system
immunology	the study of the immune system
lymph	a clear or milky-white fluid that contains lymphocytes, specialized leukocytes (white blood cells) that protect the body from infection and disease; lymphatic fluid

Key Term	Definition
lymphatic system	body system that works with the immune system to filter and destroy dead blood cells, particulate waste, and pathogens such as bacteria, viruses, toxins, and cancer cells
lymphocytes	specialized leukocytes (white blood cells) that protect the body from infection and disease by attacking foreign substances in the blood
nonspecific immunity	general protection provided by the immune system against many different types of pathogens
pathogen	a microorganism capable of causing disease; examples include bacteria, viruses, fungi, parasites, toxins, and cancer cells
phagocyte	a specialized type of disease-fighting cell that engulfs and destroys bacteria and other harmful microorganisms in the body
specific immunity	the ability of the body to recognize and respond to a specific pathogen, such as a bacterium or virus
spleen	the organ above the stomach that contains infection-fighting leukocytes, controls the amount of blood in the body, and destroys old or damaged red blood cells
thymus	small, butterfly-shaped gland in the upper chest beneath the sternum (breastbone); receives specialized leukocytes called *T lymphocytes (T cells)* from the bone marrow
tonsils	two small, oval-shaped tissue masses that lie at the back of the pharynx (throat); protect the body from infection by trapping pathogens that enter through the mouth or nose

E-Flash Card Activity: Anatomy and Physiology Vocabulary

Directions: After you have reviewed the anatomy and physiology vocabulary related to the lymphatic and immune systems, practice with the e-flash cards until you are comfortable with the spelling and definition of each term.

Identifying Major Organs of the Lymphatic System

Directions: Label the diagram of the lymphatic system.

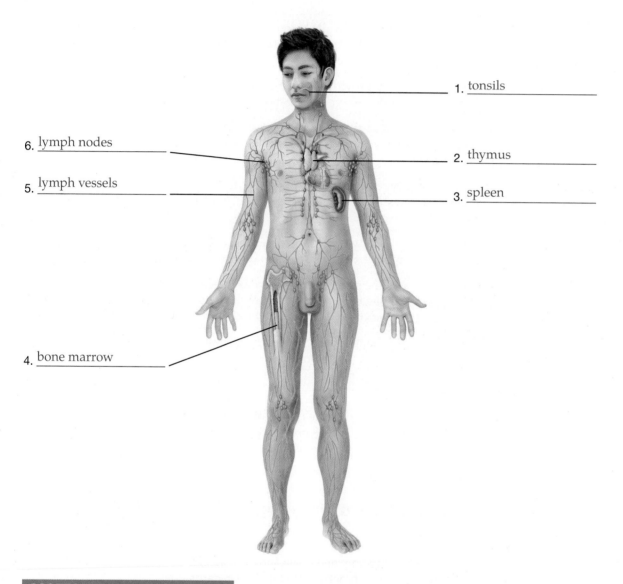

1. tonsils _____

6. lymph nodes _____

2. thymus _____

5. lymph vessels _____

3. spleen _____

4. bone marrow _____

Matching Anatomy and Physiology Vocabulary

Directions: Match the vocabulary term in Column A with its meaning in Column B.

Column A

- M 1. specific immunity
- N 2. spleen
- I 3. nonspecific immunity
- K 4. pathogen
- J 5. adenoids
- Q 6. antibody
- B 7. immune system
- C 8. lymphocytes
- E 9. immunologist
- O 10. thymus
- P 11. tonsils
- L 12. phagocyte
- H 13. lymphatic system
- F 14. immunology
- A 15. antigen
- D 16. autoimmune disorder
- G 17. lymph

Column B

A. a specific substance that, when introduced into the body, stimulates the production of an antibody

B. network of organs, tissues, and cells that work together to protect the body from disease-causing pathogens such as bacteria, viruses, toxins, and cancer cells

C. specialized leukocytes (white blood cells) that protect the body from infection and disease by attacking foreign substances in the blood

D. a disorder that arises when the immune system fails to differentiate between "self" and "non-self" cells, causing the body to attack its own cells and tissues

E. physician who specializes in the study and treatment of diseases and disorders of the immune system

F. the study of the immune system

G. a clear or milky-white fluid that contains lymphocytes, specialized white blood cells that protect the body from infection and disease; lymphatic fluid

H. body system that works with the immune system to filter and destroy dead blood cells, particulate waste, and pathogens

I. general protection provided by the immune system against many different types of foreign substances

J. small masses of lymphoid tissue located posterior to the nasal cavity; when infected, can become enlarged and interfere with breathing

K. a microorganism capable of causing disease; examples include bacteria, viruses, fungi, parasites, toxins, and cancer cells

L. a specialized type of disease-fighting cell that engulfs and destroys bacteria and other harmful microorganisms

M. the ability of the body to recognize and respond to a specific harmful substance, such as a bacterium or virus

N. the organ above the stomach that contains infection-fighting leukocytes, controls the amount of blood in the body, and destroys old or damaged cells

O. small, butterfly-shaped gland in the upper chest beneath the sternum (breastbone); produces *T lymphocytes (T cells)*

P. two small, oval-shaped tissue masses that lie at the back of the pharynx (throat); protect the body from infection by trapping pathogens that enter through the mouth or nose

Q. a special kind of protein that the body produces to destroy or inactivate an antigen

SCORECARD: How Did You Do?

Number correct (_____), divided by 17 (_____), multiplied by 100 equals _____ (your score)

Word Elements

In this section you will learn word elements—prefixes, combining forms, and suffixes—that are common to study of the lymphatic and immune systems. By learning these word elements and understanding how they are combined to build medical terms, you will be able to analyze Mr. Shumaker's health condition (described in the Intern Experience at the beginning of this chapter) and identify a large number of terms associated with the lymphatic and immune systems.

E-Flash Card Activity: Word Elements

Directions: Review the word elements in the tables that follow. Then, practice with the e-flash cards until you are able to quickly recognize the different word parts (prefixes, combining forms, and suffixes) and their meanings. The e-flash cards are grouped together by prefixes, combining forms, and suffixes, followed by a cumulative review of all the word elements that you learned in this chapter.

Prefixes

Let's start our study of word elements by looking at the prefixes listed in the table below. As you know by now, these prefixes appear not only in medical terms related to the lymphatic and immune systems but also in many terms used to describe other body systems.

Prefix	Meaning
auto-	self
hyper-	above; above normal
inter-	between
intra-	within

Combining Forms

Listed below are combining forms common in medical terminology used to describe the anatomy and physiology of the lymphatic and immune systems, as well as clinical conditions, diagnostic procedures, and therapeutic treatments related to these systems. You have already encountered some of these combining forms in previous chapters.

Root Word/Combining Vowel	Meaning
aden/o	gland
adenoid/o	adenoids
angi/o	vessel

(Continued)

Root Word/Combining Vowel	Meaning
cyt/o	cell
immun/o	protection
leuk/o	white
lymph/o	lymph
path/o	disease
phag/o	eat; swallow; engulf
splen/o	spleen
thym/o	thymus
tonsill/o	tonsils

Suffixes

Listed below are suffixes that appear in medical terms used to describe the lymphatic and immune systems. You are already familiar with these suffixes, which were introduced in previous chapters.

Suffix	Meaning
-ac	pertaining to
-ar	pertaining to
-atic	pertaining to
-cyte	cell
-ectomy	surgical removal; excision
-edema	swelling
-gen	producing; originating; causing
-ic	pertaining to
-itis	inflammation
-logist	specialist in the study and treatment of
-logy	study of
-malacia	softening
-megaly	enlargement
-oid	like; resembling
-oma	tumor; mass
-osis	abnormal condition
-pathy	disease
-pexy	surgical fixation
-rrhaphy	suture
-trophy	development

Matching Prefixes, Combining Forms, and Suffixes

Directions: In each exercise below, match the word element in Column A with its meaning in Column B. Some meanings may be used more than once.

Prefixes

Column A

C	1.	auto-
A	2.	hyper-
D	3.	inter-
B	4.	intra-

Column B

A. above; above normal

B. within

C. self

D. between

Combining Forms

Column A

G	1.	lymph/o
L	2.	tonsill/o
D	3.	cyt/o
K	4.	thym/o
A	5.	aden/o
J	6.	splen/o
C	7.	angi/o
I	8.	phag/o
B	9.	adenoid/o
E	10.	immun/o
H	11.	path/o
F	12.	leuk/o

Column B

A. gland

B. adenoids

C. vessel

D. cell

E. protection

F. white

G. lymph

H. disease

I. eat; swallow; engulf

J. spleen

K. thymus

L. tonsils

Suffixes

Column A

P	1.	-rrhaphy
A	2.	-ac
Q	3.	-trophy
A	4.	-atic
M	5.	-osis
C	6.	-ectomy

Column B

A. pertaining to

B. cell

C. surgical removal; excision

D. swelling

E. producing; originating; causing

F. inflammation

_G_ 7. -logist	G. specialist in the study and treatment of	
_L_ 8. -oma	H. study of	
_A_ 9. -ar	I. softening	
_O_ 10. -pexy	J. enlargement	
_B_ 11. -cyte	K. like; resembling	
_I_ 12. -malacia	L. tumor; mass	
_D_ 13. -edema	M. abnormal condition	
_N_ 14. -pathy	N. disease	
_F_ 15. -itis	O. surgical fixation	
_K_ 16. -oid	P. suture	
_E_ 17. -gen	Q. development	
_J_ 18. -megaly		
_A_ 19. -ic		
_H_ 20. -logy		

SCORECARD: How Did You Do?

Number correct (_____), divided by 36 (_____), multiplied by 100 equals _____ (your score)

Breaking Down and Building Terms Related to the Lymphatic and Immune Systems

Now that you have mastered the prefixes, combining forms, and suffixes for medical terminology used to describe the lymphatic and immune systems, you have the ability to dissect and build a large number of terms related to these body systems.

Below is a list of medical terms common to the study and treatment of the lymphatic and immune systems. For each term, a dissection has been provided, along with the meaning of each word element and the definition of the term as a whole.

Term	Dissection	Word Part/Meaning	Term Definition
Note: *For simplification, combining vowels have been omitted from the Word Part/Meaning column.*			
1. **adenoidectomy** (ĂD-ĕ-noy-DĔK-tō-mē)	adenoid/ectomy	adenoid = adenoids ectomy = surgical removal; excision	excision of the adenoids
2. **adenoiditis** (ĂD-ĕ-noy-DĪ-tĭs)	adenoid/itis	adenoid = adenoids itis = inflammation	inflammation of the adenoids
3. **autoimmune** (AW-tō-ĭ-MYŪN)	auto/immune	auto = self immun = protection	self-protection
Prefixes = Green Root Words = Red Suffixes = Blue			

Term	Dissection	Word Part/Meaning	Term Definition
4. **immunologist** (ĬM-yū-NŎL-ō-jĭst)	immun/o/logist	**immun** = protection **logist** = specialist in the study and treatment of	specialist in the study and treatment of protection
5. **immunology** (ĬM-yū-NŎL-ō-jē)	immun/o/logy	**immun** = protection **logy** = study of	study of protection
6. **lymphadenitis** (lĭm-FĂD-ĕ-NĪ-tĭs)	lymph/aden/itis	**lymph** = lymph **aden** = gland **itis** = inflammation	inflammation of the lymph glands
7. **lymphadenopathy** (lĭm-FĂD-ĕ-NŎP-ă-thē)	lymph/aden/o/pathy	**lymph** = lymph **aden** = gland **pathy** = disease	disease of the lymph glands
8. **lymphadenosis** (lĭm-FĂD-ĕ-NŌ-sĭs)	lymph/aden/osis	**lymph** = lymph **aden** = gland **osis** = abnormal condition	abnormal condition of the lymph glands
9. **lymphangiopathy** (lĭm-FĂN-jē-ŎP-ă-thē)	lymph/angi/o/pathy	**lymph** = lymph **angi** = vessel **pathy** = disease	disease of the lymph vessels
10. **lymphatic** (lĭm-FĂT-ĭk)	lymph/atic	**lymph** = lymph **atic** = pertaining to	pertaining to lymph
11. **lymphedema** (lĭm-fĕ-DĒ-mă)	lymph/edema	**lymph** = lymph **edema** = swelling	swelling of lymph
12. **lymphocyte** (LĬM-fō-sīt)	lymph/o/cyte	**lymph** = lymph **cyte** = cell	lymph cell
13. **lymphocytoma** (LĬM-fō-sī-TŌ-mă)	lymph/o/cyt/oma	**lymph** = lymph **cyt** = cell **oma** = tumor; mass	tumor of the lymph cells
14. **lymphoid** (LĬM-foyd)	lymph/oid	**lymph** = lymph **oid** = like; resembling	like or resembling lymph
15. **lymphoma** (lĭm-FŌ-mă)	lymph/oma	**lymph** = lymph **oma** = tumor; mass	tumor of the lymph
16. **pathogenic** (păth-ō-JĚN-ĭk)	path/o/gen/ic	**path** = disease **gen** = producing; originating; causing **ic** = pertaining to	pertaining to causing disease
17. **pathologist** (pă-THŎL-ō-jĭst)	path/o/logist	**path** = disease **logist** = specialist in the study and treatment of	specialist in the study and treatment of disease
18. **pathology** (pă-THŎL-ō-jē)	path/o/logy	**path** = disease **logy** = study of	study of disease
19. **phagocyte** (FĂG-ō-sīt)	phag/o/cyte	**phag** = eat; swallow; engulf **cyte** = cell	cell that eats, swallows, or engulfs

Prefixes = Green   Root Words = Red   Suffixes = Blue

Term	Dissection	Word Part/Meaning	Term Definition
20. **phagocytic** (făg-ō-SĬT-ĭk)	phag/o/cyt/ic	**phag** = eat; swallow; engulf **cyt** = cell **ic** = pertaining to	pertaining to a cell that eats, swallows, or engulfs
21. **splenectomy** (splē-NĔK-tō-mē)	splen/ectomy	**splen** = spleen **ectomy** = surgical removal; excision	excision of the spleen
22. **splenic** (SPLĔN-ĭk)	splen/ic	**splen** = spleen **ic** = pertaining to	pertaining to the spleen
23. **splenitis** (splē-NĪ-tĭs)	splen/itis	**splen** = spleen **itis** = inflammation	inflammation of the spleen
24. **splenoid** (SPLĒ-noyd)	splen/oid	**splen** = spleen **oid** = like; resembling	like or resembling the spleen
25. **splenoma** (splē-NŌ-mă)	splen/oma	**splen** = spleen **oma** = tumor; mass	tumor of the spleen
26. **splenomalacia** (SPLĒ-nō-mă-LĀ-shē-ă)	splen/o/malacia	**splen** = spleen **malacia** = softening	softening of the spleen
27. **splenomegaly** (SPLĒ-nō-MĔG-ă-lē)	splen/o/megaly	**splen** = spleen **megaly** = enlargement	enlargement of the spleen
28. **splenopexy** (SPLĒ-nō-PĔK-sē)	splen/o/pexy	**splen** = spleen **pexy** = surgical fixation	surgical fixation of the spleen
29. **splenorrhaphy** (splē-NOR-ă-fē)	splen/o/rrhaphy	**splen** = spleen **rrhaphy** = suture	suture of the spleen
30. **thymectomy** (thī-MĔK-tō-mē)	thym/ectomy	**thym** = thymus **ectomy** = surgical removal; excision	excision of the thymus
31. **thymic** (THĪ-mĭk)	thym/ic	**thym** = thymus **ic** = pertaining to	pertaining to the thymus
32. **thymoma** (thī-MŌ-mă)	thym/oma	**thym** = thymus **oma** = tumor; mass	tumor of the thymus
33. **tonsillar** (TŎN-sĭ-lăr)	tonsill/ar	**tonsill** = tonsils **ar** = pertaining to	pertaining to the tonsils
34. **tonsillectomy** (TŎN-sĭl-ĔK-tō-mē)	tonsill/ectomy	**tonsill** = tonsils **ectomy** = surgical removal; excision	excision of the tonsils
35. **tonsillitis** (TŎN-sĭl-Ī-tĭs)	tonsill/itis	**tonsill** = tonsils **itis** = inflammation	inflammation of the tonsils

Prefixes = Green   Root Words = Red   Suffixes = Blue

Using the pronunciation guide in the Breaking Down and Building chart, practice saying each medical term aloud. To hear the pronunciation of each term, go to the Pronounce It activity at the G-W companion website.

Audio Activity: Pronounce It

Directions: At the companion website, listen as each medical term listed below is pronounced. Practice pronouncing the terms until you are comfortable saying them aloud.

adenoidectomy
(ĂD-ĕ-noy-DĔK-tō-mē)

adenoiditis
(ĂD-ĕ-noy-DĪ-tĭs)

autoimmune
(AW-tō-ĭ-MYŪN)

immunologist
(ĬM-yū-NŎL-ō-jĭst)

immunology
(ĬM-yū-NŎL-ō-jē)

lymphadenitis
(lĭm-FĂD-ĕ-NĪ-tĭs)

lymphadenopathy
(lĭm-FĂD-ĕ-NŎP-ă-thē)

lymphadenosis
(lĭm-FĂD-ĕ-NŌ-sĭs)

lymphangiopathy
(lĭm-FĂN-jē-ŎP-ă-thē)

lymphatic
(lĭm-FĂT-ĭk)

lymphedema
(lĭm-fĕ-DĒ-mă)

lymphocyte
(LĬM-fō-sīt)

lymphocytoma
(LĬM-fō-sī-TŌ-mă)

lymphoid
(LĬM-foyd)

lymphoma
(lĭm-FŌ-mă)

pathogenic
(păth-ō-JĔN-ĭk)

pathologist
(pă-THŎL-ō-jĭst)

pathology
(pă-THŎL-ō-jē)

phagocyte
(FĂG-ō-sīt)

phagocytic
(făg-ō-SĬT-ĭk)

splenectomy
(splē-NĔK-tō-mē)

splenic
(SPLĔN-ĭk)

splenitis
(splē-NĪ-tĭs)

splenoid
(SPLĒ-noyd)

splenoma
(splē-NŌ-mă)

splenomalacia
(SPLĒ-nō-mă-LĀ-shē-ă)

splenomegaly
(SPLĒ-nō-MĔG-ă-lē)

splenopexy
(SPLĒ-nō-PĔK-sē)

splenorrhaphy
(splē-NOR-ă-fē)

thymectomy
(thī-MĔK-tō-mē)

thymic
(THĪ-mĭk)

thymoma
(thī-MŌ-mă)

tonsillar
(TŎN-sĭ-lăr)

tonsillectomy
(TŎN-sĭl-ĔK-tō-mē)

tonsillitis
(TŎN-sĭl-Ī-tĭs)

Audio Activity: Spell It

Directions: Cover the medical terms in the Pronounce It activity above with a sheet of paper. At the companion website, listen as the terms are read aloud. Correctly spell each term below.

1. adenoidectomy
2. adenoiditis
3. autoimmune
4. immunologist
5. immunology
6. lymphadenitis
7. lymphadenopathy
8. lymphadenosis
9. lymphangiopathy
10. lymphatic
11. lymphedema
12. lymphocyte
13. lymphocytoma
14. lymphoid
15. lymphoma
16. pathogenic
17. pathologist
18. pathology
19. phagocyte
20. phagocytic

21. splenectomy _____   29. splenorrhaphy _____

22. splenic _____   30. thymectomy _____

23. splenitis _____   31. thymic _____

24. splenoid _____   32. thymoma _____

25. splenoma _____   33. tonsillar _____

26. splenomalacia _____   34. tonsillectomy _____

27. splenomegaly _____   35. tonsillitis _____

28. splenopexy _____

Break It Down

Directions: Dissect each medical term below into its word elements by placing a slash between each word part (prefix, root word, combining vowel, and suffix). Then define each term.

Example:

Medical Term: lymphadenopathy

Dissection: lymph/aden/o/pathy

Definition: disease of the lymph glands

Medical Term   **Dissection**

1. tonsillectomy   t o n s i l l / e c t o m y

Definition: excision of the tonsils _____

_____

2. autoimmune   a u t o / i m m u n e

Definition: self-protection _____

_____

3. lymphadenitis   l y m p h / a d e n / i t i s

Definition: inflammation of the lymph glands _____

_____

4. pathogenic   p a t h / o / g e n / i c

Definition: pertaining to causing disease _____

_____

Medical Term	Dissection

5. splenic   s p l e n / i c

Definition: pertaining to the spleen

___

6. adenoidectomy   a d e n o i d / e c t o m y

Definition: excision of the adenoids

___

7. lymphangiopathy   l y m p h / a n g i / o / p a t h y

Definition: disease of the lymph vessels

___

8. pathology   p a t h / o / l o g y

Definition: study of disease

___

9. immunologist   i m m u n / o / l o g i s t

Definition: specialist in the study and treatment of protection

___

10. splenorrhaphy   s p l e n / o / r r h a p h y

Definition: suture of the spleen

___

11. adenoiditis   a d e n o i d / i t i s

Definition: inflammation of the adenoids

___

12. splenomegaly   s p l e n / o / m e g a l y

Definition: enlargement of the spleen

___

Medical Term	Dissection

13. tonsillitis

t o n s i l l/i t i s

Definition: inflammation of the tonsils

14. lymphocytoma

l y m p h/o/c y t/o m a

Definition: tumor of the lymph cells

15. lymphadenopathy

l y m p h/a d e n/o/p a t h y

Definition: disease of the lymph glands

16. splenitis

s p l e n/i t i s

Definition: inflammation of the spleen

17. lymphadenosis

l y m p h/a d e n/o s i s

Definition: abnormal condition of the lymph glands

18. splenopexy

s p l e n/o/p e x y

Definition: surgical fixation of the spleen

19. pathologist

p a t h/o/l o g i s t

Definition: specialist in the study and treatment of disease

SCORECARD: How Did You Do?

Number correct (_____), divided by 19 (_____), multiplied by 100 equals _____ (your score)

Build It

Directions: Build the medical term that matches each definition below by supplying the correct word elements.

P (Prefixes) = Green
RW (Root Words) = Red
S (Suffixes) = Blue
CV (Combining Vowel) = Purple

1. abnormal condition of the lymph glands

$$\underline{\quad\quad\text{lymph}\quad\quad}\qquad\underline{\quad\quad\text{aden}\quad\quad}\qquad\underline{\quad\text{osis}\quad}$$
$$\text{RW}\qquad\qquad\qquad\text{RW}\qquad\qquad\qquad\text{S}$$

2. pertaining to causing disease

$$\underline{\quad\quad\text{path}\quad\quad}\qquad\underline{\text{o}}\quad\underline{\text{gen}}\quad\underline{\text{ic}}$$
$$\text{RW}\qquad\qquad\text{CV}\quad\text{S}\quad\text{S}$$

3. study of protection

$$\underline{\quad\quad\text{immun}\quad\quad}\qquad\underline{\text{o}}\quad\underline{\text{logy}}$$
$$\text{RW}\qquad\qquad\text{CV}\quad\text{S}$$

4. inflammation of the tonsils

$$\underline{\quad\quad\text{tonsill}\quad\quad}\qquad\underline{\text{itis}}$$
$$\text{RW}\qquad\qquad\text{S}$$

5. excision of the adenoids

$$\underline{\quad\quad\text{adenoid}\quad\quad}\qquad\underline{\text{ectomy}}$$
$$\text{RW}\qquad\qquad\text{S}$$

6. disease of the lymph glands

$$\underline{\quad\quad\text{lymph}\quad\quad}\qquad\underline{\quad\quad\text{aden}\quad\quad}\qquad\underline{\text{o}}\quad\underline{\text{pathy}}$$
$$\text{RW}\qquad\qquad\qquad\text{RW}\qquad\qquad\text{CV}\quad\text{S}$$

7. self-protection

$$\underline{\text{auto}}\qquad\underline{\quad\quad\text{immune}\quad\quad}$$
$$\text{P}\qquad\qquad\text{RW}$$

8. enlargement of the spleen

$$\underline{\quad\quad\text{splen}\quad\quad}\qquad\underline{\text{o}}\quad\underline{\text{megaly}}$$
$$\text{RW}\qquad\qquad\text{CV}\quad\text{S}$$

9. tumor of the lymph

$$\frac{\text{lymph}}{\text{RW}} \qquad \frac{\text{oma}}{\text{S}}$$

10. excision of the tonsils

$$\frac{\text{tonsill}}{\text{RW}} \qquad \frac{\text{ectomy}}{\text{S}}$$

11. inflammation of the adenoids

$$\frac{\text{adenoid}}{\text{RW}} \qquad \frac{\text{itis}}{\text{S}}$$

12. suture of the spleen

$$\frac{\text{splen}}{\text{RW}} \qquad \frac{\text{o}}{\text{CV}} \quad \frac{\text{rrhaphy}}{\text{S}}$$

13. inflammation of the lymph glands

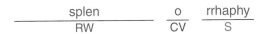

$$\frac{\text{lymph}}{\text{RW}} \qquad \frac{\text{aden}}{\text{RW}} \qquad \frac{\text{itis}}{\text{S}}$$

14. disease of the lymph vessels

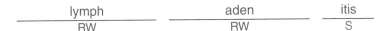

$$\frac{\text{lymph}}{\text{RW}} \qquad \frac{\text{angi}}{\text{RW}} \qquad \frac{\text{o}}{\text{CV}} \quad \frac{\text{pathy}}{\text{S}}$$

15. pertaining to the spleen

$$\frac{\text{splen}}{\text{RW}} \qquad \frac{\text{ic}}{\text{S}}$$

16. pertaining to the tonsils

$$\frac{\text{tonsill}}{\text{RW}} \qquad \frac{\text{ar}}{\text{S}}$$

17. like or resembling lymph

$$\frac{\text{lymph}}{\text{RW}} \qquad \frac{\text{oid}}{\text{S}}$$

18. excision of the spleen

$$\frac{\text{splen}}{\text{RW}} \qquad \frac{\text{ectomy}}{\text{S}}$$

19. softening of the spleen

splen	o	malacia
RW	CV	S

20. pertaining to lymph

lymph	atic
RW	S

21. specialist in the study and treatment of disease

path	o	logist
RW	CV	S

22. specialist in the study and treatment of protection

immun	o	logist
RW	CV	S

23. surgical fixation of the spleen

splen	o	pexy
RW	CV	S

24. swelling of lymph

lymph	edema
RW	S

25. tumor of the spleen

splen	oma
RW	S

SCORECARD: How Did You Do?

Number correct (_____), divided by 25 (_____), multiplied by 100 equals _____ (your score)

Diseases and Disorders

Diseases and disorders of the lymphatic and immune systems run the spectrum from the mild to the severe, and they have a number of different causes. This section presents a brief overview of some common pathological conditions of the lymphatic and immune systems.

Acquired Immunodeficiency Syndrome

Acquired immunodeficiency syndrome (AIDS) is caused by the *human immunodeficiency virus (HIV)*, which attacks the body's infection-fighting helper T cells. The first signs of HIV infection often are swollen glands and flu-like symptoms. Onset of more severe symptoms occurs months or years later (Figure 5.2). AIDS typically spreads through unprotected sexual contact with an infected person. It can also be spread through contact with the blood of an infected person or by sharing drug needles.

As we learned earlier in the chapter, specific immunity depends on helper T cells to activate an immune response. Destruction of helper T cells by HIV impairs immune function and compromises the body's ability to fight infection. Unable to defend itself against foreign invaders, the body becomes vulnerable to many different kinds of infections that a healthy immune system can easily fend off.

Allergies

An **allergy** is a hypersensitive response (exaggerated reaction) by the immune system to an **allergen**, a substance that usually is recognized by the immune system as harmless. Contact with the allergen may occur through inhalation, injection (as by a bee sting), ingestion (eating or drinking), or skin contact (Figure 5.3). Common allergens include dust, mold, pollen, pet dander, insect stings, certain kinds of foods, and drugs (over-the-counter medicines or prescription pharmaceuticals).

An allergic response is characterized as "exaggerated" because the substance that provokes the hyperreactive immune response does not cause a reaction in nonallergic individuals. During an allergic response, certain cells in the body release histamine and other allergy-mediating chemicals.

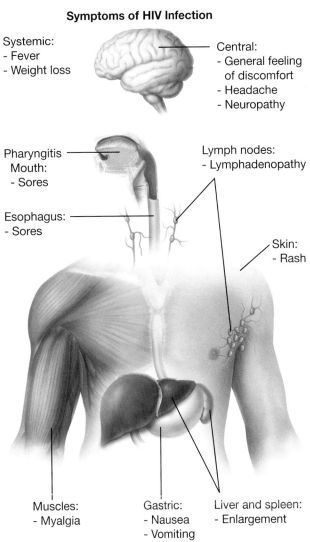

Symptoms of HIV Infection

Systemic:
- Fever
- Weight loss

Central:
- General feeling of discomfort
- Headache
- Neuropathy

Pharyngitis
Mouth:
- Sores

Lymph nodes:
- Lymphadenopathy

Esophagus:
- Sores

Skin:
- Rash

Muscles:
- Myalgia

Gastric:
- Nausea
- Vomiting

Liver and spleen:
- Enlargement

Figure 5.2 Major symptoms of acute HIV infection

Allergic Reactions

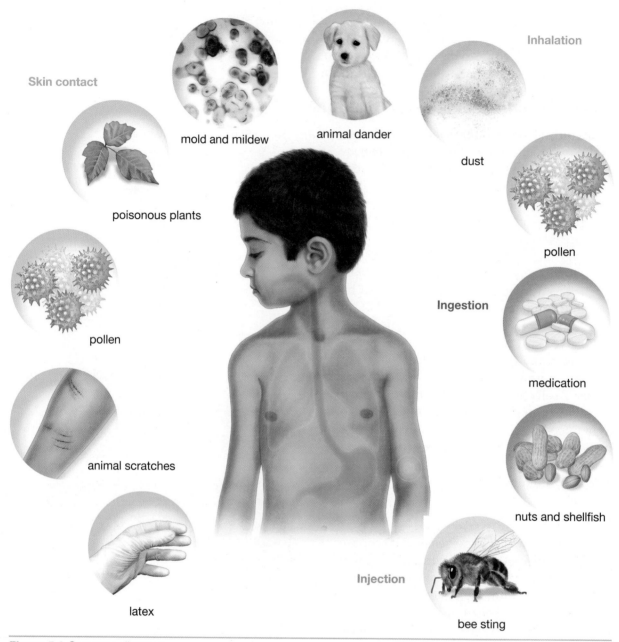

Skin contact

mold and mildew

animal dander

Inhalation

dust

poisonous plants

pollen

pollen

Ingestion

medication

animal scratches

nuts and shellfish

latex

Injection

bee sting

Figure 5.3 Common allergens

Depending on the allergen, these chemicals can cause symptoms such as nasal congestion, sneezing, coughing, wheezing, itching, burning, and swelling.

People who have allergies often are sensitive to more than one substance. Although a cure for allergies does not exist, they usually can be controlled with medication (over-the-counter or prescription) and by avoiding the allergen. However, a severe systemic (whole-body) reaction called **anaphylaxis** is life-threatening. The most serious signs of anaphylaxis are an abrupt decrease in blood pressure and difficulty breathing. Common causes of anaphylaxis include insect bites, certain foods such as shellfish, latex, and medications.

Individuals who are susceptible to systemic allergic reactions often carry an epinephrine auto-injector. Epinephrine is a chemical that constricts (narrows) the blood vessels and opens the airways in the lungs. The patient uses the device to quickly self-inject epinephrine during an anaphylactic reaction before receiving aid at an emergency facility.

Asthma

Asthma is a disorder that causes the bronchi (tubes that conduct air into the lungs) to narrow and swell and produce extra mucus. This leads to wheezing, shortness of breath, tightness in the chest, and coughing.

An asthmatic response is a hypersensitivity reaction, an exaggerated immune response to an environmental substance that the body perceives as foreign. During an asthma attack, the muscles surrounding the bronchi tighten, and the lining of the bronchial tubes becomes swollen. This tightening and swelling reduces the amount of air that can travel to the lungs. In sensitized people, asthma symptoms can be triggered by inhaling allergens. Typical asthma triggers include dust, mold, pollen, animal dander, chemicals in the air or in food, smoke, and stress. Asthma is not curable, but its symptoms can be controlled.

Autoimmune Disorders

As mentioned earlier in the chapter, an autoimmune disorder is a condition that causes the immune system to produce antibodies against its own tissues. In people with an autoimmune disorder, the immune system can't tell the difference between healthy body tissue ("self" tissue) and antigens ("non-self" substances). As a result, the immune system attacks and destroys normal body tissues. It is not yet known what mechanisms interfere with the body's ability to distinguish between healthy tissues and antigens.

There are many different types of autoimmune disorders. For example, **rheumatoid arthritis (RA)** is a chronic, systemic disease that affects the joints (Figure 5.4). This autoimmune disease causes inflammation and edema of the synovial membranes surrounding the joints. Over time, RA destroys cartilage, causes joint deformity, and erodes adjacent bone.

Autoimmune hemolytic anemia (AIHA) is a condition in which **erythrocytes** (red blood cells, or RBCs) are destroyed by antibodies. **Systemic lupus erythematosus (SLE)** is a chronic inflammatory disease that affects many different systems throughout the body. The term *erythematosus* refers to the red rash that often develops on the face of those afflicted with the disease.

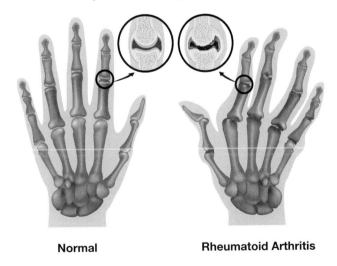

Normal **Rheumatoid Arthritis**

Alila Medical Media/Shutterstock.com

Figure 5.4 Rheumatoid arthritis is an autoimmune disease that destroys cartilage, causes joint deformity, and erodes adjacent bone.

Multiple sclerosis (MS) is an inflammatory autoimmune disease of the central nervous system (brain and spinal cord). MS is caused by damage to the myelin sheath, a layer of white fatty matter that covers most of the nerves in the brain and spinal cord. Ultimately, it causes sclerosis (hardening) that slows down or stops the transmission of nerve impulses.

Hodgkin's Disease

Hodgkin's disease (also called *Hodgkin lymphoma*) is a malignant lymphoma characterized by painless and progressive enlargement of lymphoid tissue followed by anemia, fever, persistent fatigue, and unexplained weight loss. In Hodgkin lymphoma, cells in the lymphatic system grow abnormally and may spread beyond the lymphatic system. As Hodgkin lymphoma progresses, it compromises the body's ability to fight infection. Treatment involves radiation and chemotherapy.

Mononucleosis

Mononucleosis, or **mono**, is a viral infection characterized by enlarged lymph nodes, atypical (abnormal) lymphocytes, pharyngitis (sore throat), fever, splenomegaly (enlarged spleen), and severe fatigue (Figure 5.5). Most cases of infectious mononucleosis are caused by the Epstein-Barr virus.

Mononucleosis is often called the "kissing disease" because the virus is carried in the saliva of infected individuals. Treatment includes bed rest, increased fluid intake, and acetaminophen or ibuprofen for pain and fever. The infection is generally self-limiting; that is, it resolves itself in about four to six weeks.

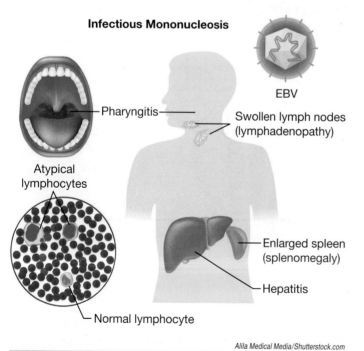

Infectious Mononucleosis

Pharyngitis

EBV

Swollen lymph nodes (lymphadenopathy)

Atypical lymphocytes

Enlarged spleen (splenomegaly)

Hepatitis

Normal lymphocyte

Alila Medical Media/Shutterstock.com

Figure 5.5 Infectious mononucleosis is characterized by atypical lymphocytes, lymphadenopathy, splenomegaly, and pharyngitis.

Sarcoidosis

Sarcoidosis is an inflammatory disease that can affect almost any body part or organ system, but it most commonly affects the lungs. The cause of the disease is unknown. Symptoms of pulmonary (lung) sarcoidosis include chest pain, dry cough, and dyspnea (difficulty breathing), along with general symptoms of fatigue, fever, and arthralgia (joint pain).

Tests used to diagnose sarcoidosis include chest X-rays, a computerized tomography (CT) scan of the chest, pulmonary function tests, and a biopsy of the lung tissue. Biopsies of other body tissues are also helpful in diagnosing the condition. In many cases, sarcoidosis abates spontaneously with no treatment. Severe symptoms may be relieved with corticosteroids (drugs that reduce inflammation) and immunosuppressants, which lower the body's immune response, preventing the immune system from attacking the body's own cells.

Tonsillitis

Tonsillitis is an inflammation of the tonsils (Figure 5.6). The condition most often occurs in childhood. While a bacterial or viral infection can cause tonsillitis, the *Streptococcus* ("strep") bacterium is the most common cause.

Symptoms of tonsillitis include sore throat, chills, fever, and pain. Lymph nodes in the jaw and throat are tender and enlarged. The tonsils usually are red and may have white spots on them. Treatment for tonsillitis includes bed rest, a liquid diet, saline irrigation for the throat, and antibiotic therapy. Surgery may be recommended for persistent, chronic tonsillitis.

Procedures and Treatments

We will now take a brief look at some common diagnostic tests and procedures used to help identify disorders and diseases of the lymphatic and immune systems, as well as some common therapeutic treatments.

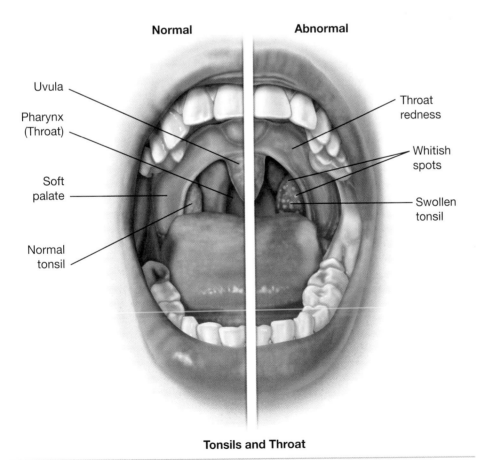

Normal   **Abnormal**

Uvula
Pharynx (Throat)
Soft palate
Normal tonsil

Throat redness
Whitish spots
Swollen tonsil

Tonsils and Throat

Figure 5.6 Symptoms of tonsillitis include redness in the throat, swollen tonsils, and white spots in the back of the throat.

Enzyme-Linked Immunosorbent Assay

Enzyme-linked immunosorbent assay (ELISA) is a common laboratory test in which a blood sample is drawn and examined for the presence of antibodies. This test is often performed to determine whether or not a person has been exposed to viruses or other substances that cause infection. It can be used to screen for current or past infections.

The ELISA test is typically the first one used to detect infection by the human immunodeficiency virus (HIV). If antibodies to HIV are present, the test is positive. The test is usually repeated to confirm the diagnosis.

The ELISA test is a good screening tool; however, it can produce "false positive" results, indicating the presence of HIV when it is nonexistent. Therefore, the ELISA test alone cannot be used to make a definitive diagnosis of HIV infection. The presence of HIV must be confirmed by a Western blot test (discussed later in this section) or other more specific tests.

Immunization

Immunization is a procedure that provides immunity against a disease-causing pathogen without inducing infection. This is accomplished through **vaccination**, the injection of a substance containing dead or attenuated (weakened) pathogens directly into the bloodstream. The substance that contains the pathogens is called a **vaccine**.

A vaccine stimulates the immune system to produce antibodies against a specific pathogen. Immunizations against measles, mumps, rubella, polio, diphtheria, and pertussis help to keep the population healthy. Vaccines are a successful, cost-effective public health tool for preventing the spread of disease that can be dangerous and even deadly.

Scratch Test

A **scratch test** is a skin test used to identify the substance causing an allergy. An extract of an allergen is applied to the skin by scratching or pricking the skin's surface so that the extract can penetrate the epidermis (outer layer of skin).

A scratch test is usually performed on the forearm or back (Figure 5.7). Areas on the skin are marked with a pen to identify each allergen that will be tested. A very small amount of extract for each potential allergen (such as pollen, animal dander, or insect venom) is placed on the corresponding mark. The reaction of the skin is then evaluated. If the scratch test is positive for a particular allergen, the skin in that area will become raised, red, and pruritic (itchy).

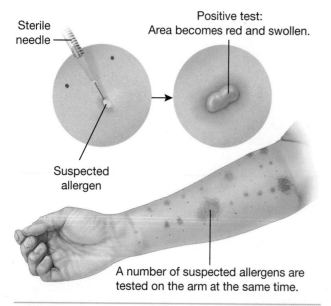

Sterile needle

Positive test: Area becomes red and swollen.

Suspected allergen

A number of suspected allergens are tested on the arm at the same time.

Figure 5.7 A scratch test is used to identify substances that provoke an allergic reaction.

Splenectomy

A **splenectomy** is the surgical removal of a diseased or damaged spleen. The spleen is located in the left upper quadrant of the abdomen, just underneath the ribs. The most common reason for splenectomy is to treat a ruptured spleen, often caused by traumatic abdominal injury, such as from an automobile accident. This procedure may also be performed to treat some blood disorders, certain cancers, infection, cysts, or tumors.

Splenectomy is most commonly performed by **laparoscopy**, also called *laparoscopic splenectomy* (Figure 5.8). The patient is placed under general anesthesia. The surgeon directs a *cannula* (hollow tube) into the abdomen, where it is inflated with carbon dioxide gas to create a space within which to operate. A **laparoscope**, a tiny telescope connected to a video camera, is inserted through the cannula and into the abdomen. The camera projects a video image of the spleen and surrounding internal organs onto a TV monitor.

During laparoscopic splenectomy, the surgeon views the operative site with the camera. Several other cannulas are placed in different locations inside the abdomen, allowing the surgeon to insert instruments, detach the spleen from other body structures, and remove it. When the spleen has been freed from surrounding tissues, it is placed in a sterile bag and then pulled out of the body through an incision.

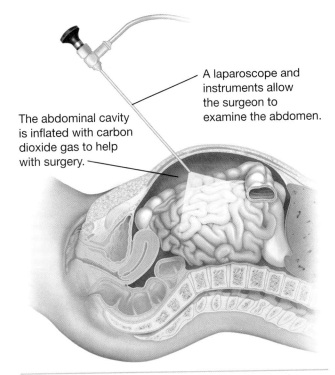

A laparoscope and instruments allow the surgeon to examine the abdomen.

The abdominal cavity is inflated with carbon dioxide gas to help with surgery.

Figure 5.8 Splenectomy is commonly performed using a laparoscopic surgical method.

Tonsillectomy

A **tonsillectomy** is the surgical removal of the tonsils. It is used to treat severe, chronic, or recurring tonsillitis or complications due to enlarged tonsils.

At one time, tonsillectomy was a common procedure for treating inflammation and infection of the tonsils. Now it is generally reserved for the removal of enlarged tonsils that interfere with breathing or cause recurrent ear infections. It is also performed to treat tonsillitis that occurs frequently and does not improve with antibiotic treatment.

Western Blot Test

A **Western blot test** is a laboratory blood test that detects the presence of antibodies to specific antigens. It is used to diagnose chronic infection with human immunodeficiency virus (HIV). It is regarded as more precise than the enzyme-linked immunosorbent assay (ELISA) and is sometimes used to check the validity of the ELISA test. A positive Western blot confirms an HIV infection.

Multiple Choice: Diseases and Disorders

Directions: Write the letter of the disease or disorder that matches each numbered definition below.

_A_ 1. an inflammatory autoimmune disease of the central nervous system
   a. multiple sclerosis
   b. rheumatoid arthritis
   c. systemic lupus erythematosus
   d. autoimmune hemolytic anemia

_C_ 2. a viral infection characterized by enlarged lymph nodes, atypical lymphocytes, sore throat, fever, splenomegaly, and severe fatigue
   a. tonsillitis
   b. sarcoidosis
   c. mononucleosis
   d. asthma

_B_ 3. a malignant lymphoma characterized by enlargement of lymphoid tissue, anemia, fatigue, fever, and weight loss
   a. asthma
   b. Hodgkin's disease
   c. multiple sclerosis
   d. sarcoidosis

_B_ 4. a condition in which erythrocytes are destroyed by antibodies
   a. rheumatoid arthritis
   b. autoimmune hemolytic anemia
   c. systemic lupus erythematosus
   d. multiple sclerosis

_D_ 5. an inflammatory disease that can affect almost any body part or organ, but most commonly affects the lungs
   a. mononucleosis
   b. tonsillitis
   c. asthma
   d. sarcoidosis

_C_ 6. inflammation of the tonsils
   a. mononucleosis
   b. sarcoidosis
   c. tonsillitis
   d. asthma

_C_ 7. a chronic inflammatory disease that affects many different body systems and often causes a red rash on the face
   a. multiple sclerosis
   b. autoimmune hemolytic anemia
   c. systemic lupus erythematosus
   d. rheumatoid arthritis

_C_ 8. an exaggerated reaction by the immune system to a substance ordinarily recognized by the immune system as harmless
   a. mononucleosis
   b. autoimmune hemolytic anemia
   c. allergy
   d. sarcoidosis

_A_ 9. a chronic, systemic autoimmune disease that causes inflammation of the joints
   a. rheumatoid arthritis
   b. systemic lupus erythematosus
   c. Hodgkin's disease
   d. sarcoidosis

_D_ 10. a life-threatening, systemic (whole-body) reaction to an allergy
   a. allergic response
   b. antigen intolerance
   c. systemic lupus erythematosus
   d. anaphylaxis

_B_ 11. a disorder that causes the bronchi to narrow, swell, and produce extra mucus
   a. mononucleosis
   b. asthma
   c. allergy
   d. anaphylaxis

SCORECARD: How Did You Do?

Number correct (_____), divided by 11 (_____), multiplied by 100 equals _____ (your score)

Multiple Choice: Procedures and Treatments

Directions: Write the letter of the diagnostic procedure or therapeutic treatment that matches each numbered definition below.

_C_   1. a procedure that provides immunity against a specific disease-causing pathogen without inducing infection
    a. scratch test
    b. Western blot test
    c. immunization
    d. enzyme-linked immunosorbent assay

_B_   2. a skin test used to identify the substance that is causing an allergy
    a. immunization
    b. scratch test
    c. enzyme-linked immunosorbent assay
    d. Western blot test

_B_   3. surgical removal of a diseased or damaged spleen
    a. splenorrhaphy   c. splenotomy
    b. splenectomy   d. splenoplasty

_C_   4. a laboratory test in which a blood sample is taken to detect the presence of antibodies; typically the first test used to detect HIV infection
    a. scratch test
    b. immunization
    c. enzyme-linked immunosorbent assay
    d. Western blot test

_B_   5. surgical removal of the tonsils
    a. tonsillotomy   c. tonsillorrhaphy
    b. tonsillectomy   d. tonsilloplasty

_C_   6. a laboratory test used to detect the presence of antibodies to specific antigens; used to definitively diagnose HIV
    a. immunization
    b. scratch test
    c. Western blot test
    d. enzyme-linked immunosorbent assay

SCORECARD: How Did You Do?

Number correct (_____), divided by 6 (_____), multiplied by 100 equals _____ (your score)

Identifying Abbreviations

Directions: Write the abbreviation for each medical term listed below.

Medical Term	Abbreviation
1. multiple sclerosis	MS
2. acquired immunodeficiency syndrome	AIDS
3. enzyme-linked immunosorbent assay	ELISA
4. human immunodeficiency virus	HIV
5. computerized tomography	CT
6. systemic lupus erythematosus	SLE
7. rheumatoid arthritis	RA
8. mononucleosis	MONO
9. autoimmune hemolytic anemia	AIHA

SCORECARD: How Did You Do?

Number correct (_____), divided by 9 (_____), multiplied by 100 equals _____ (your score)

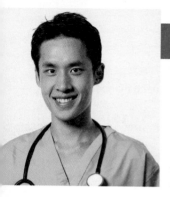

Analyzing the Intern Experience

In the Intern Experience described at the beginning of this chapter, we met Sean, an intern with the Cassel County Clinic. Sean "shadowed" (that is, followed and observed) Dr. Rymus as he interacted with William Shumaker, a 57-year-old accountant who described symptoms of extreme fatigue, persistent night sweats, weight loss, and a lump on the right side of his neck. Dr. Rymus examined William and obtained his personal and family health history. He then made a medical diagnosis and provided William with a treatment plan. Later, Dr. Rymus made a dictated recording of William's health information, which was subsequently transcribed into a chart note.

We will now learn more about William Shumaker's condition from a clinical perspective, interpreting the medical terms in his chart note as we analyze the scenario presented in the Intern Experience.

Audio Activity: William Shumaker's Chart Note

Directions: At the companion website, listen and read along as the physician dictates William Shumaker's chart note, shown below. Then do the exercise that appears after William's chart note.

CHART NOTE

Patient Name: Shumaker, William
ID Number: WS3671
Examination Date: May 2, 20xx

SUBJECTIVE
Mr. William Shumaker is a 57-year-old accountant who is new to this practice. He has noticed a painless lump on the right side of his neck. He states that he is very tired, has been experiencing night sweats, and has lost about 8 pounds in the past 2 months.

OBJECTIVE
Low-grade fever. **BP** (blood pressure), pulse, and respiration within normal limits. There are 2 firm enlarged lymph nodes on the right side of the neck, to the right and just below the **laryngeal prominence** (Adam's apple).

ASSESSMENT
Lymphadenopathy. Rule out **Hodgkin's disease**.

PLAN
CBC (complete blood count) and chest X-ray will be scheduled along with a **biopsy**.

Interpret William Shumaker's Chart Note

Directions: After listening to the dictated recording and reading the chart note on William Shumaker, provide the medical term that matches each definition below. You may encounter definitions and terms that were introduced in previous chapters.

Example: inflammation of the tonsils   *Answer:* tonsillitis

1. disease of the lymph glands   lymphadenopathy

2. Adam's apple   laryngeal prominence

3. blood pressure   BP

4. surgical removal of tissue for diagnostic examination   biopsy

5. malignant lymphoma characterized by painless and progressive enlargement of lymphoid tissue   Hodgkin's disease

6. complete blood count   CBC

SCORECARD: How Did You Do?

Number correct (_____), divided by 6 (_____), multiplied by 100 equals _____ (your score)

Working with Medical Records

In this activity, you will interpret the medical records (chart notes) of patients with health conditions related to the lymphatic and immune systems. These examples illustrate typical medical records prepared in a real-world healthcare environment. To interpret these chart notes, you will apply your knowledge of word elements (prefixes, combining forms, and suffixes), diseases and disorders, and procedures and treatments related to the lymphatic and immune systems.

Audio Activity: Sidney O'Brian's Chart Note

Directions: At the companion website, listen and read along as the physician dictates the following chart note on Sidney O'Brian. Then do the exercise that appears after Sidney's chart note.

CHART NOTE

Patient Name: O'Brian, Sidney
ID Number: SO4423
Examination Date: September 16, 20xx

SUBJECTIVE
Sidney is a 17-year-old patient who presents with a 7-day history of chills, sore throat, fatigue, fever, and headache. Over the weekend her symptoms have worsened and she is extremely tired. She states that she "shared a straw" with a friend when they were at the mall 2 weeks ago and now her friend is also sick.

OBJECTIVE
BP 120/76, temperature 102.4, respiratory rate 23, pulse 72. Lungs are clear. Lymph nodes are swollen. **Tonsils** are enlarged and have a whitish-yellow covering.

ASSESSMENT
Cervical **lymphadenopathy**. **Mononucleosis** test performed in the office is positive.

PLAN
The patient should drink plenty of fluids, gargle with warm salt water to ease sore throat pain, and get plenty of rest. She may take acetaminophen or ibuprofen for fever and discomfort.

Assessment

Interpret Sidney O'Brian's Chart Note

Directions: After listening to the dictated recording and reading the chart note on Sidney O'Brian, provide the medical term that matches each definition below.

Example: swelling of lymph   *Answer:* lymphedema

1. disease of the lymph glands

   lymphadenopathy

2. viral infection characterized by enlarged lymph nodes, atypical lymphocytes, pharyngitis, fever, splenomegaly, and severe fatigue

   mononucleosis

3. tissue structures that protect the body by trapping pathogens that enter through the mouth or nose

   tonsils

SCORECARD: How Did You Do?

Number correct (_____), divided by 3 (_____), multiplied by 100 equals _____ (your score)

Audio Activity: Carter Rosari's Chart Note

Directions: At the companion website, listen and read along as the physician dictates the following chart note on Carter Rosari. Then do the exercise that appears after Carter's chart note.

CHART NOTE

Patient Name: Rosari, Carter
ID Number: CR8062
Examination Date: November 21, 20xx

SUBJECTIVE
Carter presents with multiple raised, red, itchy welts on his left lower leg, thigh, and forearm after returning home from a camping trip with his Boy Scout troop. He states that it started about 3 days into the trip and that some of the welts seemed to get better, but then new ones began to erupt. "They seemed to move up my leg and onto my arm." He remembers something similar to this happening last year when he helped his father put up the Christmas tree.

OBJECTIVE
Wheals (welts or swellings) ranging in size from small spots on the left forearm to several large blotches about 1–2 cm in diameter on the lower leg and thigh. No fever. Vital signs are normal. History of pollen **allergy**.

ASSESSMENT
Urticaria (hives) of left leg and forearm. Allergic **contact dermatitis**.

PLAN
Apply hydrocortisone cream to the affected areas. Patient to return if condition does not improve or worsens.

Assessment

Interpret Carter Rosari's Chart Note

Directions: After listening to the dictated recording and reading the chart note on Carter Rosari, provide the medical term that matches each definition below. You may encounter definitions and terms that were introduced in previous chapters.

Example: softening of the spleen	*Answer:* splenomalacia

1. hives

    urticaria

2. edema and pruritic (itchy) skin as a result of contact with an allergen or irritant, causing edema and pruritic skin

    contact dermatitis

3. welts or swellings

    wheals

4. exaggerated response by the immune system to a substance that usually is recognized by the body as harmless

    allergy

SCORECARD: How Did You Do?

Number correct (_____), divided by 4 (_____), multiplied by 100 equals _____ (your score)

Chapter Review

Word Elements Summary

Prefixes

Prefix	Meaning
auto-	self
hyper-	above; above normal
inter-	between
intra-	within

Combining Forms

Root Word/Combining Vowel	Meaning
aden/o	gland
adenoid/o	adenoids
angi/o	vessel
cyt/o	cell
immun/o	protection
leuk/o	white
lymph/o	lymph
path/o	disease
phag/o	eat; swallow; engulf
splen/o	spleen
thym/o	thymus
tonsill/o	tonsils

Suffixes

Suffix	Meaning
-ac	pertaining to
-ar	pertaining to
-atic	pertaining to
-cyte	cell
-ectomy	surgical removal; excision

(Continued)

Suffix	Meaning
-edema	swelling
-gen	producing; originating; causing
-ic	pertaining to
-itis	inflammation
-logist	specialist in the study and treatment of
-logy	study of
-malacia	softening
-megaly	enlargement
-oid	like; resembling
-oma	tumor; mass
-osis	abnormal condition
-pathy	disease
-pexy	surgical fixation
-rrhaphy	suture
-trophy	development

More Practice: Activities and Games

The activities on the following pages will help you reinforce your skills and check your mastery of the medical terminology that you learned in this chapter. Visit the companion website for More Practice games and activities.

True or False

Directions: Indicate whether each statement below is true or false.

True or False?

    F   1. The prefix **inter-** means "through."

    F   2. The root word **path** means "pathway to a disease."

    T   3. The suffix **-cyte** means "cell."

    F   4. The suffix **-pathy** means "pertaining to the study of pathology."

    T   5. The term *adenoidectomy* contains one root word and one suffix.

    F   6. The term *lymphadenitis* contains one root word and one suffix.

    F   7. The term *autoimmune* contains a prefix and a suffix.

    T   8. Pathogens are harmful invaders such as bacteria, viruses, parasites, and antibodies.

_____F_____ 9. Nonspecific immunity is a protective mechanism that provides antibodies against a specific antigen.

_____T_____ 10. An antigen is a specific substance that, when introduced into the body, stimulates the production of an antibody.

_____T_____ 11. Tonsils help protect the body from infection by trapping pathogens that enter through the mouth or nose.

_____T_____ 12. T lymphocytes are involved in a properly functioning immune system.

_____F_____ 13. Hodgkin's disease is a disorder that causes the bronchi to narrow and swell and produce extra mucus.

_____T_____ 14. An autoimmune disorder is a condition that occurs when the immune system attacks and destroys healthy body tissue.

_____F_____ 15. There is only one type of autoimmune disorder.

_____T_____ 16. Rheumatoid arthritis is a chronic, systemic disease that affects the joints.

_____T_____ 17. Multiple sclerosis is caused by damage to the myelin sheath that covers the nerves in the brain and spinal cord.

_____F_____ 18. AIDS cannot be spread by contact with blood or bodily fluids.

_____T_____ 19. An allergy is an exaggerated reaction of the immune system in response to a substance that the body ordinarily perceives as harmless.

_____F_____ 20. *Tonsillectomy* means "inflammation of the tonsils."

_____T_____ 21. Sarcoidosis is an inflammatory disease that can affect almost any body part or organ system.

_____T_____ 22. The Western blot test is a laboratory blood test to detect the presence of antibodies to specific antigens.

Dictionary Skills

Directions: Using a medical dictionary, such as *Taber's Cyclopedic Medical Dictionary*, look up the term **lymphocele**.

For each medical term shown below, indicate whether the term appears on the same page as **lymphocele**, before the page, or after the page. Use the following abbreviations in your answers:

O = on the same page   **B** = before the page   **A** = after the page

Write the definition of each term in the space provided.

Medical Term   **O, B, A**

Answers in this
column will vary.

1. lymphorrhea   _____

Definition: flow of lymph _____

_____

2. lymphology   _____

Definition: the study of the lymph/lymphatic fluid _____

_____

Medical Term	O, B, A
	Answers in this column will vary.

3. lymphocytosis

Definition: abnormal condition of lymph cells

4. lymphoblast

Definition: an immature lymph cell

5. lymphomatosis

Definition: multiple cancerous lymph cells that are widely distributed throughout the body

6. lymphogenous

Definition: pertaining to originating from lymph or the lymphatic system

7. lymphangiography

Definition: process of recording an image of lymph vessels

8. lymphocele

Definition: tumor or swelling of lymph

9. lymphangiectomy

Definition: surgical removal of lymph vessels

10. lymphedema

Definition: swelling of tissues due to obstruction in the lymphatic vessels or lymph nodes

Break It Down

Directions: Dissect each medical term below into its word elements by placing a slash between each word part (prefix, root word, combining vowel, and suffix). Then define each term.

Example:
Medical Term: lymphangiopathy
Dissection: lymph/angi/o/pathy
Definition: disease of the lymph vessels

Medical Term	Dissection

1. adenitis   a d e n/i t i s

Definition: inflammation of a gland

2. splenocyte   s p l e n/o/c y t e

Definition: cell of the spleen

3. immunogenic   i m m u n/o/g e n/i c

Definition: pertaining to producing protection

4. tonsillopathy   t o n s i l l/o/p a t h y

Definition: disease of the tonsils

5. adenoma   a d e n/o m a

Definition: tumor of a gland

6. phagocytosis   p h a g/o/c y t/o s i s

Definition: abnormal condition of cells that eat/swallow/engulf

Medical Term	Dissection
7. pathogen	p a t h /o /g e n

Definition: producing disease

_____

8. lymphadenitis	l y m p h /a d e n /i t i s

Definition: inflammation of the lymph glands

_____

9. splenogenic	s p l e n /o /g e n /i c

Definition: pertaining to originating in the spleen

_____

10. adenolymphoma	a d e n /o /l y m p h /o m a

Definition: tumor of the glands and lymph

_____

Spelling

Directions: Circle the correctly spelled term in each row.

1.	(lymphadenitis)	lymphedenitis	lymphodenitis	lymphadynitis
2.	pathagenic	pathogenec	(pathogenic)	pathegenic
3.	splennopexy	splenopexxy	splaenopexy	(splenopexy)
4.	tonsilar	(tonsillar)	tonsiller	tonsillor
5.	(anaphylaxis)	anyphalaxis	anephylaxis	anaphalaxis
6.	reumatoid	(rheumatoid)	rhuematoid	rheumetoid
7.	(antigen)	antagen	antegen	antogen
8.	sarcoydosis	sarkoydosis	sarcoidossis	(sarcoidosis)
9.	splenorraphy	splenorhaphy	(splenorrhaphy)	splenoraphy
10.	lymphodema	(lymphedema)	lymphedemia	lymphadema
11.	tonsilitis	(tonsillitis)	tonsylitis	tonsolitis
12.	splenomelacia	(splenomalacia)	splenomalaysia	splenomalatia

Audio Activity: Kim Lee's Chart Note

Directions: At the companion website, listen and read along as the physician dictates the following chart note on Kim Lee. Then do the exercise that appears after Kim's chart note.

CHART NOTE

Patient Name: Lee, Kim
ID Number: KL7214
Examination Date: May 14, 20xx

SUBJECTIVE
This 9-year-old patient presents with chronic nasal congestion, sore throat, and enlarged **tonsils**. Mother states that Kim always breathes through her mouth and snores at night. Also, mother said it is getting to the point where she is having difficulty understanding her since word formation is poor. Patient has a chronic history of strep throat.

OBJECTIVE
Temperature is 101. **Tympanic membranes** (eardrums) are clear. Exam of the **pharynx** reveals markedly enlarged tonsils, almost touching. **Erythema** is present. Nasal mucosa is edematous. Neck is supple without lymphadenopathy. Chest is clear.

ASSESSMENT
Tonsillitis and probable **hypertrophy** of the adenoids.

PLAN
Refer to **ENT** (ear, nose, and throat specialist) for possible **tonsillectomy** and **adenoidectomy**.

Interpret Kim Lee's Chart Note

Directions: After listening to the dictated recording and reading the chart note on Kim Lee, provide the medical term that matches each definition below. You may encounter definitions and terms that were introduced in previous chapters.

Example: tumor of the lymph cells   *Answer:* lymphocytoma

1. excision of the tonsils   tonsillectomy

2. eardrums   tympanic membranes

3. excision of the adenoids   adenoidectomy

4. the throat   pharynx

5. inflammation of the tonsils   tonsillitis

6. tissue structures that protect the body from infection by trapping pathogens that enter through the mouth or nose   tonsils

7. above-normal development   hypertrophy

8. ear, nose, and throat specialist   ENT

9. redness   erythema

Chapter 6
Special Sensory Organs: Eye and Ear

ophthalm / o / logy = the study of the eye

ot / o / logy = the study of the ear

Chapter Organization

- Intern Experience
- Overview of Anatomy and Physiology of the Eye and Ear
- Word Elements
- Breaking Down and Building Terms Related to the Eye and Ear
- Diseases and Disorders
- Procedures and Treatments
- Analyzing the Intern Experience
- Working with Medical Records
- Chapter Review

Chapter Objectives

After completing this chapter, you will be able to

1. label anatomical diagrams of the eye and the ear;
2. dissect and define common medical terminology related to the special sensory organs of vision and hearing;
3. build terms used to describe diseases and disorders of the eye and ear, as well as diagnostic procedures and therapeutic treatments;
4. pronounce and spell common medical terminology related to the special sensory organs of vision and hearing;
5. understand that the processes of building and dissecting a medical term based on its prefix, word root, and suffix enable you to analyze an extremely large number of medical terms beyond those presented in this chapter;
6. interpret the meaning of abbreviations associated with the special sensory organs of vision and hearing; and
7. interpret medical records containing terminology and abbreviations related to these special sensory organs.

You will see this icon ⬈ at various points throughout this chapter. The icon indicates that you will find interactive activities and games on the Medical Terminology Companion Website. These activities and games will help you learn, practice, and expand your medical terminology knowledge and skills. Some of these activities are also available on the Medical Terminology Mobile Website.

 Companion Website
www.g-wlearning.com/healthsciences

 Mobile Site
www.m.g-wlearning.com/5800

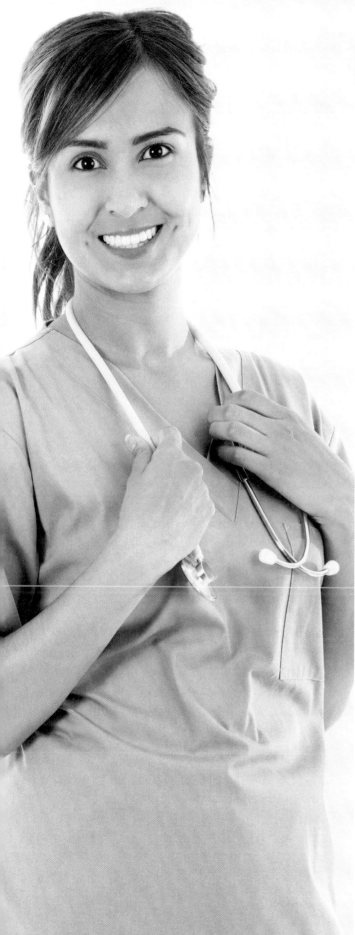

Debra is in the second week of her internship with University Eye and Ear Specialists, Inc. Sofia Rodriguez had called the office as soon as it opened, expressing concern for her four-year-old son, Juan. At their designated appointment time, Debra greets Mrs. Rodriguez and her son in the waiting room and escorts them to an exam room.

Mrs. Rodriguez appears fatigued. She states that she was awakened early that morning by her son's anguished screams. She informs Debra that Juan's face felt hot to the touch, and he was tugging at his left ear. Because Juan has had recurrent ear infections, Mrs. Rodriguez is worried about possible hearing loss. Debra notes the mother's concerns in Juan's chart, obtains his vital signs, and, using her laptop computer, electronically signals to the physician that the patient is ready to be seen.

To help you understand Juan's health condition, this chapter will present word elements (combining forms, prefixes, and suffixes) that make up medical terminology related to the ear, the sensory organ that controls hearing and equilibrium (balance). You will also learn word elements and medical terminology related to the eye, the sensory organ of sight.

Let's begin our study with a brief anatomical and physiological overview of both the eye and the ear. We will cover major structures of these special sensory organs, along with their primary functions. Later in the chapter, you will learn about some common pathological conditions of the eye and ear, tests and procedures used to diagnose those conditions, and common methods for treating them.

Overview of Anatomy and Physiology of the Eye and Ear

The special sensory organs contain receptors that receive information about stimuli outside the body (the external environment) and transmit neural impulses about these stimuli to the brain for interpretation. The special sensory organs also process and interpret information about external stimuli to help maintain internal *homeostasis*, a condition of stable physiological equilibrium (balance) that allows the body to function normally. (You will learn more about homeostasis in your study of Chapter 7: The Nervous System.) Organs of the sensory system play a vital role in homeostasis by alerting the body to potential danger.

For example, two college students are walking down a dark, windy street late at night after seeing a movie with some friends. They hear the muffled crunching of stones from behind them, as if someone is following them. The students quickly dart into a nearby convenience store and text their roommates, asking whether one of them can give them a ride back to their dormitory.

In this scenario, both the ears and the eyes—two of the special sensory organs—play a crucial role in alerting the body to potential danger.

Sensory systems of the body include the five commonly recognized sensory organs:

Organ	Function(s)
Eye	Sight (visual)
Ear	Hearing (auditory); equilibrium, or balance (vestibular)
Nose	Smell (olfactory)
Tongue	Taste (gustatory)
Skin	Touch (tactile or somatic)

For the purposes of this chapter, we will limit our discussion of special sensory organs to the eye and the ear.

The Eye

The eye operates much like a camera. Incoming light passes through the **cornea**, similar in function to the aperture (adjustable opening) of a camera (Figure 6.1). The cornea is the clear, outer layer of the eye that covers the iris and pupil; it allows light to travel to the interior of the eye. The amount of light that enters the eye is controlled by the **iris**, the colored portion of the anterior eye. Within the iris is an opening called the **pupil**, which contracts (narrows) and dilates (expands) to regulate the amount of light entering the eye, much like a camera shutter.

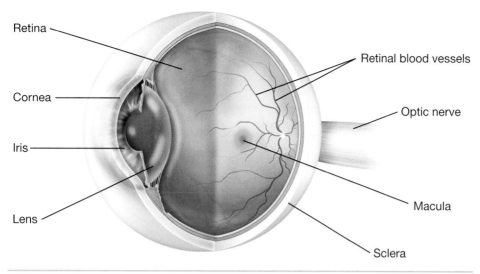

Figure 6.1 Major structures of the eye

The **lens**, located behind the pupil, focuses the light onto the retina. The **retina** (RĔT-ĭ-nă), the innermost layer of the eye, receives images formed by the lens. It contains light-sensing cells responsible for color vision and fine detail. The retina acts much like camera film—or, in today's technology, the memory card inside a cell phone that carries information about the subscriber's identity. The retina sends information via the **optic nerve** to the brain for interpretation. The **sclera** (SKLĒ-ră) is the white, outer protective layer of the eye.

The Ear

The ear has three main parts: the **external** (outer) **ear**, the **middle ear**, and the **internal** (inner) **ear** (Figure 6.2 on the next page). Sound waves enter the external ear, or **external auditory meatus** (mē-ĂT-ŭs), and pass through the middle ear to the **tympanic** (tĭm-PĂN-ĭk) **membrane** (eardrum), causing it to vibrate. Vibrations in the eardrum are transmitted to the internal ear by three very small bones called **ossicles**. The vibrations are detected by sensory receptors in the inner ear, where the information is transmitted by nerve impulses to the brain. The brain interprets these neural impulses as sound.

Besides the function of hearing, the ear is responsible for your sense of equilibrium, or balance. Fluid in the **semicircular canals**, tiny channels within the inner ear, control orientation and balance. They help you maintain steadiness while standing or walking.

Anatomy and Physiology Vocabulary

Now that you have been introduced to the basic anatomy and physiology of the eye and the ear, we will explore in more detail the key terms presented in the introduction (see table on the next page).

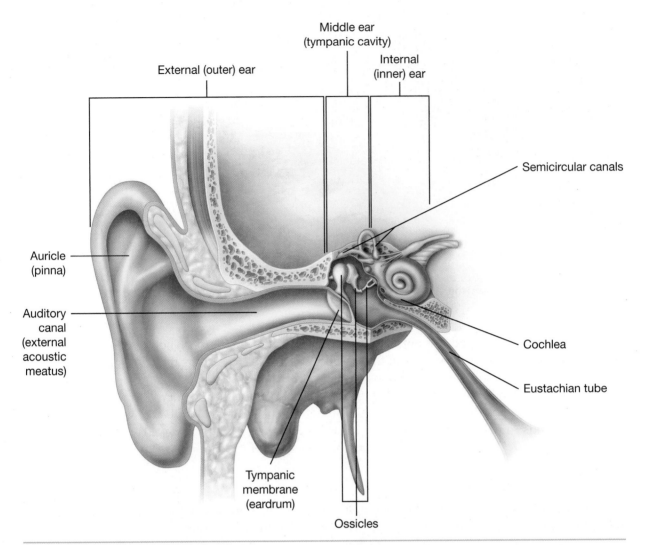

Figure 6.2 Major structures of the ear

Key Term	Definition
cornea	transparent outer layer of the eye that covers the iris and pupil and allows light to enter
external auditory meatus	external (outer) ear
internal ear	inner ear
iris	colored portion of the anterior eye
lens	structure of the eye that focuses light onto the retina
middle ear	central cavity of the ear
optic nerve	nerve that carries impulses for the sense of sight from the retina to the brain

(Continued)

Key Term	Definition
ossicles	three small bones of the ear that transmit vibrations from the eardrum to the internal ear
pupil	opening in the iris that contracts and dilates, regulating the amount of light that enters the eye
retina	innermost layer of the eye that receives images formed by the lens
sclera	white, outer protective layer of the eye
semicircular canals	tiny channels in the inner ear that control balance
tympanic membrane	eardrum

E-Flash Card Activity: Anatomy and Physiology Vocabulary

Directions: After you have reviewed the anatomy and physiology vocabulary related to the sensory organs of sight and hearing, practice with the e-flash cards until you are comfortable with the spelling and definition of each term.

Assessment

Identifying Major Structures of the Eye

Directions: Label the anatomical diagram of the eye.

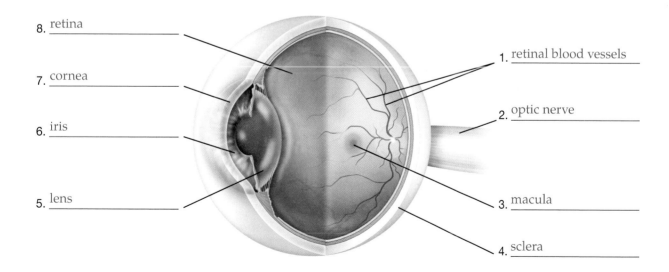

8. retina

7. cornea

6. iris

5. lens

1. retinal blood vessels

2. optic nerve

3. macula

4. sclera

SCORECARD: How Did You Do?

Number correct (_____), divided by 8 (_____), multiplied by 100 equals _____ (your score)

Identifying Major Structures of the Ear

Directions: Label the anatomical diagram of the ear.

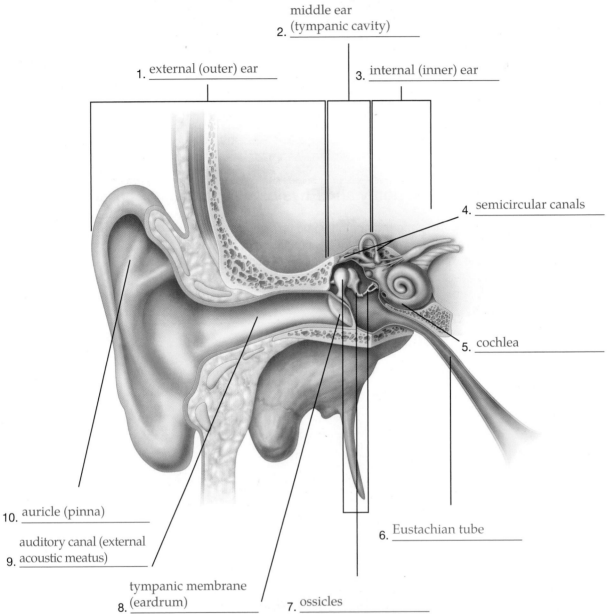

middle ear
2. (tympanic cavity) _____

1. external (outer) ear _____

3. internal (inner) ear _____

4. semicircular canals _____

5. cochlea _____

10. auricle (pinna) _____

auditory canal (external
9. acoustic meatus) _____

6. Eustachian tube _____

tympanic membrane
8. (eardrum) _____

7. ossicles _____

Matching Anatomy and Physiology Vocabulary

Directions: Match the vocabulary term in Column A with its meaning in Column B. The meanings can be used more than once.

Column A

_G_ 1. internal ear

_F_ 2. lens

_J_ 3. middle ear

_B_ 4. optic nerve

_E_ 5. retina

_I_ 6. tympanic membrane

_M_ 7. cornea

_K_ 8. semicircular canals

_L_ 9. pupil

_H_ 10. sclera

_D_ 11. ossicles

_A_ 12. iris

_C_ 13. external auditory meatus

Column B

A. colored portion of the anterior eye

B. nerve that carries impulses for the sense of sight from the retina to the brain

C. external (outer) ear

D. three small bones of the ear that transmit vibrations from the eardrum to the internal ear

E. innermost layer of the eye that receives images formed by the lens

F. structure of the eye that focuses light onto the retina

G. inner ear

H. white, outer protective layer of the eye

I. eardrum

J. central cavity of the ear

K. tiny channels in the inner ear that control balance

L. opening in the iris that contracts and dilates, regulating the amount of light that enters the eye

M. transparent outer layer of the eye that covers the iris and pupil and allows light to enter

SCORECARD: How Did You Do?

Number correct (_____), divided by 13 (_____), multiplied by 100 equals _____ (your score)

Word Elements

In this section you will learn word elements—prefixes, combining forms, and suffixes—that are common to the special senses. By learning these word elements and understanding how they are combined to build medical terms, you will be able to analyze Juan's health problem (described in the Intern Experience at the beginning of this chapter) and identify a large number of terms associated with the special senses.

E-Flash Card Activity: Word Elements

Directions: Review the word elements in the tables that follow. Then, practice with the e-flash cards until you are able to quickly recognize the different word parts (prefixes, combining forms, and suffixes) and their meanings. The e-flash cards are grouped together by prefixes, combining forms, and suffixes, followed by a cumulative review of all the word elements that you learned in this chapter.

Prefixes

This chapter presents terms that contain the prefixes listed below.

Prefix	Meaning
an-	not; without
extra-	outside
hemi-	half
intra-	inside; within
para-	near; beside
peri-	around

Combining Forms

Listed below are common combining forms used in medical terms pertaining to the sensory organs of vision and hearing.

Root Word/Combining Vowel	Meaning
audi/o	hearing
blephar/o	eyelid
ir/o	iris
irid/o	iris
kerat/o	cornea
myc/o	fungus
myring/o	tympanic membrane; eardrum
ocul/o	eye
ophthalm/o	eye
opt/o	eye; vision
optic/o	eye; vision
ot/o	ear
pleg/o	paralysis
presby/o	old age
retin/o	retina
scler/o	sclera (white of the eye)
tympan/o	tympanic membrane; eardrum

Suffixes

Listed below are suffixes used in medical terms related to the special sensory organs. You have already learned many of these suffixes.

Suffix	Meaning
-al	pertaining to
-algia	pain
-ar	pertaining to
-ectomy	surgical removal; excision
-gram	record; image
-ia	condition
-ic	pertaining to
-itis	inflammation
-logist	specialist in the study of
-logy	study of
-meter	instrument used to measure
-metry	measurement
-opia	vision
-osis	abnormal condition
-pexy	surgical fixation
-plasty	surgical repair
-ptosis	drooping; downward displacement
-rrhea	discharge; flow
-rrhexis	rupture
-scope	instrument used to observe
-scopy	process of observing
-spasm	involuntary muscle contraction
-stomy	new opening
-tomy	incision; cut into

Matching Prefixes, Combining Forms, and Suffixes

Directions: In each exercise below, match the word element in Column A with its meaning in Column B. Some meanings may be used more than once.

Prefixes

Column A

D	1. extra-
E	2. para-
B	3. an-
F	4. peri-
C	5. hemi-
A	6. intra-

Column B

A. inside; within

B. not; without

C. half

D. outside

E. near; beside

F. around

Combining Forms

Column A

K	1. retin/o
A	2. ir/o
J	3. myring/o
F	4. kerat/o
J	5. tympan/o
E	6. audi/o
B/G	7. opt/o
H	8. blephar/o
I	9. myc/o
D	10. scler/o
C	11. ot/o
A	12. irid/o
B	13. ophthalm/o
B	14. ocul/o
L	15. pleg/o
M	16. presby/o

Column B

A. iris

B. eye

C. ear

D. sclera

E. hearing

F. cornea

G. vision

H. eyelid

I. fungus

J. tympanic membrane; eardrum

K. retina

L. paralysis

M. old age

Suffixes

Column A

__V__	1.	-stomy
__K__	2.	-metry
__Q__	3.	-ia
__M__	4.	-tomy
__A__	5.	-al
__N__	6.	-osis
__D__	7.	-ectomy
__C__	8.	-rrhea
__B__	9.	-algia
__F__	10.	-scopy
__A__	11.	-ar
__P__	12.	-plasty
__A__	13.	-ic
__U__	14.	-scope
__H__	15.	-logist
__J__	16.	-meter
__S__	17.	-spasm
__E__	18.	-gram
__T__	19.	-rrhexis
__G__	20.	-itis
__R__	21.	-ptosis
__I__	22.	-logy
__O__	23.	-pexy
__L__	24.	-opia

Column B

A. pertaining to

B. pain

C. discharge; flow

D. surgical removal; excision

E. record; image

F. process of observing

G. inflammation

H. specialist in the study of

I. study of

J. instrument used to measure

K. measurement

L. vision

M. incision; cut into

N. abnormal condition

O. surgical fixation

P. surgical repair

Q. condition

R. drooping; downward displacement

S. involuntary muscle contraction

T. rupture

U. instrument used to observe

V. new opening

SCORECARD: How Did You Do?

Number correct (_____), divided by 46 (_____), multiplied by 100 equals _____ (your score)

Breaking Down and Building Terms Related to the Eye and Ear

Now that you have mastered the prefixes, combining forms, and suffixes for medical terminology used to describe the special sensory organs of sight and hearing, you have the ability to dissect and build a large number of terms related to these special sensory systems.

Below is a list of common medical terms related to the study and treatment of the eye and the ear. For each term, a dissection has been provided, along with the meaning of each word element and the definition of the term as a whole.

Term	Dissection	Word Part/Meaning	Term Meaning
Note: *For simplification, combining vowels have been omitted from the Word Part/Meaning column.*			
1. **audiogram** (AW-dē-ō-grăm)	audi/o/gram	**audi** = hearing **gram** = record; image	record of hearing
2. **audiologist** (AW-dē-ŎL-ō-jĭst)	audi/o/logist	**audi** = hearing **logist** = specialist in the study and treatment of	specialist in the study and treatment of hearing
3. **audiology** (AW-dē-ŎL-ō-jē)	audi/o/logy	**audi** = hearing **logy** = study of	study of hearing
4. **audiometer** (AW-dē-ŎM-ĕ-ter)	audi/o/meter	**audi** = hearing **meter** = instrument used to measure	instrument used to measure hearing
5. **audiometry** (AW-dē-ŎM-ĕ-trē)	audi/o/metry	**audi** = hearing **metry** = measurement	measurement of hearing
6. **blepharitis** (BLĔF-ă-RĪ-tĭs)	blephar/itis	**blephar** = eyelid **itis** = inflammation	inflammation of the eyelid
7. **blepharoplasty** (BLĔF-ă-rō-PLĂS-tē)	blephar/o/plasty	**blephar** = eyelid **plasty** = surgical repair	surgical repair of the eyelid
8. **blepharoplegia** (BLĔF-ă-rō-PLĒ-jē-ă)	blephar/o/pleg/ia	**blephar** = eyelid **pleg** = paralysis **ia** = condition	condition of eyelid paralysis
9. **blepharoptosis** (BLĔF-ă-rŏp-TŌ-sĭs)	blephar/o/ptosis	**blephar** = eyelid **ptosis** = drooping; downward displacement	drooping of the eyelid
10. **blepharospasm** (BLĔF-ă-rō-SPĂZM)	blephar/o/spasm	**blephar** = eyelid **spasm** = involuntary muscle contraction	involuntary muscle contraction of the eyelid

Prefixes = **Green**   Root Words = **Red**   Suffixes = **Blue**

Term	Dissection	Word Part/Meaning	Term Meaning
11. **extraocular** (ĔKS-tră-ŎK-yū-lăr)	extra/ocul/ar	**extra** = outside **ocul** = eye **ar** = pertaining to	pertaining to the outside of the eye
12. **iridectomy** (ĬR-ĭ-DĔK-tō-mē)	irid/ectomy	**irid** = iris **ectomy** = surgical removal; excision	excision of the iris
13. **iridoplasty** (ĬR-ĭd-ō-PLĂS-tē)	irid/o/plasty	**irid** = iris **plasty** = surgical repair	surgical repair of the iris
14. **iridoplegia** (ĬR-ĭd-ō-PLĒ-jē-ă)	irid/o/pleg/ia	**irid** = iris **pleg** = paralysis **ia** = condition	condition of iris paralysis
15. **iridopexy** (ĬR-ĭd-ō-PĔK-sē)	irid/o/pexy	**irid** = iris **pexy** = surgical fixation	surgical fixation of the iris
16. **iritis** (ĭr-Ī-tĭs)	ir/itis	**ir** = iris **itis** = inflammation	inflammation of the iris
17. **keratometer** (kĕr-ă-TŎM-ĕ-ter)	kerat/o/meter	**kerat** = cornea **meter** = instrument used to measure	instrument used to measure the cornea
18. **keratometry** (kĕr-ă-TŎM-ĕ-trē)	kerat/o/metry	**kerat** = cornea **metry** = measurement	measurement of the cornea
19. **myringectomy** (mĭr-ĭn-JĔK-tō-mē)	myring/ectomy	**myring** = tympanic membrane; eardrum **ectomy** = surgical removal; excision	excision of the eardrum
20. **myringitis** (mĭr-ĭn-JĪ-tĭs)	myring/itis	**myring** = eardrum **itis** = inflammation	inflammation of the eardrum
21. **myringoplasty** (mĭr-ĬNG-gō-plăst-ē)	myring/o/plasty	**myring** = tympanic membrane; eardrum **plasty** = surgical repair	surgical repair of the eardrum
22. **myringotomy** (mĭr-ĭng-GŎT-ō-mē)	myring/o/tomy	**myring** = tympanic membrane; eardrum **tomy** = incision; cut into	incision to the eardrum
23. **ocular** (ŎK-yū-lăr)	ocul/ar	**ocul** = eye **ar** = pertaining to	pertaining to the eye
24. **oculomycosis** (ŎK-yū-lō-mī-KŌ-sĭs)	ocul/o/myc/osis	**ocul** = eye **myc** = fungus **osis** = abnormal condition	abnormal condition of fungus in the eye
25. **ophthalmic** (ŏf-THĂL-mĭk)	ophthalm/ic	**ophthalm** = eye **ic** = pertaining to	pertaining to the eye

Prefixes = Green   Root Words = Red   Suffixes = Blue

Term	Dissection	Word Part/Meaning	Term Meaning
26. **ophthalmologist** (ŎF-thăl-MŎL-ō-jĭst)	ophthalm/o/logist	**ophthalm** = eye **logist** = specialist in the study and treatment of	specialist in the study and treatment of the eye
27. **ophthalmology** (ŎF-thăl-MŎL-ō-jē)	ophthalm/o/logy	**ophthalm** = eye **logy** = study of	study of the eye
28. **ophthalmoscope** (ŏf-THĂL-mō-skōp)	ophthalm/o/scope	**ophthalm** = eye **scope** = instrument used to observe	instrument used to observe the eye
29. **optic** (ŎP-tĭk)	opt/ic	**opt** = eye; vision **ic** = pertaining to	pertaining to the eye or vision
30. **otalgia** (ō-TĂL-jē-ă)	ot/algia	**ot** = ear **algia** = pain	pain in the ear
31. **otitis** (ō-TĪ-tĭs)	ot/itis	**ot** = ear **itis** = inflammation	inflammation of the ear
32. **otologist** (ō-TŎL-ō-jĭst)	ot/o/logist	**ot** = ear **logist** = specialist in the study and treatment of	specialist in the study and treatment of the ear
33. **otology** (ō-TŎL-ō-jē)	ot/o/logy	**ot** = ear **logy** = study of	study of the ear
34. **otomycosis** (Ō-tō-mī-KŌ-sĭs)	ot/o/myc/osis	**ot** = ear **myc** = fungus **osis** = abnormal condition	abnormal condition of fungus in the ear
35. **otoplasty** (Ō-tō-PLĂS-tē)	ot/o/plasty	**ot** = ear **plasty** = surgical repair	surgical repair of the ear
36. **otorrhea** (ō-tō-RĒ-ă)	ot/o/rrhea	**ot** = ear **rrhea** = discharge; flow	discharge from the ear
37. **otoscope** (Ō-tō-skōp)	ot/o/scope	**ot** = ear **scope** = instrument used to observe	instrument used to observe the ear
38. **otoscopy** (ō-TŎS-kō-pē)	ot/o/scopy	**ot** = ear **scopy** = process of observing	process of observing the ear
39. **paraocular** (PĂR-ă-ŎK-yū-lăr)	para/ocul/ar	**para** = near; beside **ocul** = eye **ar** = pertaining to	pertaining to near the eye
40. **periocular** (PĔR-ē-ŎK-yū-lăr)	peri/ocul/ar	**peri** = around **ocul** = eye **ar** = pertaining to	pertaining to around the eye

Prefixes = **Green**   Root Words = **Red**   Suffixes = **Blue**

Term	Dissection	Word Part/Meaning	Term Meaning
41. **retinal** (RĔT-ĭ-năl)	retin/al	**retin** = retina **al** = pertaining to	pertaining to the retina
42. **retinitis** (RĔT-ĭ-NĪ-tĭs)	retin/itis	**retin** = retina **itis** = inflammation	inflammation of the retina
43. **scleral** (SKLĔR-ăl)	scler/al	**scler** = sclera **al** = pertaining to	pertaining to the sclera
44. **scleritis** (sklĕ-RĪ-tĭs)	scler/itis	**scler** = sclera itis = inflammation	inflammation of the sclera
45. **sclerotomy** (sklĕ-RŎT-ō-mē)	scler/o/tomy	**scler** = sclera **tomy** = incision; cut into	incision to the sclera
46. **tympanectomy** (tĭm-păn-ĔK-tō-mē)	tympan/ectomy	**tympan** = eardrum **ectomy** = excision; surgical removal	excision of the eardrum
47. **tympanic** (tĭm-PĂN-ĭk)	tympan/ic	**tympan** = tympanic membrane; eardrum **ic** = pertaining to	pertaining to the eardrum
48. **tympanometer** (TĬM-pă-NŎM-ĕ-tĕr)	tympan/o/meter	**tympan** = tympanic membrane; eardrum **meter** = instrument used to measure	instrument used to measure the eardrum
49. **tympanometry** (TĬM-pă-NŎM-ĕ-trē)	tympan/o/metry	**tympan** = tympanic membrane; eardrum **metry** = measurement	measurement of the eardrum
50. **tympanoplasty** (TĬM-păn-ō-PLĂS-tē)	tympan/o/plasty	**tympan** = tympanic membrane; eardrum **plasty** = surgical repair	surgical repair of the eardrum
51. **tympanorrhexis** (TĬM-păn-ŏr-RĔKS-ĭs)	tympan/o/rrhexis	**tympan** = tympanic membrane; eardrum **rrhexis** = rupture	rupture of the eardrum
52. **tympanostomy** (TĬM-păn-ŎS-tō-mē)	tympan/o/stomy	**tympan** = tympanic membrane; eardrum **stomy** = new opening	new opening in the eardrum

Prefixes = Green   Root Words = Red   Suffixes = Blue

Using the pronunciation guide from the Break It Down chart above, practice saying each medical term aloud. To hear the pronunciation of each term, go to the Pronounce It activity at the G-W companion website.

Audio Activity: Pronounce It

Directions: At the companion website, listen as each medical term listed below is pronounced. Practice pronouncing the terms until you are comfortable saying them aloud.

audiogram
(AW-dē-ō-grăm)

audiologist
(AW-dē-ŎL-ō-jĭst)

audiology
(AW-dē-ŎL-ō-jē)

audiometer
(AW-dē-ŎM-ĕ-ter)

audiometry
(AW-dē-ŎM-ĕ-trē)

blepharitis
(BLĔF-ă-RĪ-tĭs)

blepharoplasty
(BLĔF-ă-rō-PLĂS-tē)

blepharoplegia
(BLĔF-ă-rō-PLĒ-jē-ă)

blepharoptosis
(BLĔF-ă-rŏp-TŌ-sĭs)

blepharospasm
(BLĔF-ă-rō-SPĂZM)

extraocular
(ĔKS-tră-ŎK-yū-lăr)

iridectomy
(ĬR-ĭ-DĔK-tō-mē)

iridoplasty
(ĬR-ĭd-ō-PLĂS-tē)

iridoplegia
(ĬR-ĭd-ō-PLĒ-jē-ă)

iridopexy
(ĬR-ĭd-ō-PĔK-sē)

iritis
(ĭr-Ī-tĭs)

keratometer
(kĕr-ă-TŎM-ĕ-ter)

keratometry
(kĕr-ă-TŎM-ĕ-trē)

myringectomy
(mĭr-ĭn-JĔK-tō-mē)

myringitis
(mĭr-ĭn-JĪ-tĭs)

myringoplasty
(mĭr-ĬNG-gō-plăst-ē)

myringotomy
(mĭr-ĭng-GŎT-ō-mē)

ocular
(ŎK-yū-lăr)

oculomycosis
(ŎK-yū-lō-mī-KŌ-sĭs)

ophthalmic
(ŏf-THĂL-mĭk)

ophthalmologist
(ŎF-thăl-MŎL-ō-jĭst)

ophthalmology
(ŎF-thăl-MŎL-ō-jē)

ophthalmoscope
(ŏf-THĂL-mō-skōp)

optic
(ŎP-tĭk)

otalgia
(ō-TĂL-jē-ă)

otitis
(ō-TĪ-tĭs)

otologist
(ō-TŎL-ō-jĭst)

otology
(ō-TŎL-ō-jē)

otomycosis
(Ō-tō-mī-KŌ-sĭs)

otoplasty
(Ō-tō-PLĂS-tē)

otorrhea
(ō-tō-RĒ-ă)

otoscope
(Ō-tō-skōp)

otoscopy
(ō-TŎS-kō-pē)

paraocular
(PĂR-ă-ŎK-yū-lăr)

periocular
(PĔR-ē-ŎK-yū-lăr)

retinal
(RĔT-ĭ-năl)

retinitis
(RĔT-ĭ-NĪ-tĭs)

scleral
(SKLĔR-ăl)

scleritis
(sklĕ-RĪ-tĭs)

sclerotomy
(sklĕ-RŎT-ō-mē)

tympanectomy
(tĭm-păn-ĔK-tō-mē)

tympanic
(tĭm-PĂN-ĭk)

tympanometer
(TĬM-pă-NŎM-ĕ-tĕr)

tympanometry
(TĬM-pă-NŎM-ĕ-trē)

tympanoplasty
(TĬM-păn-ō-PLĂS-tē)

tympanorrhexis
(TĬM-păn-ŏr-RĔKS-ĭs)

tympanostomy
(TĬM-păn-ŌS-tō-mē)

Audio Activity: Spell It

Directions: Cover the medical terms in the Pronounce It activity with a sheet of paper. At the companion website, listen as the terms are read aloud. Correctly spell each term below.

1. audiogram
2. audiologist
3. audiology
4. audiometer
5. audiometry
6. blepharitis
7. blepharoplasty
8. blepharoplegia
9. blepharoptosis
10. blepharospasm
11. extraocular
12. iridectomy
13. iridoplasty
14. iridoplegia
15. iridopexy
16. iritis
17. keratometer
18. keratometry
19. myringectomy
20. myringitis
21. myringoplasty
22. myringotomy
23. ocular
24. oculomycosis
25. ophthalmic
26. ophthalmologist

27. ophthalmology
28. ophthalmoscope
29. optic
30. otalgia
31. otitis
32. otologist
33. otology
34. otomycosis
35. otoplasty
36. otorrhea
37. otoscope
38. otoscopy
39. paraocular
40. periocular
41. retinal
42. retinitis
43. scleral
44. scleritis
45. sclerotomy
46. tympanectomy
47. tympanic
48. tympanometer
49. tympanometry
50. tympanoplasty
51. tympanorrhexis
52. tympanostomy

Break It Down

Directions: Dissect each medical term below into its word elements by placing a slash between each word part (prefix, root word, combining vowel, and suffix). Then define each term.

Example:

Medical Term: oculomycosis

Dissection: ocul/o/mycosis

Definition: abnormal condition of fungus in the eye

Medical Term	Dissection
1. blepharoptosis	b l e p h a r/o/p t o s i s

Definition: drooping of the eyelid

| 2. scleritis | s c l e r/i t i s |

Definition: inflammation of the sclera

| 3. opthalmoscope | o p t h a l m/o/s c o p e |

Definition: instrument used to observe the eye

| 4. tympanic | t y m p a n/i c |

Definition: pertaining to the eardrum

| 5. audiometry | a u d i/o/m e t r y |

Definition: measurement of hearing

| 6. iridoplasty | i r i d/o/p l a s t y |

Definition: surgical repair of the iris

Medical Term	Dissection

7. paraocular

p a r a/o c u l/a r

Definition: pertaining to near the eye
_____

_____

8. myringectomy

m y r i n g/e c t o m y

Definition: excision of the eardrum
_____

_____

9. optic

o p t/i c

Definition: pertaining to the eye or vision
_____

_____

10. otorrhea

o t/o/r r h e a

Definition: discharge from the ear
_____

_____

11. extraocular

e x t r a/o c u l/a r

Definition: pertaining to outside the eye
_____

_____

12. iridectomy

i r i d/e c t o m y

Definition: excision of the iris
_____

_____

13. retinal

r e t i n/a l

Definition: pertaining to the retina
_____

_____

14. periocular

p e r i/o c u l/a r

Definition: pertaining to around the eye
_____

_____

Medical Term	Dissection

15. tympanorrhexis   t y m p a n/o/r r h e x i s

Definition: rupture of the eardrum

16. blepharoplegia   b l e p h a r/o/p l e g/i a

Definition: condition of eyelid paralysis

17. iridopexy   i r i d/o/p e x y

Definition: surgical fixation of the iris

18. keratometry   k e r a t/o/m e t r y

Definition: measurement of the cornea

19. otitis   o t/i t i s

Definition: inflammation of the ear

20. otoscope   o t/o/s c o p e

Definition: instrument used to observe the ear

SCORECARD: How Did You Do?

Number correct (_____), divided by 20 (_____), multiplied by 100 equals _____ (your score)

Build It

Directions: Build the medical terms that match the definitions provided below by supplying the correct word elements.

P (Prefixes) = Green
RW (Root Words) = Red
S (Suffixes) = Blue
CV (Combining Vowel) = Purple

1. record of hearing

audi	o	gram
RW	CV	S

2. excision of the eardrum **(two possible answers)**

myring	ectomy
RW	S

tympan	ectomy
RW	S

3. instrument used to measure hearing

audi	o	meter
RW	CV	S

4. rupture of the eardrum

tympan	o	rrhexis
RW	CV	S

5. surgical repair of the eyelid

blephar	o	plasty
RW	CV	S

6. excision of the iris

irid	ectomy
RW	S

7. study of the eye

ophthalm	o	logy
RW	CV	S

8. inflammation of the iris

$$\frac{\text{ir}}{\text{RW}} \quad \frac{\text{itis}}{\text{S}}$$

9. new opening in the eardrum

$$\frac{\text{tympan}}{\text{RW}} \quad \frac{\text{o}}{\text{CV}} \quad \frac{\text{stomy}}{\text{S}}$$

10. instrument used to measure the cornea

$$\frac{\text{kerat}}{\text{RW}} \quad \frac{\text{o}}{\text{CV}} \quad \frac{\text{meter}}{\text{S}}$$

11. involuntary muscle contraction of the eyelid

$$\frac{\text{blephar}}{\text{RW}} \quad \frac{\text{o}}{\text{CV}} \quad \frac{\text{spasm}}{\text{S}}$$

12. inflammation of the eardrum

$$\frac{\text{myring}}{\text{RW}} \quad \frac{\text{itis}}{\text{S}}$$

13. condition of eyelid paralysis

$$\frac{\text{blephar}}{\text{RW}} \quad \frac{\text{o}}{\text{CV}} \quad \frac{\text{pleg}}{\text{RW}} \quad \frac{\text{ia}}{\text{S}}$$

14. pain in the ear

$$\frac{\text{ot}}{\text{RW}} \quad \frac{\text{algia}}{\text{S}}$$

15. specialist in the study and treatment of the ear

$$\frac{\text{ot}}{\text{RW}} \quad \frac{\text{o}}{\text{CV}} \quad \frac{\text{logist}}{\text{S}}$$

SCORECARD: How Did You Do?

Number correct (_____), divided by 15 (_____), multiplied by 100 equals _____ (your score)

Diseases and Disorders

Diseases and disorders of the special sensory organs range from the mild to the severe, and they have a wide variety of causes. We will briefly examine some problems that commonly affect the eye and the ear.

The Eye

The eyes are among the most delicate organs of the body. Some eye conditions, such as minor infections, are short lived. Others require corrective treatment such as eyeglasses, contact lenses, or surgery. Left untreated, serious eye conditions—especially those linked with systemic pathology (for example, diabetic retinopathy)—can result in permanent loss of vision.

Astigmatism

Astigmatism (ă-STĬG-mă-tĭzm) is a common condition that causes blurred vision due either to an irregularly shaped cornea or curvature of the lens (Figure 6.3). An irregular-shaped cornea or lens prevents light from properly focusing on the retina. As a result, vision becomes distorted or blurred at any distance, causing eye discomfort and headaches.

Astigmatism is often present at birth and may occur in conjunction with myopia or hyperopia (Figure 6.4, on the next page). **Myopia** (mī-ŌP-ē-ă), more commonly known as *nearsightedness*, is a condition in which close objects are seen clearly, but objects farther away appear blurred. **Hyperopia** (HĪ-pĕr-ŌP-ē-ă), or *farsightedness*, is a condition in which distant objects are usually seen clearly, but close ones do not come into proper focus. Together, myopia and hyperopia are referred to as *refractive errors* because they affect how the eyes *refract*, or bend, light. The specific cause of astigmatism is unknown.

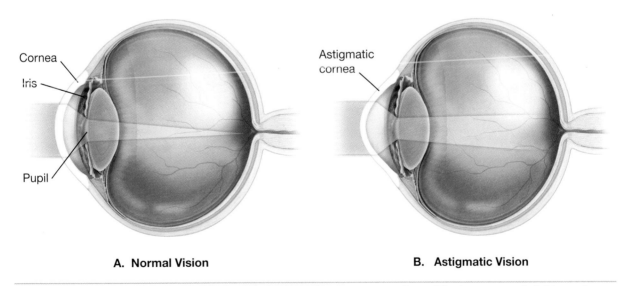

A. Normal Vision   **B. Astigmatic Vision**

Figure 6.3 Astigmatism, the result of an irregularly shaped cornea or curvature of the lens, prevents light rays from properly focusing on the retina, causing blurred or distorted vision.

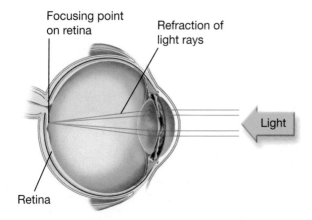

A. **Normal vision:**
Light rays focus on the retina.

Cataract

A **cataract** (KĂT-ă-răct) is a clouding of the lens of the eye (Figure 6.5). The lens of the eye is normally clear. It functions like the lens of a camera, focusing light as it travels to the retina at the back of the eye. Normally, the shape of the lens is able to change, allowing the eye to focus on an object, whether it is close or far away. With age, the lens begins to break down and becomes cloudy. As a result, vision may become blurred.

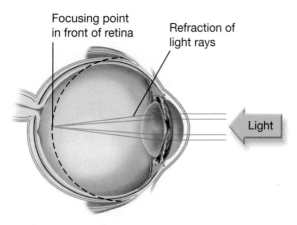

B. **Myopia (nearsightedness):**
Light rays focus in front of the retina.

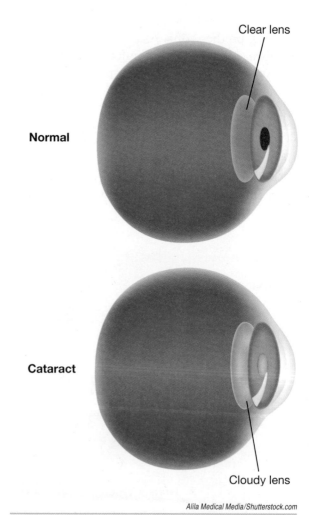

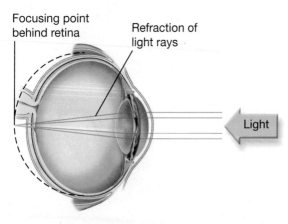

C. **Hyperopia (farsightedness):**
Light rays focus beyond the retina.

Figure 6.4 Myopia and hyperopia

Alila Medical Media/Shutterstock.com

Figure 6.5 A cataract is a clouding of the lens of the eye. Cataracts are typically associated with aging.

Diabetic Retinopathy

Diabetic retinopathy (RĔT-ĭ-NŎP-ă-thē) is a serious complication of diabetes marked by progressive damage to the blood vessels of the retina. It is a chronic condition that can develop in patients with uncontrolled diabetes. In the early stages of diabetic retinopathy, patients are often asymptomatic (without symptoms). As the condition progresses, it may result in blurred or fluctuating vision (sight that "comes and goes"), floaters (small spots or specks that float around in the field of vision), dark or empty areas in the vision, or difficulty with color perception. Typically, diabetic retinopathy affects both eyes.

Glaucoma

Glaucoma (glaw-KŌ-mă) is a group of eye conditions that cause optic nerve damage, which may lead to loss of vision. The optic nerve carries visual information from the eye to the brain. In most cases, damage to this nerve is the result of abnormally high *intraocular pressure (IOP)*, or pressure within the eye. Because glaucoma damage is gradual, the patient may not notice any loss of vision until the disease has reached an advanced stage. Glaucoma is a major cause of blindness in the United States.

Macular Degeneration

Macular degeneration is a leading cause of vision loss among Americans 60 years of age and older. In macular degeneration, the central portion of the retina, called the *macular area*, degenerates over time, resulting in loss of central vision (Figure 6.6). Varying degrees of peripheral vision remain, but those afflicted with macular degeneration are often unable to read or drive, and other activities of daily living are severely restricted due to the loss of full, clear vision.

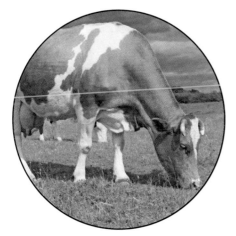

How a scene appears with normal vision

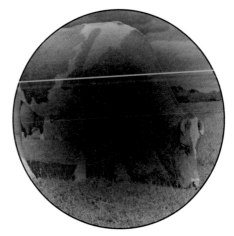

How a scene appears with vision affected by macular degeneration

Photo credit: Smereka/Shutterstock.com. Concept adapted from Lighthouse International; http://lighthouse.org/about-low-vision-blindness/vision-disorders/age-related-macular-degeneration-amd/

Figure 6.6 Macular degeneration

Presbyopia

Presbyopia (PRĔZ-bē-ŌP-ē-ă) is a condition in which the lens of the eye gradually loses its elasticity, or the ability to change its shape, making it difficult to see objects up close. Presbyopia occurs naturally with age; thus, it is often called the "aging eye condition." As the lens of the eye becomes less flexible, it no longer can change shape to focus on images at close range. As a result, objects appear out of focus.

The Ear

Infection or disease of the ear can affect hearing, balance, or both. Certain conditions of the ear can cause hearing disorders or deafness. We will take a brief look at some of the more common conditions.

Ménière's Disease

Ménière's (měn-YĚRZ) **disease** is a chronic inner-ear disorder that affects balance and hearing (Figure 6.7). The inner ear contains semicircular canals, small fluid-filled tubes that help your body maintain its position and balance. Every time you move your head, the fluid within the canals stimulates tiny hairs lining each canal. These hairs interpret the movement of the fluid and transmit neural impulses to the brain. The cause of Ménière's disease is unknown. Symptoms include dizziness or a sensation of spinning called **vertigo** (VĔR-tĭ-gō or vĕr-TĒ-gō); **tinnitus** (TĬN-ĭ-tŭs or tĭ-NĪ-tŭs), commonly known as "ringing in the ears"; pressure within the ear; and hearing loss.

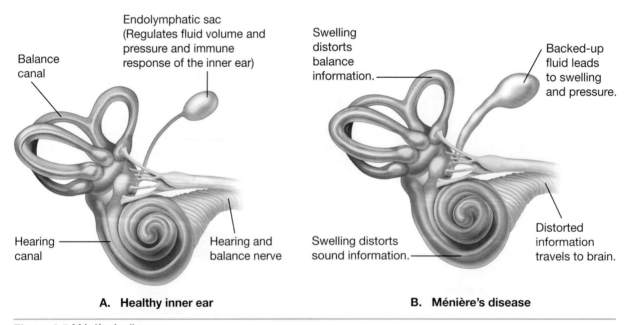

A. **Healthy inner ear**   B. **Ménière's disease**

Figure 6.7 Ménière's disease

Otitis Media

Otitis media (ō-TĪ-tĭs MĒ-dē-ă) is a bacterial or viral infection of the middle ear (Figure 6.8). It is more common in children than adults. The *otalgia* (ō-TĂL-gē-ă), or ear pain, that accompanies otitis media is due to inflammation and buildup of fluid in the middle ear. Persistent ear infections can cause hearing problems and other serious complications.

Presbycusis

Presbycusis (PRĔZ-bē-KŪ-sĭs) is the gradual loss of hearing that occurs as people age. Although there is no single known cause for presbycusis, it is most commonly associated with degenerative changes to the inner ear. One of the hallmarks of presbycusis is difficulty hearing high-frequency sound, such as that produced by someone talking, particularly amid background noise. Genetic factors as well as repeated or prolonged exposure to loud noises can contribute to age-related hearing loss.

Procedures and Treatments

We will now briefly review common diagnostic tests and procedures used to help identify disorders and diseases of the eyes and ears, as well as some common therapeutic treatments.

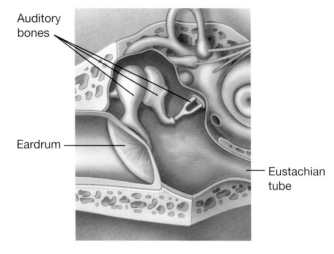

A. Normal middle ear

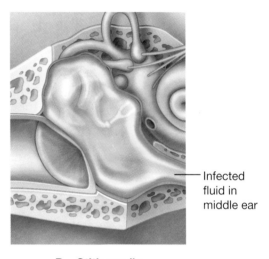

B. Otitis media

Figure 6.8 Middle ear infection

The Eye

A variety of procedures are used to test visual acuity and help diagnose diseases and disorders of the eye, and rapidly developing technologies have brought about cutting-edge treatments. For the purpose of this brief overview, we will present a few common procedures and treatments.

Visual Acuity Test

The **visual acuity** (ă-KYŪ-ĭ-tē) **test** is a routine part of an eye examination. The Snellen chart, a standardized eye chart, is used to assess eyesight clarity and detect problems with vision (Figure 6.9).

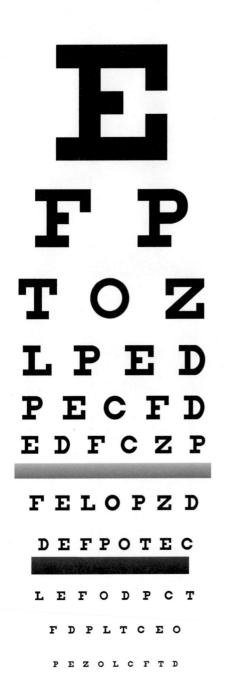

Figure 6.9 The Snellen chart is used to test visual acuity.

Radu Bercan/Shutterstock.com

During an eye exam, the patient covers one eye at a time and reads aloud the smallest line of letters that he or she can see on the Snellen chart. Visual acuity is expressed as a fraction. The top number refers to the distance from which the patient reads the chart, typically 20 feet. The bottom number indicates the distance from which a person with normal vision can read the line. Vision of 20/20 is considered normal. A reading of 20/30 indicates that the line read by the patient read at a distance of 20 feet away can be read by a person with normal vision at a distance of 30 feet away.

Abnormal results of a visual acuity test may indicate a need for glasses or contact lenses due to an eye condition that needs further evaluation by an ophthalmologist, such as astigmatism, myopia, or hyperopia. Besides attempting to read the smallest line of type on the Snellen chart, the patient may be asked to read letters or numbers from a card held 14 inches from the face in a test of near vision. For very young children or patients who cannot read, visual acuity is tested with pictures instead of letters.

Blepharoplasty

Blepharoplasty (BLĔF-ă-rō-PLĂS-tē) is the surgical repair of drooping eyelids (Figure 6.10). It can be both a functional (necessary) and a cosmetic surgery. During the procedure, excess skin and fat are removed or repositioned, and surrounding muscles and tendons may be reinforced.

With age, the eyelids stretch and muscular support weakens, resulting in excess fat above and below the eyelids. This causes sagging eyebrows, drooping upper lids, and puffy "bags" under the eyes. Severely sagging skin around the eyes can impair peripheral (side) vision. Blepharoplasty can reduce or eliminate impaired vision and improve appearance.

Fluorescein Angiography

Fluorescein (flor-ĔS-ē-ĭn) **angiography** (ĂN-jē-ŎG-ră-fē) is a photographic method of imaging the retina. A fluorescein dye (an orange fluorescent dye) is injected into a vein in the patient's arm. As the dye circulates throughout the body, multiple photographs are taken of the blood vessels in the eye. Fluorescein angiography is used to diagnose and document eye disease and to monitor response to therapy. It aids the physician in diagnosing retinal and vascular disease, diabetes, macular degeneration, intraocular tumors, and other conditions.

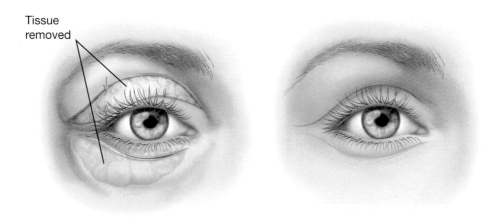

Tissue removed

Figure 6.10 Blepharoplasty is the surgical repair of drooping eyelids.

LASIK

LASIK is an acronym for **laser-assisted in situ** (SĪ-tū) **keratomileusis** (KĔR-ă-tō-mī-LŪ-sĭs), a type of refractive surgery performed to correct myopia, hyperopia, or astigmatism (Figure 6.11). Other common names for LASIK include *laser eye surgery* and *laser vision correction*. The procedure changes the shape of the cornea so that light rays entering the eye focus more precisely on the retina rather than at some point before or beyond the retina. LASIK eliminates or reduces the need for eyeglasses or contact lenses.

Tonometry

Tonometry (tō-NŎM-ĕ-trē) is a test for measuring pressure within the eyes. It is used to screen for glaucoma. There are several tonometric methods of glaucoma testing. In one method, the surface of the eye is numbed with eyedrops to prevent discomfort. Then an orange or yellow fluorescein dye is applied to the eye with drops or a special strip of paper. A low-power microscope called a *slit lamp* is moved toward the

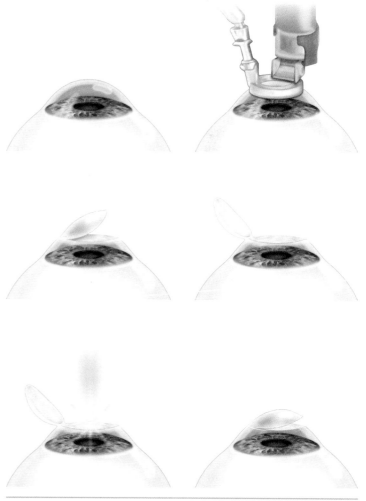

Figure 6.11 Laser-assisted in situ keratomileusis, more commonly known as LASIK surgery.

eye until it makes very light contact with the cornea, where it records a pressure reading. Another form of tonometric testing is a noncontact method that uses a puff of air to record eye pressure. A tiny device barely touches the outside of the eye and instantly records eye pressure by analyzing how the light reflections change as the air strikes the eye.

The Ear

In this section, you will learn about some common diagnostic technologies and treatment methods related to the special sensory organ of hearing and balance.

Audiometry

An **audiometry** exam is a hearing test that measures a person's ability to hear different sounds, pitches, and frequencies (Figure 6.12). Sounds vary based on their *intensity* (loudness) and *tone* (the speed of sound-wave vibrations). Hearing occurs when sound waves stimulate the nerves of the inner ear and then travel along neural pathways to the brain, where they are interpreted.

During an audiometry test, the patient wears headphones that cover both ears to eliminate outside noise. The headphones are connected to an **audiometer** (AW-dē-ŎM-ĕ-ter) that produces a series of tones at different frequencies (high or low pitches) and varying intensities (loud or soft). The patient presses a button or raises a hand to indicate when a tone is heard. Audiometry measures the ability of the patient to discriminate between different sound intensities,

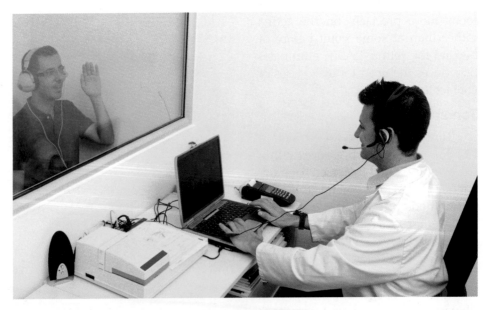

Maica/istockphoto.com

Figure 6.12 Audiometry

recognize different pitches, and distinguish speech from background noise. The test evaluates hearing loss and aids the physician in determining whether a patient needs a hearing aid.

Myringotomy

A **myringotomy** (mĭr-ĭng-GŎT-ō-mē), also called a **tympanostomy** (TĬM-păn-ŎS-tō-mē), is a surgical procedure in which a small incision is made in the *tympanic membrane* (eardrum) to relieve pressure and inflammation caused by fluid accumulation in the middle ear (Figure 6.13). Tympanostomy tubes, small tubes that are open at both ends, are inserted into the surgically created opening. The procedure allows drainage of fluid or pus (*effusion*) and provides ventilation to the middle ear in patients suffering from otitis media. The tubes are left in place until they fall out by themselves or are removed by a physician.

Myringoplasty

Myringoplasty (mĭr-ĬNG-gō-plăst-ē), also known as **tympanoplasty** (TĬM-păn-ō-PLĂS-tē), is the surgical repair of a perforated tympanic membrane (hole in the eardrum). A perforated eardrum is usually caused by an infection in the middle ear that burst through the eardrum, but it may also result from trauma. A perforated tympanic membrane may lead to repeated ear infections and hearing loss. Surgery can prevent recurring ear infection and sometimes improve hearing.

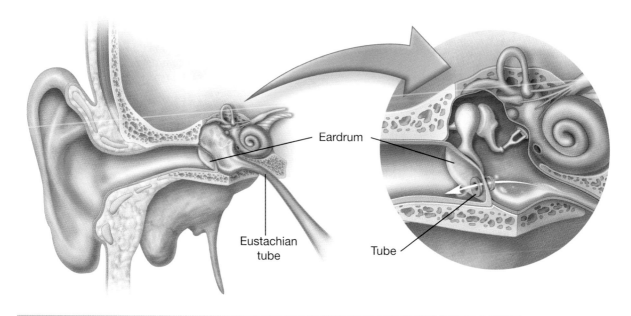

Eardrum

Eustachian tube

Tube

Figure 6.13 Myringotomy

Multiple Choice: Diseases and Disorders

Directions: Write the letter of the disease or disorder that matches each numbered definition below.

B 1. nearsightedness
   a. tinnitus   c. hyperopia
   b. myopia   d. vertigo

B 2. bacterial or viral infection of the middle ear
   a. presbycusis
   b. otitis media
   c. presbyopia
   d. Ménière's disease

A 3. ringing in the ears
   a. tinnitus   c. hyperopia
   b. myopia   d. vertigo

D 4. complication of diabetes that affects the eyes
   a. cataract
   b. glaucoma
   c. astigmatism
   d. diabetic retinopathy

D 5. chronic inner ear disorder that affects balance and hearing
   a. presbycusis
   b. otitis media
   c. presbyopia
   d. Ménière's disease

D 6. dizziness or sensation of spinning
   a. tinnitus   c. hyperopia
   b. myopia   d. vertigo

A 7. ear pain due to inflammation and buildup of fluid in the middle ear
   a. otalgia
   b. otitis media
   c. presbyopia
   d. Ménière's disease

C 8. farsightedness
   a. tinnitus   c. hyperopia
   b. myopia   d. vertigo

B 9. a group of eye conditions that cause optic nerve damage, which may lead to loss of vision
   a. cataract
   b. glaucoma
   c. astigmatism
   d. diabetic retinopathy

A 10. gradual loss of hearing that occurs as people age
   a. presbycusis
   b. otitis media
   c. presbyopia
   d. Ménière's disease

A 11. clouding of the lens of the eye
   a. cataract
   b. glaucoma
   c. astigmatism
   d. diabetic retinopathy

C 12. condition in which the lens of the eye naturally loses its elasticity or its ability to change its shape, making it difficult to see objects up close
   a. presbycusis
   b. otitis media
   c. presbyopia
   d. Ménière's disease

C 13. a common condition that causes blurred vision due to an irregularly shaped cornea or curvature of the lens
   a. cataract
   b. glaucoma
   c. astigmatism
   d. diabetic retinopathy

SCORECARD: How Did You Do?

Number correct (_____), divided by 13 (_____), multiplied by 100 equals _____ (your score)

Multiple Choice: Procedures and Treatments

Directions: Write the letter of the diagnostic procedure or therapeutic treatment that matches each numbered definition below.

B   1. laser eye surgery
  a. blepharoplasty
  b. LASIK
  c. myringotomy
  d. myringoplasty

A   2. surgical repair of drooping eyelids
  a. blepharoplasty
  b. LASIK
  c. myringotomy
  d. myringoplasty

C   3. surgical procedure in which a small incision is made in the tympanic membrane to relieve pressure and inflammation caused by accumulation of fluid in the middle ear
  a. blepharoplasty
  b. LASIK
  c. myringotomy
  d. myringoplasty

B   4. glaucoma screening test that measures pressure within the eyes
  a. audiometry
  b. tonometry
  c. visual acuity testing
  d. fluorescein angiography

A   5. hearing test that measures a person's ability to hear different sounds, pitches, and frequencies
  a. audiometry
  b. tonometry
  c. visual acuity testing
  d. fluorescein angiography

D   6. surgical repair of a perforated tympanic membrane
  a. blepharoplasty
  b. LASIK
  c. myringotomy
  d. myringoplasty

C   7. a routine part of an eye exam to detect vision problems
  a. audiometry
  b. tonometry
  c. visual acuity testing
  d. fluorescein angiography

D   8. photographic technique for imaging the retina
  a. audiometry
  b. tonometry
  c. visual acuity testing
  d. fluorescein angiography

SCORECARD: How Did You Do?

Number correct (_____), divided by 8 (_____), multiplied by 100 equals _____ (your score)

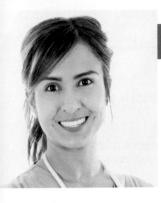

Analyzing the Intern Experience

In the Intern Experience described at the beginning of this chapter, we met Debra, an intern with University Eye and Ear Specialists. Debra met Mrs. Rodriguez and her four-year-old son, Juan, when the young boy was brought to the doctor's office because of severe otalgia (ear pain).

A physician examined Juan and obtained his personal and family health history from Mrs. Rodriguez. The doctor then made a medical diagnosis and provided Juan's mother with a treatment plan. Later, the physician made a dictated recording of the patient's health information, which was subsequently transcribed into a chart note.

We will now learn more about Juan's condition from a clinical perspective, interpreting the medical terms in his chart note as we analyze the scenario presented in the Intern Experience.

Audio Activity: Juan Rodriguez's Chart Note

Directions: At the companion website, listen and read along as the physician dictates Juan Rodriguez's chart note, shown below. Then do the exercise that appears after the chart note.

CHART NOTE

Patient Name: Rodriguez, Juan
ID Number: JR4239
Examination Date: February 6, 20xx

SUBJECTIVE
This 4-year-old male patient was brought in by his mother, who states he had a cold last week. He woke up this morning screaming, felt hot, and was tugging on his left ear. This is the third episode this year. Mother concerned with potential hearing loss.

OBJECTIVE
Temperature is 102.5° F and pulse is 100. Left **tympanic membrane** is dull, red, and bulging. Eyes are clear. Nose and throat clear. Neck is supple without **adenopathy** (disease of gland tissue). Lungs are clear.

ASSESSMENT
Left acute **otitis media**.

PLAN
Augmentin® (penicillin) 250 mg t.i.d. (three times a day) x 10 days. Recheck at end of treatment. Due to her concern with a hearing loss, I discussed a **tympanometry** evaluation and/or referral to an **otorhinolaryngologist (ENT)**, an ear, nose, and throat specialist.

Interpret Juan Rodriguez's Chart Note

Directions: After listening to the dictated recording and reading the chart note on Juan Rodriguez, provide the medical term that matches each definition below.

Example: discharge from the ear   *Answer*: otorrhea

1. specialist in the study of the ears, nose, and throat   otorhinolaryngologist (ENT)

2. pertaining to the eardrum   tympanic

3. measurement of the eardrum   tympanometry

4. bacterial or viral infection of the middle ear   otitis media

---

SCORECARD: How Did You Do?

Number correct (_____), divided by 4 (_____), multiplied by 100 equals _____ (your score)

Working with Medical Records

In this activity, you will interpret the medical records (chart notes) of patients with health conditions related to the special senses system. These examples illustrate typical medical records prepared in a real-world healthcare environment. To interpret these chart notes, you will apply your knowledge of word elements (prefixes, combining forms, and suffixes), diseases and disorders, and procedures and treatments related to the special sensory organs.

Audio Activity: Maria Jacobowitz's Chart Note

Directions: At the companion website, listen and read along as the physician dictates the following chart note on Maria Jacobowitz. Then do the exercise that appears after the chart note.

CHART NOTE

Patient Name: Jacobowitz, Maria
ID Number: MJ3321
Examination Date: August 12, 20xx

SUBJECTIVE
This 32-year-old female was struck in the left eye by the slats of a mini-blind, lacerating (scratching or tearing) the **sclera**. Mild pain was noted but no immediate visual problems, no **photophobia** (extreme sensitivity to light), and no blurred vision.

OBJECTIVE
There appears to be an abrasion of the left sclera with surrounding **subconjunctival** (below the membrane that lines the eyelids) hematoma. Pupils are equal, regular, and reactive to light. There does not appear to be any involvement of the **cornea**. Fluorescein stain shows some mild uptake over the injury site.

ASSESSEMENT
Scleral abrasion, left eye.

PLAN
Patient should apply Garamycin® **ophthalmic** solution (antibiotic medication), 1–2 drops to left eye every 4 hours for 3 days. Recheck if problem continues or symptoms worsen.

Assessment

Interpret Maria Jacobowitz's Chart Note

Directions: After listening to the dictated recording and reading the chart note on Maria Jacobowitz, provide the medical term that matches each definition below.

Example: inflammation of the retina   *Answer:* retinitis

1. clear, outer layer of the eye that covers the iris and pupil, and admits light

   cornea

2. extreme sensitivity to light

   photophobia

3. below the membrane that lines the eyelids

   subconjunctival

4. white, outer protective layer of the eye

   sclera

5. pertaining to the eye

   ophthalmic

SCORECARD: How Did You Do?

Number correct (_____), divided by 5 (_____), multiplied by 100 equals _____ (your score)

Chapter Review

Word Elements Summary

Prefixes

Prefix	Meaning
an-	not; without
extra-	outside
hemi-	half
intra-	inside; within
para-	near; beside
peri-	around

Combining Forms

Root Word/Combining Vowel	Meaning
audi/o	hearing
blephar/o	eyelid
ir/o	iris
irid/o	iris
kerat/o	cornea
myc/o	fungus
myring/o	tympanic membrane; eardrum
ocul/o	eye
ophthalm/o	eye
opt/o	eye; vision
optic/o	eye; vision
ot/o	ear
pleg/o	paralysis
presby/o	old age
retin/o	retina
scler/o	sclera (white of the eye)
tympan/o	tympanic membrane; eardrum

Suffixes

Suffix	Meaning
-al	pertaining to
-algia	pain
-ar	pertaining to
-ectomy	surgical removal; excision
-gram	record; image
-ia	condition
-ic	pertaining to
-itis	inflammation
-logist	specialist in the study of
-logy	study of
-meter	instrument used to measure
-metry	measurement
-opia	vision
-osis	abnormal condition
-pexy	surgical fixation
-plasty	surgical repair
-ptosis	drooping; downward displacement
-rrhea	discharge; flow
-rrhexis	rupture
-scope	instrument used to observe
-scopy	process of observing
-spasm	involuntary muscle contraction
-stomy	new opening
-tomy	incision; cut into

More Practice: Activities and Games

The activities on the following pages will help you reinforce your skills and check your mastery of the medical terminology that you learned in this chapter. Visit the companion website for More Practice games and activities.

Break It Down

Directions: Dissect each medical term below into its word elements by placing a slash between each word part (prefix, root word, combining vowel, and suffix). Then define each term.

Example:
Medical Term: blepharoptosis
Dissection: blephar/o/ptosis
Definition: drooping of the eyelid

Medical Term	Dissection

1. hemiplegia   h e m i/p l e g/i a

Definition: condition of half paralysis
_____

2. intraocular   i n t r a/o c u l/a r

Definition: pertaining to within the eye
_____

3. intraretinal   i n t r a/r e t i n/a l

Definition: pertaining to within the retina
_____

4. periophthalmic   p e r i/o p h t h a l m/i c

Definition: pertaining to the area around the eye
_____

5. periotic   p e r i/o t/i c

Definition: pertaining to the area around the ear
_____

6. blepharal   b l e p h a r/a l

Definition: pertaining to the eyelid
_____

Medical Term	Dissection
7. blepharectomy	b l e p h a r / e c t o m y

Definition: surgical removal of the eyelid

| 8. iridorrhexis | i r i d / o / r r h e x i s |

Definition: rupture of the iris

| 9. iridotomy | i r i d / o / t o m y |

Definition: incision to the iris

| 10. keratitis | k e r a t / i t i s |

Definition: inflammation of the cornea

Spelling

Directions: Each medical term listed below is misspelled. Rewrite each term with the correct spelling.

1. otomychosis — otomycosis
2. iridiplexy — iridopexy
3. presbycosis — presbycusis
4. miryngitis — myringitis
5. occular — ocular
6. otagia — otalgia
7. otorhea — otorrhea
8. blepharplegea — blepharoplegia
9. perocular — periocular
10. ophtaloscope — ophthalmoscope
11. sclarotomy — sclerotomy
12. optomology — ophthalmology

Audio Activity: Phuong Tao's Chart Note

Directions: At the companion website, listen and read along as the physician dictates the following chart note on Phuong Tao. Then do the exercise that appears after the chart note.

CHART NOTE

Patient Name: Tao, Phuong
ID Number: TP9231
Examination Date: January 7, 20xx

SUBJECTIVE
This 58-year-old female patient presents with declining vision. She states that she failed her driver's license eye exam two weeks ago. She wants a "solution" because she drives herself and her mother to the grocery store and to doctor appointments on a monthly basis.

OBJECTIVE
Vision is **20/50** in the right eye and 20/70 in the left eye.

ASSESSMENT
Senile cataracts.

PLAN
Slight improvement in left eye can be obtained by increasing the prescription. Copy of prescription for left eye **lens** change was given to the patient. Driver's license form completed. Patient instructed to drive only during the daytime. I informed the patient that **cataract** surgery is warranted in the near future. I discussed the need for the procedure and its risks and benefits. She was given a pamphlet explaining the procedure and will follow up.

Assessment

Interpret Phuong Tao's Chart Note

Directions: After listening to the dictated recording and reading the chart note on Phuong Tao, provide the medical term that matches each definition below.

Example: pertaining to near the eye   *Answer*: paraocular

1. clouding of the lens of the eye

   cataract

2. fractional number that represents visual acuity (In this case, the line read by the patient read from a distance of 20 feet can be read by a person with normal vision from a distance of 50 feet.)

   20/50

3. structure of the eye that focuses light onto the retina

   lens

Chapter 7

The Nervous System

neur / o / logy: the study of the nervous system

Chapter Organization

- Intern Experience
- Overview of Nervous System Anatomy and Physiology
- Word Elements
- Breaking Down and Building Nervous System Terms
- Diseases and Disorders
- Procedures and Treatments
- Analyzing the Intern Experience
- Working with Medical Records
- Chapter Review

Chapter Objectives

After completing this chapter, you will be able to

1. label an anatomical diagram of the nervous system;
2. dissect and define common medical terminology related to the nervous system;
3. build terms used to describe nervous system diseases and disorders, diagnostic procedures, and therapeutic treatments;
4. pronounce and spell common medical terminology related to the nervous system;
5. understand that the processes of building and dissecting a medical term based on its prefix, word root, and suffix enable you to analyze an extremely large number of medical terms beyond those presented in this chapter;
6. interpret the meaning of abbreviations associated with the nervous system; and
7. interpret medical records containing terminology and abbreviations related to the nervous system.

You will see this icon at various points throughout this chapter. The icon indicates that you will find interactive activities and games on the Medical Terminology Companion Website. These activities and games will help you learn, practice, and expand your medical terminology knowledge and skills. Some of these activities are also available on the Medical Terminology Mobile Website.

Companion Website
www.g-wlearning.com/healthsciences

Mobile Site
www.m.g-wlearning.com/5800

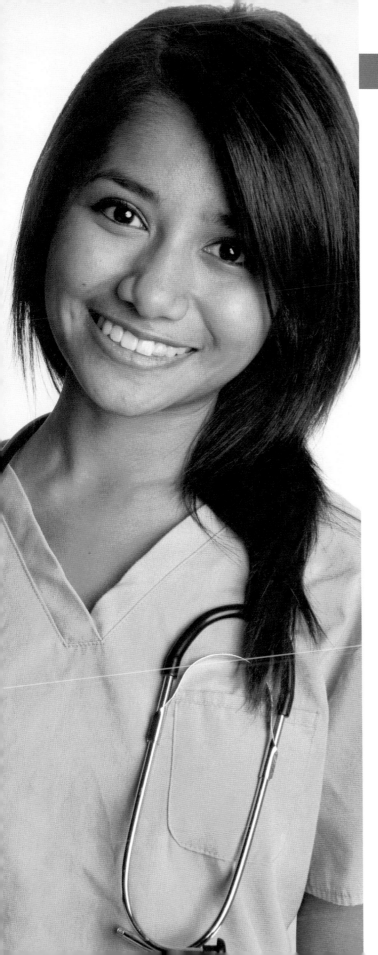

Intern Experience

Today is Nancy Chang's second day as an intern with Egan Immediate Care Center. Nancy has been assigned to "shadow" Beth, a medical assistant who works with Dr. Gangliola. Nancy and Beth escort their first patient, Steven Rutter, to the examination room. Mr. Rutter, 84 years of age, lives with his daughter, who brought him to the immediate care center. Mr. Rutter is agitated, angry, and frightened. His daughter explains that he left a pot of soup cooking on the stove while he went to get the mail, and he "almost burned down the house." Mr. Rutter found himself wandering along the street and did not know how he got there.

Steven Rutter is suffering from a disorder that has affected his nervous system, a complex network of nerve fibers and organs that carry messages to and from the brain, coordinating voluntary and involuntary muscular action, thought, sensation, and emotion. To help you understand what is happening to Mr. Rutter, this chapter will present word elements (combining forms, prefixes, and suffixes) that make up medical terms related to the nervous system.

By now, you know that many of the same medical word elements appear in terms used to describe different body systems. This systematic use of combining forms, prefixes, and suffixes helps make the study of medical terminology logical, consistent, and predictable.

We will begin our study of the nervous system with a brief overview of its anatomy and physiology. Later in the chapter, you will learn about some common pathological conditions of the nervous system, tests and procedures used to diagnose these conditions, and common methods for treating them.

Overview of Nervous System Anatomy and Physiology

The **nervous system** consists of the brain, spinal cord, and nerves (Figure 7.1). As the body's "command" center, the nervous system sends, receives, and interprets messages both from the body (internal stimuli) and from the environment (external stimuli).

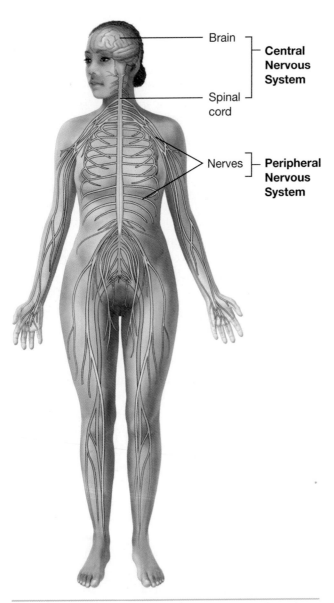

The nervous system is divided into two branches: the **central nervous system (CNS)**, which consists of the brain and spinal cord, and the **peripheral nervous system (PNS)**, which is made up of all nerve tissue outside the brain and spinal cord. The peripheral nervous system transmits sensory and motor information to and from the central nervous system. The central nervous system receives, processes, and interprets this information.

Major Functions and Structures of the Nervous System

The primary functions of the nervous system include

- coordinating the body's responses to internal and external stimuli; and

- regulating body systems to maintain *homeostasis*, a condition of stable internal balance that allows the body to function normally. To achieve homeostasis, your body is constantly working to keep physiological processes such as heart rate, blood pressure, body temperature, glucose levels, and hormonal activity within normal limits.

The human brain is a complex, multifaceted organ, composed of multiple regions and subregions with interrelated functions. For the purposes of this overview, we will discuss four major parts of the brain: the cerebrum, cerebellum, brain stem, and diencephalon (Figure 7.2 on the next page).

- The **cerebrum** is the largest part of the brain, located in the anterior (upper) part of the skull. It controls voluntary

Figure 7.1 The nervous system is divided into two branches: the central nervous system, consisting of the brain and spinal cord, and the peripheral nervous system, which includes all nerve tissue outside the brain and spinal cord.

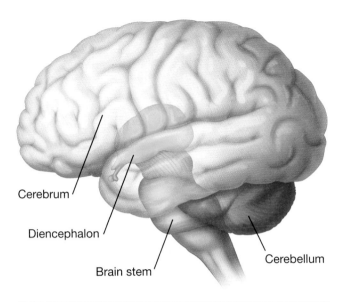

Cerebrum

Diencephalon

Brain stem

Cerebellum

Figure 7.2 Four major parts of the brain

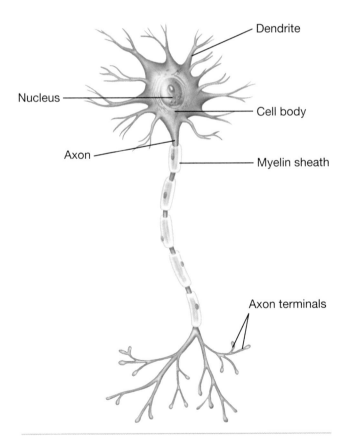

Dendrite

Nucleus

Cell body

Axon

Myelin sheath

Axon terminals

Figure 7.3 Simplified anatomy of a neuron, the basic functional cell of the nervous system

movement and is the "seat" of higher-level mental processes, such as thinking, speaking, imagining, remembering, and planning.

- The **cerebellum** (Latin for "little brain") is located posterior to the cerebrum, behind the brain stem. It coordinates voluntary muscle activity, including fine-motor movement and equilibrium (balance).

- The **brain stem**, situated in the most inferior part of the brain, connects the brain to the spinal cord. It is composed of the *midbrain, pons,* and *medulla oblongata.* The brain stem controls life-sustaining cardiovascular and respiratory activities, such as heart rate, blood pressure, and breathing. It also relays sensory and motor information to and from the cerebellum.

- The **diencephalon** is located superior and anterior to the midbrain. It serves as a "relay station" by directing nerve impulses to and from the cerebrum.

The diencephalon contains three glands: the thalamus, hypothalamus, and pineal gland. The *thalamus* routes sensory input to the correct areas of the brain. The *hypothalamus* controls involuntary homeostatic functions such as heart rate, blood pressure, temperature, and hormone production as well as the senses of sight, hearing, smell, taste, and touch. The *pineal gland* produces the hormone melatonin, which regulates sleep.

The brain and spinal cord are protected by the *cranium, vertebral column,* and three membranous layers collectively called the *meninges.*

Neurons are the basic functional cells of the nervous system (Figure 7.3). They conduct electrical impulses that carry critical information between the CNS and the body. Neurons do not touch each other; instead, they have a gap between them called a *synaptic cleft* (Figure 7.4). Chemical messengers called **neurotransmitters** carry electrical impulses across this gap.

Neurology is the study of the nervous system. A **neurologist** is a physician who specializes in the study and treatment of nervous system diseases and disorders. Neurologists may also treat patients with muscular conditions caused by a nervous system disorder.

Anatomy and Physiology Vocabulary

Now that you have been introduced to the basic structure and functions of the nervous system, we will explore in more detail the key terms presented in the introduction.

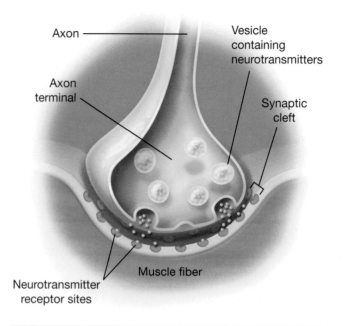

Figure 7.4 Neurotransmitters transport electrical impulses across the synaptic cleft between neurons.

Key Term	Definition
brain stem	structure that connects the brain to the spinal cord; relays sensory and motor information to and from the cerebellum; also controls life-sustaining, involuntary functions such as heart rate, blood pressure, and breathing
central nervous system (CNS)	the part of the nervous system consisting of the brain and spinal cord
cerebellum	the part of the brain that coordinates voluntary muscle activity and equilibrium (balance)
cerebrum	the largest part of the brain; controls higher-level mental processes and voluntary movement
diencephalon	"relay station" of the brain, which directs nerve impulses to and from the cerebrum and also controls involuntary homeostatic activity
nervous system	the system of the body that transmits nerve impulses between parts of the body and regulates the body's responses to internal and external stimuli
neurologist	physician who specializes in the study and treatment of nervous system diseases and disorders
neurology	the study of the nervous system
neuron	the basic functional cell of the nervous system; responsible for sending and receiving nerve impulses between parts of the body and the brain
peripheral nervous system (PNS)	the part of the nervous system made up of all nerve tissue outside the brain and spinal cord

E-Flash Card Activity: Anatomy and Physiology Vocabulary

Directions: After you have reviewed the anatomy and physiology vocabulary related to the nervous system, practice with the e-flash cards until you are comfortable with the spelling and definition of each term.

Identifying Major Structures of the Nervous System

Directions: Label the diagram of the nervous system.

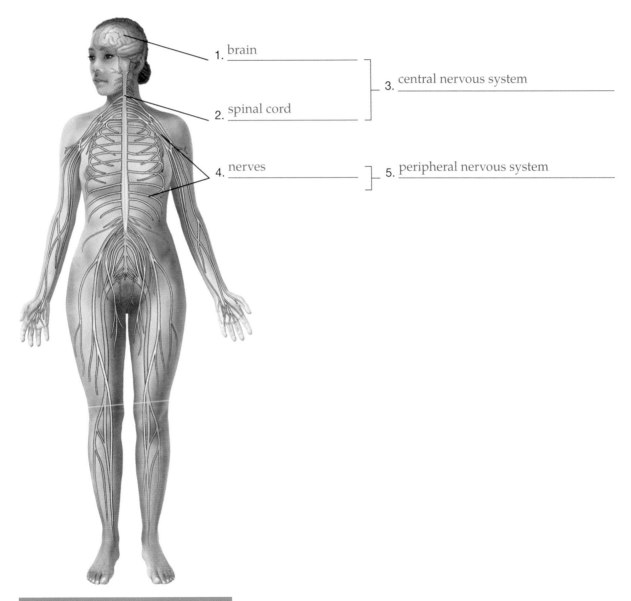

1. brain _____

2. spinal cord _____

3. central nervous system _____

4. nerves _____

5. peripheral nervous system _____

SCORECARD: How Did You Do?

Number correct (_____), divided by 5 (_____), multiplied by 100 equals _____ (your score)

Identifying Major Parts of the Brain

Directions: Label the four major parts of the brain.

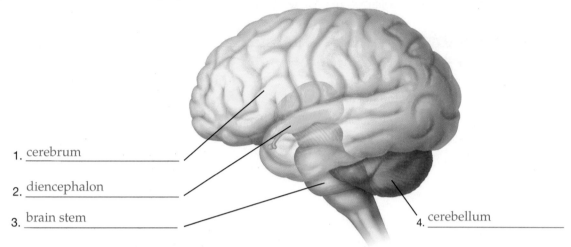

1. cerebrum

2. diencephalon

3. brain stem

4. cerebellum

Matching Anatomy and Physiology Vocabulary

Directions: Match the vocabulary term in Column A with its meaning in Column B.

Column A

___J___ 1. nervous system

___I___ 2. neurology

___E___ 3. diencephalon

___A___ 4. brain stem

___C___ 5. cerebellum

___H___ 6. cerebrum

___G___ 7. neuron

___D___ 8. neurologist

___F___ 9. central nervous system

___B___ 10. peripheral nervous system

Column B

A. connects the brain and spinal cord

B. contains all nerve tissue outside the brain and spinal cord

C. controls muscle activity and balance

D. physician who specializes in the study and treatment of the nervous system

E. directs nerve impulses to and from the cerebrum

F. part of the nervous system made up of the brain and spinal cord

G. basic functional cell of the nervous system

H. largest part of the brain; controls mental processes and voluntary movement

I. the study of the nervous system

J. transmits nerve impulses and controls responses to stimuli

Word Elements

In this section you will learn word elements—prefixes, combining forms, and suffixes—that are common to the study of the nervous system. By learning these word elements and understanding how they are combined to build medical terms, you will be able to analyze Mr. Rutter's health condition (described in the Intern Experience at the beginning of this chapter) and identify a large number of terms associated with the nervous system.

E-Flash Card Activity: Word Elements

Directions: Review the word elements in the tables that follow. Then, practice with the e-flash cards until you are able to quickly recognize the different word parts (prefixes, combining forms, and suffixes) and their meanings. The e-flash cards are grouped together by prefixes, combining forms, and suffixes, followed by a cumulative review of all the word elements that you learned in this chapter.

Prefixes

Let's start our study of word elements by looking at the prefixes listed in the table below. As you know by now, these prefixes appear not only in medical terms related to the nervous system but also in many terms used to describe other body systems.

Prefix	Meaning
a-	not; without
an-	not; without
dys-	painful; difficult
hemi-	half
hyper-	above; above normal
poly-	many; much
quadri-	four

Combining Forms

Listed below are combining forms that appear in medical terms used to describe the anatomy and physiology of the nervous system, as well as pathological conditions, diagnostic procedures, and therapeutic treatments related to this body system. Some of these combining forms also appear in medical terms related to other body systems.

Root Word/Combining Vowel	Meaning
angi/o	blood vessel
cephal/o	head
cerebr/o	cerebrum
cerebell/o	cerebellum

(Continued)

Root Word/Combining Vowel	Meaning
cran/o, crani/o	skull; cranium
encephal/o	brain
hydr/o	water
mening/o, meningi/o	meninges (membranes covering the brain and spinal cord)
myel/o	spinal cord
neur/o	nerve
path/o	disease
pleg/o	paralysis
psych/o	mind
radicul/o	nerve root
spin/o	spine; backbone
vascul/o	blood vessel

Suffixes

Listed below are suffixes that appear in medical terms used to describe the nervous system. You are already familiar with these suffixes, which were introduced in previous chapters.

Suffix	Meaning
-al	pertaining to
-algia	pain
-ar	pertaining to
-ary	pertaining to
-asthenia	weakness
-cele	hernia; swelling; protrusion
-eal	pertaining to
-esthesia	sensation; feeling
-gram	record; image
-graphy	process of recording an image
-ia	condition
-ic	pertaining to
-ical	pertaining to
-itis	inflammation
-logist	specialist in the study and treatment of
-logy	study of
-malacia	softening
-metry	process of measuring

(Continued)

Suffix	Meaning
-oma	tumor; mass
-osis	abnormal condition
-pathy	disease
-phasia	speech
-plasty	surgical repair
-rrhaphy	suture
-sclerosis	hardening
-tomy	incision; cut into
-us	structure; thing

Matching Prefixes, Combining Forms, and Suffixes

Directions: In each exercise below, match the word element in Column A with its meaning in Column B. Some meanings may be used more than once.

Prefixes

Column A

_C_ 1. poly-

_F_ 2. hemi-

_B_ 3. quadri-

_A_ 4. a-

_E_ 5. dys-

_A_ 6. an-

_D_ 7. hyper-

Column B

A. not; without

B. four

C. many; much

D. above; above normal

E. painful; difficult

F. half

Combining Forms

Column A

_F_ 1. neur/o

_B_ 2. encephal/o

_D_ 3. radicul/o

_K_ 4. cerebr/o

_L_ 5. myel/o

_I_ 6. angi/o

_C_ 7. mening/o, meningi/o

_G_ 8. cephal/o

Column B

A. water

B. brain

C. meninges (membranes covering the brain and spinal cord)

D. nerve root

E. spine; backbone

F. nerve

G. head

H. cerebellum

N	9. psych/o	I. blood vessel
H	10. cerebell/o	J. disease
I	11. vascul/o	K. cerebrum
M	12. cran/o, crani/o	L. spinal cord
J	13. path/o	M. skull; cranium
A	14. hydr/o	N. mind
E	15. spin/o	O. paralysis
O	16. pleg/o	

Suffixes

Column A

R	1. -sclerosis	
A	2. -ical	
I	3. -esthesia	
H	4. -pathy	
C	5. -us	
A	6. -al	
B	7. -metry	
M	8. -rrhaphy	
A	9. -ary	
E	10. -osis	
Q	11. -tomy	
F	12. -cele	
P	13. -algia	
A	14. -ar	
G	15. -ia	
J	16. -asthenia	
A	17. -ic	
A	18. -eal	
K	19. -logy	
N	20. -graphy	
D	21. -oma	
L	22. -plasty	
O	23. -gram	

Column B

A. pertaining to

B. process of measuring

C. structure; thing

D. tumor; mass

E. abnormal condition

F. hernia; swelling; protrusion

G. condition

H. disease

I. sensation; feeling

J. weakness

K. study of

L. surgical repair

M. suture

N. process of recording an image

O. record; image

P. pain

Q. incision; cut into

R. hardening

SCORECARD: How Did You Do?

Number correct (_____), divided by 46 (_____), multiplied by 100 equals _____ (your score)

Breaking Down and Building Nervous System Terms

Now that you have mastered the prefixes, combining forms, and suffixes for medical terminology used to describe the nervous system, you have the ability to dissect and build a large number of terms related to these body systems.

Below is a list of common medical terms related to the study and treatment of the nervous system. For each term, a dissection has been provided, along with the meaning of each word element and the definition of the term as a whole.

Term	Dissection	Word Part/Meaning	Term Definition
Note: For simplification, combining vowels have been omitted from the Word Part/Meaning column.			
1. **anesthesia** (ĂN-ĕs-THĒ-zē-ă)	an/esthesia	an = not; without esthesia = sensation; feeling	without sensation or feeling
2. **aphasia** (ă-FĀ-zē-ă)	a/phasia	a = not; without phasia = speech	condition of without speech
3. **cephalalgia** (SĔF-ă-LĂL-jē-ă)	cephal/algia	cephal = head algia = pain	pain in the head (headache)
4. **cephalic** (sĕ-FĂL-ĭk)	cephal/ic	cephal = head ic = pertaining to	pertaining to the head
5. **cerebral** (SĔR-ĕ-brăl) (sĕ-RĒ-brăl)	cerebr/al	cerebr = cerebrum al = pertaining to	pertaining to the cerebrum
6. **cerebrospinal** (SĔR-ĕ-brō-SPĪ-năl)	cerebr/o/spin/al	cerebr = cerebrum spin = spine; backbone al = pertaining to	pertaining to the cerebrum and spine
7. **cerebrovascular** (SĔR-ĕ-brō-VĂS-kū-lăr)	cerebr/o/vascul/ar	cerebr = cerebrum vascul = blood vessel ar = pertaining to	pertaining to the blood vessels in the cerebrum
8. **cranial** (KRĀ-nē-ăl)	crani/al	crani = skull; cranium al = pertaining to	pertaining to the skull/cranium
9. **craniotomy** (KRĀ-nē-ŎT-ō-mē)	crani/o/tomy	crani = skull; cranium tomy = incision; cut into	incision to the skull/cranium
10. **dysphasia** (dĭs-FĀ-zē-ă)	dys/phasia	dys = painful; difficult phasia = speech	condition of difficult speech
11. **encephalitis** (ĕn-SĔF-ă-LĪ-tĭs)	encephal/itis	encephal = brain itis = inflammation	inflammation of the brain
12. **encephalomyelopathy** (ĕn-SĔF-ă-lō-MĪ-ĕ-LŎP-ă-thē)	encephal/o/myel/o/ pathy	encephal = brain myel = spinal cord pathy = disease	disease of the brain and spinal cord
Prefixes = Green Root Words = Red Suffixes = Blue			

Term	Dissection	Word Part/Meaning	Term Definition
13. **hemiplegia** (HĔM-ē-PLĒ-jē-ă)	hemi/pleg/ia	**hemi** = half **pleg** = paralysis **ia** = condition	condition of half paralysis (paralysis of two extremities)
14. **hydrocephalus** (HĪ-drō-SĔF-ă-lŭs)	hydr/o/cephal/us	**hydr** = water **cephal** = head **us** = structure; thing	pertaining to water in the head*
15. **meningeal** (mĕ-NĬN-jē-ăl)	mening/eal	**mening** = meninges **eal** = pertaining to	pertaining to the meninges
16. **meningitis** (MĔN-ĭn-JĪ-tĭs)	mening/itis	**mening** = meninges **itis** = inflammation	inflammation of the meninges
17. **myelogram** (MĪ-ĕ-lō-grăm)	myel/o/gram	**myel** = spinal cord **gram** = record; image	record or image of the spinal cord
18. **neural** (NŪ-răl)	neur/al	**neur** = nerve **al** = pertaining to	pertaining to the nerves
19. **neuralgia** (nū-RĂL-jē-ă)	neur/algia	**neur** = nerve **algia** = pain	pain in the nerve (nerve pain)
20. **neurologist** (nū-RŎL-ō-jĭst)	neur/o/logist	**neur** = nerve **logist** = specialist in the study and treatment of	specialist in the study and treatment of the nerves
21. **neurology** (nū-RŎL-ō-jē)	neur/o/logy	**neur** = nerve **logy** = study of	study of the nerves
22. **neuropathy** (nū-RŎP-ă-thē)	neur/o/pathy	**neur** = nerve **pathy** = disease	disease of the nerves
23. **psychology** (sī-KŎL-ō-jē)	psych/o/logy	**psych** = mind **logy** = study of	study of the mind
24. **quadriplegia** (KWAH-drĭ-PLĒ-jē-ă)	quadri/pleg/ia	**quadri** = four **pleg** = paralysis **ia** = condition	condition of paralysis of four (paralysis of all four extremities)
25. **radiculitis** (ră-DĬK-ū-LĪ-tĭs)	radicul/itis	**radicul** = nerve root **itis** = inflammation	inflammation of the nerve root

Prefixes = Green   Root Words = Red   Suffixes = Blue

*Hydrocephalus comes from two Greek words: *hydros*, which means "water," and *cephalus*, which means "head."
The suffix -us is a Latin noun form that means "structure or thing." In this case, -us refers to an anatomical structure.

Using the pronunciation guide in the Breaking Down and Building chart, practice saying each medical term aloud. To hear the pronunciation of each term, go to the Pronounce It activity at the G-W companion website.

Audio Activity: Pronounce It

Directions: At the companion website, listen as each medical term shown below is pronounced. Practice pronouncing the terms until you are comfortable saying them aloud.

anesthesia
(ĂN-ĕs-THĒ-zē-ă)

aphasia
(ă-FĀ-zē-ă)

cephalalgia
(SĔF-ă-LĂL-jē-ă)

cephalic
(sĕ-FĂL-ĭk)

cerebral
(SĔR-ĕ-brăl)
(sĕ-RĒ-brăl)

cerebrospinal
(SĔR-ĕ-brō-SPĪ-năl)

cerebrovascular
(SĔR-ĕ-brō-VĂS-kū-lăr)

cranial
(KRĀ-nē-ăl)

craniotomy
(KRĀ-nē-ŎT-ō-mē)

dysphasia
(dĭs-FĀ-zē-ă)

encephalitis
(ĕn-SĔF-ă-LĪ-tĭs)

encephalomyelopathy
(ĕn-SĔF-ă-lō-MĪ-ĕ-LŎP-ă-thē)

hemiplegia
(HĔM-ē-PLĒ-jē-ă)

hydrocephalus
(HĪ-drō-SĔF-ă-lŭs)

meningeal
(mĕ-NĬN-jē-ăl)

meningitis
(MĔN-ĭn-JĪ-tĭs)

myelogram
(MĪ-ĕ-lō-grăm)

neural
(NŪ-răl)

neuralgia
(nū-RĂL-jē-ă)

neurologist
(nū-RŎL-ō-jĭst)

neurology
(nū-RŎL-ō-jē)

neuropathy
(nū-RŎP-ă-thē)

psychology
(sī-KŎL-ō-jē)

quadriplegia
(KWAH-drĭ-PLĒ-jē-ă)

radiculitis
(ră-DĬK-ū-LĪ-tĭs)

Audio Activity: Spell It

Directions: Cover the medical terms in the Pronounce It activity with a sheet of paper. At the companion website, listen as the terms are read aloud. Correctly spell each term below.

1. anesthesia
2. aphasia
3. cephalalgia
4. cephalic
5. cerebral
6. cerebrospinal
7. cerebrovascular
8. cranial
9. craniotomy
10. dysphasia
11. encephalitis
12. encephalomyelopathy
13. hemiplegia
14. hydrocephalus
15. meningeal
16. meningitis
17. myelogram
18. neural
19. neuralgia
20. neurologist
21. neurology
22. neuropathy
23. psychology
24. quadriplegia
25. radiculitis

Break It Down

Directions: Dissect each medical term below into its word elements by placing a slash between each word part (prefix, root word, combining vowel, and suffix). Then define each term.

Example:

Medical Term: meningitis

Dissection: mening/itis

Definition: inflammation of the meninges

Medical Term	Dissection

1. anesthesia   a n/e s t h e s i a

Definition: without sensation or feeling

2. radiculitis   r a d i c u l/i t i s

Definition: inflammation of the nerve root

3. quadriplegia   q u a d r i/p l e g/i a

Definition: condition of paralysis of four (paralysis of all four extremities)

4. cerebrospinal   c e r e b r/o/s p i n/a l

Definition: pertaining to the cerebrum and spine

5. encephalitis   e n c e p h a l/i t i s

Definition: inflammation of the brain

6. myelogram   m y e l/o/g r a m

Definition: record or image of the spinal cord

Medical Term	Dissection
7. psychology	p s y c h/o/l o g y

Definition: study of the mind

_____

| 8. hydrocephalus | h y d r/o/c e p h a l/u s |

Definition: pertaining to water in the head

_____

| 9. cranial | c r a n i/a l |

Definition: pertaining to the skull/cranium

_____

| 10. hemiplegia | h e m i/p l e g/i a |

Definition: condition of half paralysis (paralysis of two extremities)

_____

| 11. meningeal | m e n i n g/e a l |

Definition: pertaining to the meninges

_____

| 12. dysphasia | d y s/p h a s i a |

Definition: condition of difficult speech

_____

| 13. craniotomy | c r a n i/o/t o m y |

Definition: incision to the skull/cranium

_____

| 14. neuralgia | n e u r/a l g i a |

Definition: pain in the nerve (nerve pain)

_____

SCORECARD: How Did You Do?

Number correct (_____), divided by 14 (_____), multiplied by 100 equals _____ (your score)

Build It

Directions: Build the medical term that matches each definition below by supplying the correct word elements.

P (Prefixes) = Green
RW (Root Words) = Red
S (Suffixes) = Blue
CV (Combining Vowel) = Purple

1. pertaining to the head

cephal	ic
RW	S

2. condition of without speech

a	phasia
P	S

3. study of the nerves

neur	o	logy
RW	CV	S

4. specialist in the study and treatment of the nerves

neur	o	logist
RW	CV	S

5. without sensation or feeling

an	esthesia
P	S

6. record or image of the spinal cord

myel	o	gram
RW	CV	S

7. pertaining to water in the head

hydr	o	cephal	us
P	CV	RW	S

8. pertaining to the skull/cranium

crani	al
RW	S

9. pertaining to the blood vessels in the cerebrum

cerebr	o	vascul	ar
RW	CV	RW	S

10. pertaining to the nerves

neur	al
RW	S

11. pertaining to the meninges

mening	eal
RW	S

12. condition of paralysis of four (paralysis of all four extremities)

quadri	pleg	ia
P	RW	S

13. pertaining to the cerebrum

cerebr	al
RW	S

14. pain in the head

cephal	algia
RW	S

15. incision to the skull/cranium

crani	o	tomy
RW	CV	S

16. inflammation of the meninges

mening	itis
RW	S

17. inflammation of the nerve root

radicul	itis
RW	S

18. condition of difficult speech

dys	phasia
P	S

19. condition of half paralysis (paralysis of two extremities)

hemi	pleg	ia
P	RW	S

20. disease of the nerves

neur	o	pathy
RW	CV	S

21. inflammation of the brain

encephal	itis
RW	S

22. disease of the brain and spinal cord

encephal	o	myel	o	pathy
RW	CV	RW	CV	S

SCORECARD: How Did You Do?

Number correct (_____), divided by 22 (_____), multiplied by 100 equals _____ (your score)

Diseases and Disorders

Diseases and disorders of the nervous system run the spectrum from the mild to the severe in nature and etiology (cause). In this section, we will briefly explore some common pathological conditions of this body system.

Cerebral Aneurysm

A **cerebral aneurysm** is a bulge or ballooning of an artery in the brain due to thinning and weakening of the arterial wall (Figure 7.5). Aneurysms can appear anywhere in the brain, but they are more common in arteries at the base of the brain. A cerebral aneurysm can leak or rupture, causing bleeding into the brain. A sudden, extremely severe headache is the key symptom of a ruptured aneurysm. Patients often describe this event as "the worst headache they have ever had." However, a cerebral aneurysm that is small and intact may produce no symptoms.

Cerebral Embolism

Cerebral embolism is the sudden blockage of an artery in the brain due to a thrombus or other foreign matter (Figure 7.6). A stationary blood clot is called a *thrombus*. When the thrombus breaks away from the site at which it has lodged, it becomes an *embolism*.

Emboli (plural of *embolus*) can move through the bloodstream from their original location to another part of the body, where they can obstruct arterial blood flow. An embolism can develop anywhere within the cardiovascular (circulatory) system. When an embolism obstructs a cerebral artery, it is called a **cerebral embolism**.

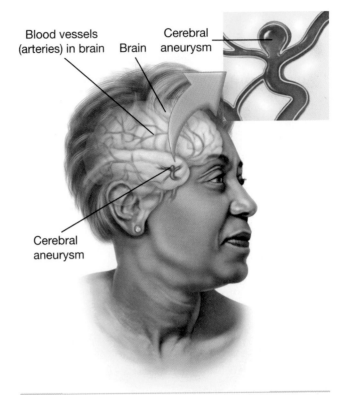

Figure 7.5 Cerebral aneurysm. Note the ballooning of the weakened artery.

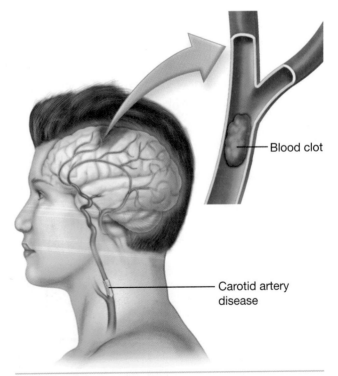

Figure 7.6 Cerebral embolism

Cerebral Palsy

Cerebral palsy (CP) is a group of neurological disorders caused by damage to the brain and nervous system during embryonic development or soon after birth. CP impairs muscle movement and is associated with intellectual disabilities, vision and hearing problems, and, in some cases, seizures. The effect of cerebral palsy on functional abilities varies greatly from one patient to the next. It is not yet known what triggers the abnormality in brain development that leads to CP.

Cerebral Vascular Attack

A **cerebral vascular attack (CVA)** is a sudden interruption in blood flow to a part of the brain (Figure 7.7). An embolism travels from another part of the body and lodges within an artery in the brain. The blocked artery deprives the brain of oxygen, damaging the surrounding brain tissue. If blood flow is cut off for longer than a few seconds, the brain cannot receive blood and oxygen. Brain cells die, causing permanent damage to brain function. A cerebral vascular attack is more commonly known as a "brain attack" or "stroke."

Concussion

A **concussion** is a *traumatic brain injury (TBI)* caused by a severe blow or jolt to the head. The force of impact causes the brain to slide back and forth inside the skull (Figure 7.8). The result is a brief or prolonged loss of consciousness that affects normal brain function.

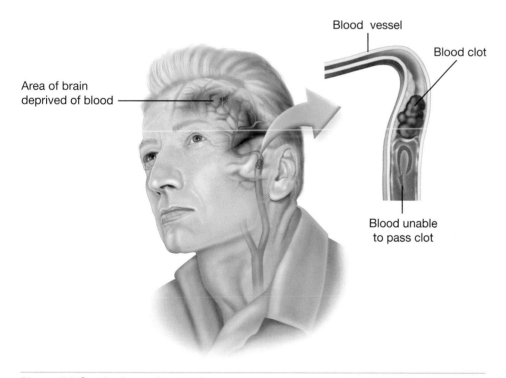

Blood vessel

Blood clot

Area of brain deprived of blood

Blood unable to pass clot

Figure 7.7 Cerebral vascular attack

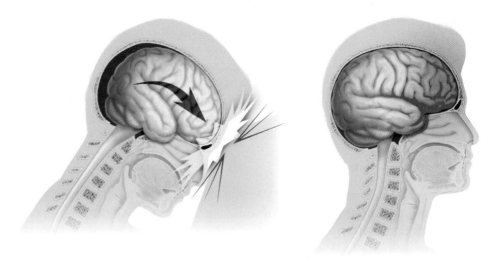

Figure 7.8 A concussion is a traumatic brain injury caused by a severe blow or jolt to the head.

Concussions are often caused by head trauma sustained during car accidents, contact sports, or falls. According to the Centers for Disease Control and Prevention (CDC), they are also a leading cause of child abuse deaths due to Shaken Baby Syndrome in the United States. The head trauma associated with Shaken Baby Syndrome is the result of violently shaking an infant by the shoulders, arms, or legs.

Because some head injuries produce no loss of consciousness, some patients who experience a concussion may not be aware of it. Aftermath of concussion may include problems with headache, concentration, memory, judgment, balance, or coordination. The person must be closely watched for signs of disorientation, sleepiness, irritability, and impaired speech or muscle coordination. The patient must get sufficient rest so that the injured brain can heal.

Dementia

Dementia is a broad term for a group of cognitive disorders caused by the slow, progressive death of cerebral neurons manifested in deteriorating mental function. It is attributed to brain trauma, substance abuse, or any of a number of neurodegenerative diseases. Common signs of dementia include impaired memory, motor activity, and language processing skills. **Alzheimer's disease** is the most common form of dementia. It is a hereditary dementia associated with certain inherited chromosomal mutations.

Encephalitis

Encephalitis is inflammation of the brain due to a bacterial or viral infection. Abrupt fever, severe headache, muscle weakness, restlessness, and lethargy are typical symptoms. Blood tests can identify the causative bacterium or virus.

Encephalitis may also be diagnosed through an electroencephalogram (EEG), a lumbar puncture to evaluate the cerebrospinal fluid (CSF) for infection, and brain imaging tests such as computerized tomography (CT) or magnetic resonance imaging (MRI). CT and MRI technologies were discussed in Chapter 4: Musculoskeletal System.

Epilepsy

Epilepsy is a disorder in which nerve cells in the brain send out abnormal signals, producing seizures. In milder cases of epilepsy, seizures may take the form of staring spells or strange sensations. More severe cases are marked by convulsions (seizures), violent muscle spasms, and loss of consciousness. Repeated seizures can result in long-term memory loss and personality changes. Prior to a seizure, some patients experience an *aura*, a strange sensation such as a tingling or buzzing sound, an unusual odor, or a flashing light, which signals the impending seizure.

The type of epileptic seizure that a patient experiences depends on the cause of the epilepsy and the part of the brain that is affected. Common causes include illness, brain injury, or abnormal brain development. In many cases, though, its cause is *idiopathic* (unknown). Electroencephalograms (EEGs) and brain scans are used to diagnose epilepsy.

Meningitis

Meningitis is inflammation of the meninges, the three-layer membrane that surrounds and protects the brain and spinal cord. It may be caused by a virus, bacterium, or other microorganism such as a fungus or parasite.

Because of the proximity of the meninges to the brain and spinal cord, this disease is often considered a medical emergency. The swelling associated with meningitis produces symptoms of high fever, stiff neck, severe headache, nausea, and vomiting. A lumbar puncture may be performed to diagnose or exclude meningitis. Treatment involves immediate administration of antibiotics, corticosteroids (inflammation-reducing steroid drugs), and, in some cases, antiviral drugs. Some forms of meningitis may be prevented by immunization.

Migraine Headache

A **migraine headache** (commonly called a **migraine**) is a recurring episode of moderate or severe throbbing pain, typically on one side of the head. The pain is accompanied by sensitivity to light and sound, as well as nausea and vomiting in some cases. Migraines can be triggered by any of a number of factors, including stress, anxiety, hunger, sleep deprivation, and, in women, hormonal changes. Before the onset of a migraine, some patients experience an aura that produces visual disturbances. This aura serves as a warning sign that a severe headache is imminent. Medications can help prevent migraines or relieve symptoms when they occur.

Parkinson's Disease

Parkinson's disease is a chronic, degenerative neurological disorder marked by muscle tremor and rigidity (Figure 7.9). Bradykinesia (slow movement) is common, along with stiff posture and gait. Patients often have speech problems and display an immobile, mask-like face that shows little or no expression.

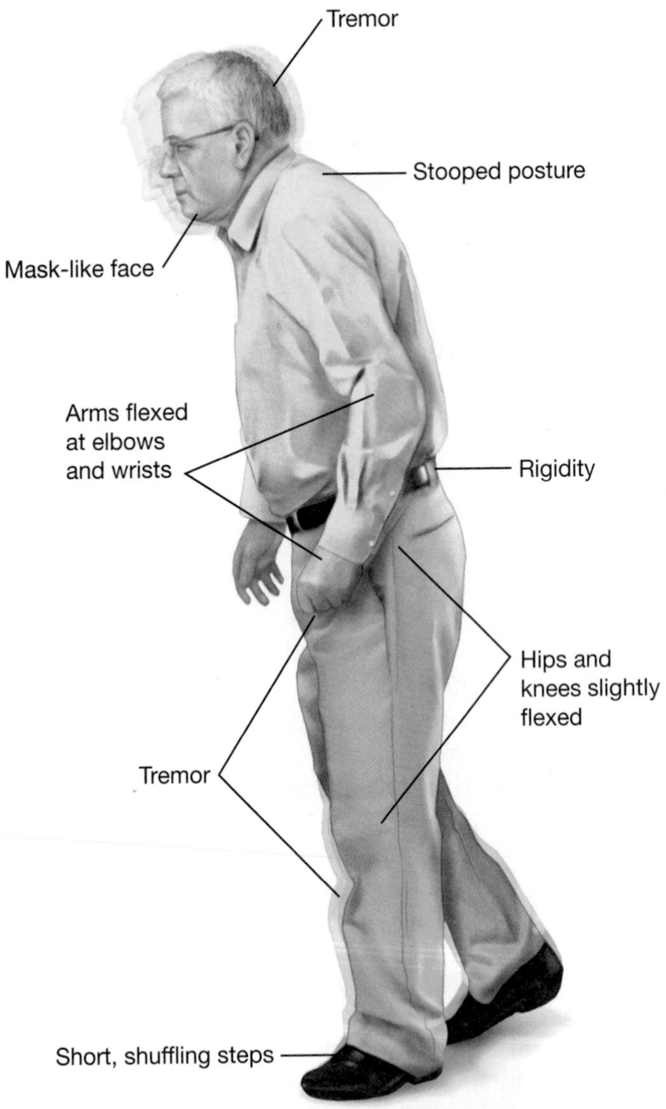

Parkinson's disease develops when neural cells in the brain fail to produce enough dopamine, a neurotransmitter involved in regulating bodily movement. While it may be genetic or environmental, the etiology (cause) of Parkinson's disease is unknown, and symptoms worsen over time.

Transient Ischemic Attack

A **transient ischemic attack (TIA)** occurs when blood flow to a section of the brain is briefly interrupted. A TIA, or "mini stroke," produces signs and symptoms similar to those of a stroke; however, it usually lasts only a few minutes and causes no permanent damage. A TIA is a warning sign that a stroke might occur and provides an opportunity for preventive measures.

Procedures and Treatments

We will now take a brief look at some diagnostic tests and procedures used to help identify disorders and diseases of the nervous system, as well as common therapeutic methods for treating some of these conditions.

Babinski Reflex

A *reflex* is a predictable, involuntary response to a stimulus. A *stimulus* is an action that produces a reaction from a muscle, nerve, or other body tissue.

The **Babinski reflex** (also called **Babinski's sign**) is a reflex that happens in infants. It is evoked during a physical examination by a healthcare specialist.

Figure 7.9 Signs and symptoms of Parkinson's disease

Labels: Tremor; Stooped posture; Mask-like face; Arms flexed at elbows and wrists; Rigidity; Hips and knees slightly flexed; Tremor; Short, shuffling steps

The doctor or other medical specialist stimulates the heel of the foot with a small object and then moves the object along the outer edge of the sole, to the base of the toes. The great (big) toe moves toward the top surface of the foot, and the other toes fan out after the sole of the foot has been firmly stroked (Figure 7.10).

The Babinski reflex is normal between infancy and two years of age. The presence of this reflex in children older than two years or in adults indicates damage to the nerve pathways that connect the brain and spinal cord. The Babinski reflex may be a sign of tumor, defect, or injury to the brain or spinal cord, multiple sclerosis, or other neurological disorder.

Cerebral Angiography

Cerebral angiography is a diagnostic procedure that uses a contrast agent ("dye") and X-rays to evaluate the vessels that supply blood to the brain. A thin, flexible catheter (tube) is inserted into the femoral artery in the groin. The physician threads the catheter past the heart into an artery of the brain. Then the contrast agent is injected into the catheter, through which it travels to selected cerebral arteries. Cerebral angiography can identify or confirm cerebral vascular abnormalities or pathologies that may indicate an aneurysm, brain tumor, or stenosis (abnormal narrowing of blood vessels).

Computerized Tomography

Computerized tomography (CT), also called *computed tomography*, is a diagnostic imaging procedure that uses X-rays and a computer to scan and display cross-sectional images of internal body structures in multiple planes. A radiopaque (RĀ-dē-ō-PĀK) contrast agent (a dye that sharpens X-ray detail) is sometimes injected into the patient to enhance anatomical imagery during the scanning process.

Because of its ability to "image" body structures in multiple planes, CT technology can detect tumors, masses, and diseases that otherwise could go undetected if they were visualized in only one plane, as is the case with radiographs. A more detailed explanation of computerized tomography is presented in chapter 4.

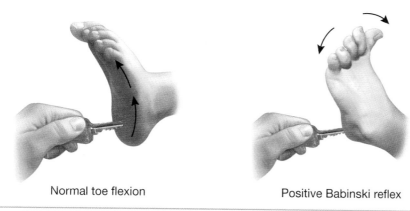

Normal toe flexion

Positive Babinski reflex

Figure 7.10 In a positive Babinski reflex, the great toe moves toward the top surface of the foot, and the other toes fan out.

Electroencephalogram

An **electroencephalogram (EEG)** is a test that measures the electrical activity of the brain. A series of flat, metal disks called *electrodes* are affixed to the scalp. The electrodes are held in place with a sticky substance and are connected by wires to a recording device (Figures 7.11A and 7.11B). The device translates electrical signals from the brain into waveforms (wavy patterns), which are interpreted by a neurologist (Figure 7.11C).

The EEG test is used to confirm an epilepsy diagnosis. It is also used to diagnose sleep disorders, dementia, and other brain disorders.

Finger-to-Nose Test

The **finger-to-nose test** is a neurological test used to evaluate physical coordination. The patient is asked to close his or her eyes, extend the arms outward, and then slowly touch the nose with an index finger. Inability to do so may indicate cerebellar dysfunction.

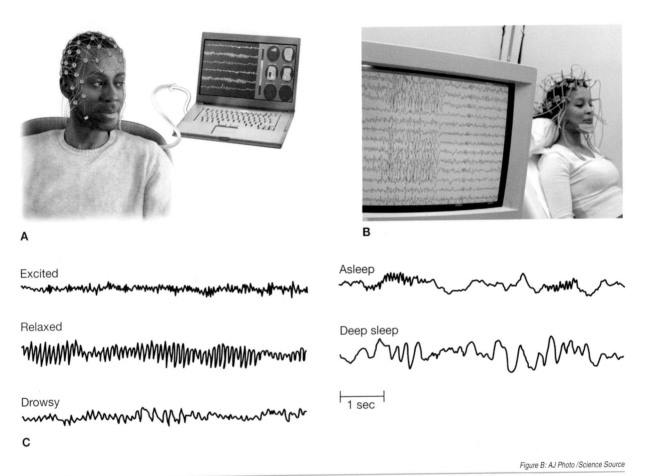

Figure B: AJ Photo /Science Source

Figure 7.11 An electroencephalogram measures the electrical activity of the brain. A—Electrodes are placed on the scalp and connected by wires to a recording device. B—The device translates electrical signals from the brain into waveforms. C—Waveforms, which signify different types of brain activity, are interpreted by a neurologist.

Kernig's Sign

Kernig's sign (also called **Kernig sign**) is a test that facilitates the diagnosis of meningitis. The maneuver is usually performed with the patient in a supine position (lying face upward) with the hips and knees flexed to 90 degrees (Figure 7.12). Inability to extend the legs beyond 135 degrees without experiencing pain, stiffness, and involuntary contraction of the hamstrings (the group of muscles in the back of the thigh) constitutes a positive test for Kernig's sign. A positive Kernig's sign indicates meningeal inflammation.

Lumbar Puncture

A **lumbar puncture (LP)**, sometimes called a *spinal tap*, is a diagnostic or therapeutic procedure that involves inserting a needle into the lumbar region (lower back) to extract cerebrospinal fluid (Figure 7.13). Cerebrospinal fluid (CSF) is the protective fluid that surrounds and cushions the brain and spinal column. The CSF obtained from a lumbar puncture is analyzed for the presence of infection, injury, or other pathological condition of the brain or spinal cord.

Magnetic Resonance Angiogram

A **magnetic resonance angiogram (MRA)** is a type of magnetic resonance imaging (MRI) scan. MRA provides critical information about the condition and function of blood vessels that cannot be obtained from X-rays, ultrasound tests, or CT scans. It can detect an aneurysm (blood-filled bulge in an artery), vascular stenosis (narrowing of a blood vessel), and other disorders and diseases of the blood vessels. (For more detailed information on MRI technology, see the Procedures and Treatments section of chapter 4.)

Romberg's Sign

Romberg's sign (also called **Romberg sign** or **Romberg test**) is a measure of *sensory ataxia*, defective muscle coordination resulting from loss of input from the senses of sight and equilibrium (balance). The patient is asked to stand erect with the eyes closed and the feet close together. If the patient sways and falls when the eyes are closed, the Romberg's sign is positive, indicating sensory ataxia.

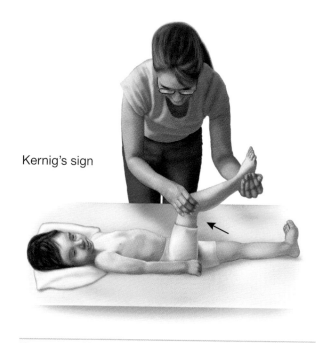

Kernig's sign

Figure 7.12 Kernig's sign helps diagnose meningitis.

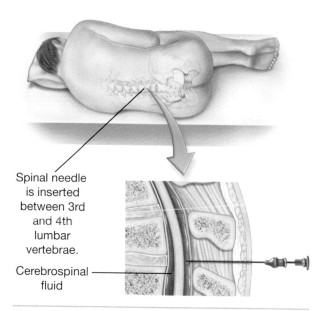

Spinal needle is inserted between 3rd and 4th lumbar vertebrae.

Cerebrospinal fluid

Figure 7.13 Cerebrospinal fluid extracted during a lumbar puncture helps detect infection, injury, or disease of the brain or spinal cord.

Multiple Choice: Diseases and Disorders

Directions: Write the letter of the disease or disorder that matches each numbered definition below.

__A__   1. a bulge or ballooning of an artery in the brain due to thinning and weakening of the arterial wall
   a. cerebral aneurysm
   b. cerebral embolism
   c. cerebral vascular attack
   d. cerebral palsy

__B__   2. the sudden blockage of an artery in the brain due to a thrombus or other foreign matter
   a. cerebral palsy
   b. cerebral embolism
   c. cerebral aneurysm
   d. cerebral vascular attack

__A__   3. a sudden interruption in blood flow to a part of the brain; caused by an embolism that lodges in an artery of the brain after traveling from another part of the body
   a. cerebral vascular attack
   b. cerebral aneurysm
   c. cerebral palsy
   d. cerebral embolism

__A__   4. a disorder in which nerve cells in the brain send out abnormal signals, producing seizures
   a. epilepsy
   b. dementia
   c. transient ischemic attack
   d. encephalitis

__D__   5. a group of neurological disorders caused by damage to the brain and nervous system during embryonic development or soon after birth; characterized in part by impaired muscle movement and intellectual disabilities
   a. cerebral vascular attack
   b. cerebral embolism
   c. cerebral aneurysm
   d. cerebral palsy

__B__   6. broad term for a group of cognitive disorders caused by the slow, progressive death of cerebral neurons and marked by deteriorating mental function
   a. epilepsy
   b. dementia
   c. transient ischemic attack
   d. encephalitis

__A__   7. inflammation of the brain due to a bacterial or viral infection
   a. encephalitis
   b. dementia
   c. transient ischemic attack
   d. epilepsy

__B__   8. a traumatic brain injury (TBI) caused by a severe blow or jolt to the head, resulting in brief or prolonged loss of consciousness
   a. migraine headache   c. epilepsy
   b. concussion   d. dementia

__A__   9. a symptom of an aneurysm is
   a. sudden, extremely severe headache
   b. repeated seizures
   c. muscle tremor
   d. mini stroke

__B__   10. a recurring headache characterized by moderate or severe pain, usually on one side of the head
   a. concussion   c. meningitis
   b. migraine headache   d. encephalitis

__D__   11. an interruption in blood flow to the brain that lasts only a few minutes and causes no permanent damage; mini stroke
   a. cerebral embolism
   b. cerebral aneurysm
   c. migraine headache
   d. transient ischemic attack

SCORECARD: How Did You Do?

Number correct (_____), divided by 11 (_____), multiplied by 100 equals _____ (your score)

Multiple Choice: Procedures and Treatments

Directions: Write the letter of the diagnostic procedure or therapeutic treatment that matches each numbered definition below.

B   1. a diagnostic or therapeutic procedure that involves inserting a needle into the lumbar region (lower back) to extract cerebrospinal fluid
a. electroencephalogram
b. lumbar puncture
c. magnetic resonance angiography
d. cerebral angiography

A   2. a test that measures the electrical activity of the brain by means of electrodes connected to a recording device that generates waveforms
a. electroencephalogram
b. magnetic resonance angiography
c. cerebral angiography
d. computerized tomography

B   3. a test that facilitates the diagnosis of meningitis
a. Babinski reflex   c. Romberg's sign
b. Kernig's sign   d. finger-to-nose test

A   4. a test in which the outer edge of the sole of the foot is firmly stroked
a. Babinski reflex   c. Romberg's sign
b. Kernig's sign   d. sole test

D   5. a neurological test used to evaluate physical coordination and test for cerebellar dysfunction
a. Babinski reflex   c. Romberg's sign
b. Kernig's sign   d. finger-to-nose test

C   6. measure of *sensory ataxia,* defective muscle coordination resulting from loss of input from the senses of sight and balance
a. Babinski reflex   c. Romberg's sign
b. Kernig's sign   d. finger-to-nose test

C   7. a form of MRI that can detect aneurysms, vascular stenosis, and other blood vessel diseases and disorders
a. electroencephalogram
b. lumbar puncture
c. magnetic resonance angiography
d. cerebral angiography

D   8. a diagnostic procedure that uses a contrast agent and X-rays to evaluate the vessels that supply blood to the brain
a. electroencephalogram
b. lumbar puncture
c. magnetic resonance angiography
d. cerebral angiography

B   9. a diagnostic procedure involving the use of X-rays and a computer to scan and display cross-sectional images of internal body structures in multiple planes
a. electroencephalogram
b. computerized tomography
c. magnetic resonance angiogram
d. lumbar puncture

SCORECARD: How Did You Do?

Number correct (_____), divided by 9 (_____), multiplied by 100 equals _____ (your score)

Identifying Abbreviations

Directions: Write the abbreviation for each medical term listed below.

Medical Term	Abbreviation
1. central nervous system	CNS
2. cerebral palsy	CP
3. cerebrospinal fluid	CSF
4. cerebral vascular attack	CVA
5. magnetic resonance imaging	MRI
6. computerized tomography	CT
7. electroencephalogram	EEG
8. lumbar puncture	LP
9. traumatic brain injury	TBI
10. magnetic resonance angiography	MRA
11. peripheral nervous system	PNS
12. transient ischemic attack	TIA

SCORECARD: How Did You Do?

Number correct (_____), divided by 12 (_____), multiplied by 100 equals _____ (your score)

Spelling

Directions: Write the correct spelling next to each misspelled medical term.

1. cerabellum	cerebellum	
2. diencepholon	diencephalon	
3. nuerologist	neurologist	
4. encephylitis	encephalitis	
5. neuralgea	neuralgia	
6. hydracephalis	hydrocephalus	

SCORECARD: How Did You Do?

Number correct (_____), divided by 6 (_____), multiplied by 100 equals _____ (your score)

Analyzing the Intern Experience

In the Intern Experience described at the beginning of this chapter, we met Nancy, an intern with the Egan Immediate Care Center. Nancy was assigned to shadow (follow and observe) Beth, medical assistant to Dr. Gangliola. Their first patient was Steven Rutter, a 84-year-old man brought to the clinic by his daughter, who explained that her father had nearly "burned down the house." He had left a pot of soup cooking on the stove while he walked outside to the mailbox. He found himself wandering along the street with no awareness of how he had gotten there. During his physical exam in the doctor's office, Mr. Rutter appeared agitated, angry, and frightened.

Dr. Gangliola examined Mr. Rutter and obtained his personal and family health history. He then made a medical diagnosis and provided Mr. Rutter and his daughter with a treatment plan. Later, Dr. Gangliola made a dictated recording of the patient's health information, which was subsequently transcribed into a chart note.

We will now learn more about Steven Rutter's condition from a clinical perspective, interpreting the medical terms in his chart note as we analyze the scenario presented in the Intern Experience.

Audio Activity: Steven Rutter's Chart Note

Directions: At the companion website, listen and read along as the physician dictates Steven Rutter's chart note, shown below. Then do the exercise that appears after the chart note.

CHART NOTE

Patient Name: Rutter, Steven
ID Number: 257RS
Examination Date: December 6, 20xx

SUBJECTIVE
Mr. Rutter is an anxious 84-year-old gentleman who appears older than his stated age. He states that he has been experiencing increasing episodes of memory loss.

OBJECTIVE
Physical exam reveals an agitated but depressed-appearing male who is underweight but in no acute distress. He denies any falls or head injuries. He has a history of **TIAs** and a **CVA** that occurred 3 years ago. Vital signs normal. **Cranial** nerves II through XII are intact in detail to visual fields and ophthalmoscopic (pertaining to an instrument used to visualize the eyes) examination. Motor and sensory exams and reflexes within normal limits.

ASSESSMENT
Patient has memory loss without objective findings relating to organic (causing a change in physical structure) **etiology**. Depression may be a key factor. Rule out **dementia**.

PLAN
I will order a **CT** scan of the brain. Pending results may necessitate a neurology consult.

Interpret Steven Rutter's Chart Note

Directions: After listening to the dictated recording and reading the chart note on Steven Rutter, provide the medical term that matches each definition below. You may encounter terms that were introduced in previous chapters.

Example: inflammation of the meninges   *Answer:* meningitis

1. sudden interruption in blood flow to a part of the brain

   CVA _____

2. cause of a disorder or disease

   etiology _____

3. diagnostic imaging procedure that uses X-rays and a computer to scan and display cross-sectional images of internal body structures in multiple planes; computerized tomography

   CT _____

4. brief interruptions in blood flow to a section of the brain; also called "mini strokes"

   TIA _____

5. pertaining to the skull or cranium

   cranial _____

6. term used to describe a group of cognitive disorders caused by the slow, progressive death of cerebral neurons and marked by deteriorating mental function

   dementia _____

SCORECARD: How Did You Do?

Number correct (_____), divided by 6 (_____), multiplied by 100 equals _____ (your score)

Working with Medical Records

In this activity, you will interpret the medical records (chart notes) of patients with nervous system disorders. These examples illustrate typical medical records prepared in a real-world healthcare environment. To interpret these chart notes, you will apply your knowledge of word elements (prefixes, combining forms, and suffixes), diseases and disorders, and procedures and treatments related to the nervous system.

Audio Activity: Ellen Wyamback's Chart Note

Directions: At the companion website, listen and read along as the physician dictates the following emergency department (ED) report on Ellen Wyamback. Then do the exercise that appears after the chart note.

Emergency Department Report

Patient Name: Wyamback, Ellen
ID Number: 138EW
Examination Date: August 25, 20xx

SUBJECTIVE
16-year-old patient presents with a history of falling off her bike. While performing "tricks," she fell into a fence. She complains of head, neck, and left knee pain. A brief loss of consciousness was observed by a friend. She is slow to answer questions and repeats questions about the accident.

OBJECTIVE
Patient presents on a rigid backboard with a **C-collar** (cervical spine brace) in place. Pupils equal and reactive to light. No blood in the ears. There is tenderness over the mid-posterior **C-spine** (cervical spine) without obvious swelling or deformity. Heart and chest exam normal. Patient moves all 4 extremities well. Mild tenderness over the left patella (kneecap) but no instability or limited **ROM** (range of motion) noted. Cranial nerves II–VII intact. C-spine X-rays and **CT** scan of head are negative.

ASSESSMENT
Mild **concussion**.

PLAN
Patient sent home with treatment instructions. She should follow up with her physician in 1–2 days or return **PRN*** (as needed) or if any change in mental status.

*The abbreviation **PRN** comes from the Latin phrase *pro re nata* (prō rā NÄ-tä), which means "as the circumstances require" (as needed).

Interpret Ellen Wyamback's Chart Note

Directions: After listening to the dictated recording and reading the chart note on Ellen Wyamback, provide the medical term that matches each definition below.

Example: pain in the head   *Answer:* cephalalgia

1. cervical spine

   C-spine

2. procedure that uses X-rays and a computer to scan and display cross-sectional images

   CT

3. neck brace worn to stabilize the cervical spine

   C-collar

4. as needed

   PRN

5. range of motion

   ROM

6. traumatic brain injury caused by a severe blow or jolt to the head

   concussion

SCORECARD: How Did You Do?

Number correct (_____), divided by 6 (_____), multiplied by 100 equals _____ (your score)

Audio Activity: Lucy Carmel's Chart Note

Directions: At the companion website, listen and read along as the physician dictates the following emergency department (ED) report on Lucy Carmel. Then do the exercise that appears after the chart note.

Emergency Department Report

Patient Name: Carmel, Lucy
ID Number: 495LC
Examination Date: February 19, 20xx

CHIEF COMPLAINT
Nausea, vomiting, and headache.

HISTORY OF PRESENT ILLNESS
This is an 18-year-old female who was seen by her **PCP** (primary care physician) early this morning. She has a 5-day history of nausea, vomiting, headache, and elevated temperature with increasing lethargy. She was evaluated and sent to the emergency department for a **lumbar puncture** to rule out **meningitis**.

ALLERGIES
None known.

PHYSICAL EXAMINATION
Physical examination reveals a well-developed, well-nourished, somewhat lethargic young female. **BP** is 110/74, pulse 94, respirations 25, and temperature 101.2. Examination of the neck revealed marked stiffness with rigidity and positive **Babinski reflex** and **Kernig's sign**. Cardiac exam is regular in rate and rhythm with no murmurs (atypical, extra sounds heard while examining heartbeat). Lungs are clear bilaterally. During the course of the exam the patient became profoundly lethargic and did not respond appropriately to pain stimuli.

LABORATORY DATA
Lumbar puncture revealed gram-negative cocci (type of bacteria). A **CBC** (complete blood count) is also consistent for a bacterial process.

IMPRESSION
Acute bacterial meningitis.

PLAN
Request **neurological** consult for probable acute bacterial meningitis.

Interpret Lucy Carmel's Chart Note

Directions: After listening to the dictated recording and reading the chart note on Lucy Carmel, provide the medical term that matches each definition below. You may encounter definitions and terms that were introduced in previous chapters.

Example: condition of difficult speech   *Answer:* dysphasia

1. test that facilitates the diagnosis of meningitis   Kernig's sign

2. complete blood count   CBC

3. pertaining to study of the nerves   neurological

4. inflammation of the meninges   meningitis

5. diagnostic or therapeutic procedure that involves inserting a needle into the lumbar region (lower back) to extract cerebrospinal fluid; also called a *spinal tap*   lumbar puncture

6. procedure that involves stimulating the heel of the foot with a small object and then moving the object along the outer edge of the sole, to the base of the toes   Babinski reflex

7. blood pressure   BP

8. primary care physician   PCP

SCORECARD: How Did You Do?

Number correct (_____), divided by 8 (_____), multiplied by 100 equals _____ (your score)

Chapter Review

Word Elements Summary

Prefixes

Prefix	Meaning
a-	not; without
an-	not; without
dys-	painful; difficult
hemi-	half
hyper-	above; above normal
poly-	many; much
quadri-	four

Combining Forms

Root Word/Combining Vowel	Meaning
angi/o	blood vessel
cephal/o	head
cerebr/o	cerebrum
cerebell/o	cerebellum
cran/o, crani/o	skull; cranium
encephal/o	brain
hydr/o	water
mening/o, meningi/o	meninges (membranes covering the brain and spinal cord)
myel/o	spinal cord
neur/o	nerve
path/o	disease
pleg/o	paralysis
psych/o	mind
radicul/o	nerve root
spin/o	spine; backbone
vascul/o	blood vessel

Suffixes

Suffix	Meaning
-al	pertaining to
-algia	pain
-ar	pertaining to
-ary	pertaining to
-asthenia	weakness
-cele	hernia; swelling; protrusion
-eal	pertaining to
-esthesia	sensation; feeling
-gram	record; image
-graphy	process of recording an image
-ia	condition
-ic	pertaining to
-ical	pertaining to
-itis	inflammation
-logist	specialist in the study and treatment of
-logy	study of
-malacia	softening
-metry	process of measuring
-oma	tumor; mass
-osis	abnormal condition
-pathy	disease
-phasia	speech
-plasty	surgical repair
-rrhaphy	suture
-sclerosis	hardening
-tomy	incision; cut into
-us	structure; thing

More Practice: Activities and Games

The activities on the following pages will help you reinforce your skills and check your mastery of the medical terminology that you learned in this chapter. Visit the companion website for More Practice games and activities.

Audio Activity: Nigel Dixon's Chart Note

Directions: At the companion website, listen and read along as the physician dictates the following chart note on Nigel Dixon. Then do the exercise that appears after the chart note.

CHART NOTE

Patient Name: Dixon, Nigel
ID Number: 602DN
Examination Date: April 7, 20xx

SUBJECTIVE
Nigel is now 5 weeks post (after) completion of radiation therapy. He is alert, cooperative, and responsive to questions. He is often tired and sleepy.

OBJECTIVE
Neurological assessment reveals pupils equal, round, and reactive to light. Normal fundoscopic examination (of the inner part of the eye). Extraocular (pertaining to outside the eye) movements still show limitations on the right. The face is symmetric, including eye and lip closure. Nigel continues to have a mild right **hemiplegia** that is unchanged from his examination 5 weeks ago. Sensory exam is normal to touch, pinprick, and position. **Cerebellar** examination is normal with a negative **Romberg test** and a good **finger-to-nose test**.

ASSESSMENT
The repeated **MRA** study indicates a diminished brain stem lesion. Sustained clinical improvement over the course of his radiation therapy treatments.

PLAN
Patient will return in 6 weeks for follow-up.

Interpret Nigel Dixon's Chart Note

Directions: After listening to the dictated recording and reading the chart note on Nigel Dixon, provide the medical term that matches each definition below. You may encounter terms that were introduced in previous chapters.

Example: inflammation   *Answer:* radiculitis

1. condition of half paralysis (paralysis of two extremities)

   hemiplegia

2. neurological test used to evaluate physical coordination

   finger-to-nose test

3. type of magnetic resonance imaging test that provides information about the condition and function of blood vessels

   MRA

4. test used to measure sensory ataxia

   Romberg test

5. pertaining to the study of the nerves

   neurological

6. pertaining to the cerebellum

   cerebellar

True or False

Directions: Indicate whether each statement below is true or false.

True or False?

F	1.	The prefix hemi- means "full."
T	2.	The prefix quadri- means "four."
F	3.	The root word cerebr means "cerebellum."
F	4.	The root word neur means "nervous."
T	5.	The root word pleg means "paralysis."
T	6.	The suffix -ical means "pertaining to."
T	7.	A CVA is also called a *stroke*.
F	8.	A positive Romberg's sign is a failure to maintain balance while sitting.
T	9.	A stationary blood clot is called a *thrombus*.
F	10.	A TIA causes permanent damage to the brain.
F	11.	All patients who get migraine headaches have warning symptoms.
T	12.	Alzheimer's disease is the most common form of dementia.

Break It Down

Directions: Dissect each medical term into its word elements by placing a slash between each word part (prefix, root word, combining vowel, and suffix). Then define each term.

Example:
Medical Term: polyneuritis
Dissection: poly/neur/itis
Definition: inflammation of many nerves

Medical Term	Dissection

1. encephalomalacia   e n c e p h a l/o/m a l a c i a

Definition: softening of the brain
_____

2. meningioma   m e n i n g i/o m a

Definition: tumor of the meninges
_____

3. polyneuritis   p o l y/n e u r/i t i s

Definition: inflammation of many nerves
_____

4. quadriplegic   q u a d r i/p l e g/i c

Definition: pertaining to paralysis of four (paralysis of all four extremities)
_____

5. radiculopathy   r a d i c u l/o/p a t h y

Definition: disease of the nerve root
_____

6. hemicerebrum   h e m i/c e r e b r u m

Definition: half of the cerebrum
_____

Medical Term	Dissection
7. neurorrhaphy	n e u r / o / r r h a p h y

Definition: suture of the nerve

| 8. neurasthenia | n e u r / a s t h e n i a |

Definition: weakness of the nerve

| 9. meningocele | m e n i n g / o / c e l e |

Definition: swelling of the meninges

Spelling

Directions: Circle the correctly spelled term in each row.

1.	(aphasia)	aphaesia	aphasea	aphazia
2.	craneal	(cranial)	craenial	chranial
3.	cerebovasular	cerebralvascolar	(cerebrovascular)	cerebrovascullar
4.	disphasia	(dysphasia)	disphasea	dysphasea
5.	(polyneuritis)	polynuritis	polynueritis	polineuritis
6.	hemipeglia	(hemiplegia)	hemaplegia	hemipledgia
7.	menyngitis	menangitis	meninghitis	(meningitis)
8.	(meningocele)	meningiocele	meningecele	meningacele
9.	nueral	nural	(neural)	neureal
10.	neurosthenia	neuresthenia	neuresthaenia	(neurasthenia)
11.	quodriplegia	quadroplegia	(quadriplegia)	quodreplegia
12.	ridiculopathy	(radiculopathy)	radicculopathy	rediculapathy

Cumulative Review

Chapters 5–7: Lymphatic and Immune Systems, Special Sensory Organs, and Nervous System

Directions: Check your mastery of common word elements used in medical terminology related to the lymphatic and immune systems, special sensory organs (eyes and ears), and nervous system. Write the definition of each prefix, combining form, and suffix listed in this section. For more cumulative review practice, visit the companion website.

Prefixes

a-	not; without
an-	not; without
auto-	self
dys-	painful; difficult
extra-	outside
hemi-	half
hyper-	above; above normal
inter-	between
intra-	inside; within
para-	near; beside
peri-	around
poly-	many; much
quadri-	four

Combining Forms

aden/o	gland
adenoid/o	adenoids
angi/o	blood vessel
audi/o	hearing
blephar/o	eyelid
cephal/o	head

cerebell/o	cerebellum
cerebr/o	cerebrum
cran/o, crani/o	skull; cranium
cyt/o	cell
encephal/o	brain
hydr/o	water
immun/o	protection
ir/o	iris
irid/o	iris
kerat/o	cornea
leuk/o	white
lymph/o	lymph
mening/o, meningi/o	meninges
myc/o	fungus
myel/o	spinal cord
myring/o	tympanic membrane; eardrum
neur/o	nerve
ocul/o	eye
ophthalm/o	eye
opt/o	eye; vision
optic/o	eye; vision
ot/o	ear
path/o	disease
pleg/o	paralysis
phag/o	eat; swallow; engulf
psych/o	mind
radicul/o	nerve root
retin/o	retina

scler/o	sclera (white of the eye)
spin/o	spine; backbone
splen/o	spleen
thym/o	thymus
tonsill/o	tonsils
tympan/o	tympanic membrane; eardrum
vascul/o	blood vessel

Suffixes

-ac	pertaining to
-al	pertaining to
-algia	pain
-ar	pertaining to
-ary	pertaining to
-asthenia	weakness
-atic	pertaining to
-cele	hernia; swelling; protrusion
-cyte	cell
-eal	pertaining to
-ectomy	surgical removal; excision
-edema	swelling
-esthesia	sensation; feeling
-gen	producing; originating; causing
-gram	record; image
-graphy	process of recording an image
-ia	condition
-ic	pertaining to
-ical	pertaining to
-itis	inflammation

-logist	specialist in the study and treatment of
-logy	study of
-malacia	softening
-megaly	large; enlargement
-meter	instrument used to measure
-metry	process of measuring; measurement
-oid	like; resembling
-oma	tumor; mass
-opia	vision
-osis	abnormal condition
-pathy	disease
-pexy	surgical fixation
-phasia	speech
-plasty	surgical repair
-ptosis	drooping; downward displacement
-rrhaphy	suture
-rrhea	discharge; flow
-rrhexis	rupture
-sclerosis	hardening
-scope	instrument used to observe
-scopy	process of observing
-spasm	involuntary muscle contraction
-stomy	new opening
-tomy	incision; cut into
-trophy	development
-us	structure; thing

Chapter 8

The Male and Female Reproductive Systems

gynec / o / logy: the study of the woman (female reproductive system)

ur / o / logy: the study of the urinary tract (male reproductive system)

Chapter Organization

- Intern Experience
- Overview of Reproductive System Anatomy and Physiology
- Word Elements
- Breaking Down and Building Reproductive System Terms
- Diseases and Disorders
- Procedures and Treatments
- Analyzing the Intern Experience
- Working with Medical Records
- Chapter Review

Chapter Objectives

After completing this chapter, you will be able to

1. label anatomical diagrams of the male and female reproductive systems;

2. dissect and define common medical terminology related to the male and female reproductive systems;

3. build terms used to describe reproductive system diseases and disorders, diagnostic procedures, and therapeutic treatments;

4. pronounce and spell common medical terminology related to the male and female reproductive systems;

5. understand that the processes of building and dissecting a medical term based on its prefix, word root, and suffix enable you to analyze an extremely large number of medical terms beyond those presented in this chapter;

6. interpret the meaning of abbreviations associated with the reproductive systems; and

7. interpret medical records containing terminology and abbreviations related to the reproductive systems.

You will see this icon ⬈ at various points throughout this chapter. The icon indicates that you will find interactive activities and games on the Medical Terminology Companion Website. These activities and games will help you learn, practice, and expand your medical terminology knowledge and skills. Some of these activities are also available on the Medical Terminology Mobile Website.

 Companion Website
www.g-wlearning.com/healthsciences

 Mobile Site
www.m.g-wlearning.com/5800

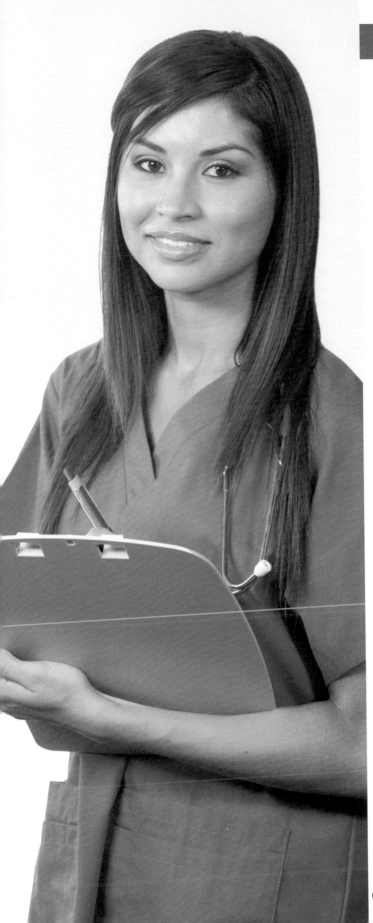

Emily is serving an internship with the Village Square Institute. She is delighted about the opportunity because the medical facility has an excellent reputation in the healthcare community. Emily had heard that the Institute has an opening for a medical assistant; she hopes that her internship experience will result in an employment offer.

On her first day, Emily reports to Pam Masters, RN. She escorts her first patient, Nancy Hopps, to the examination room. Mrs. Hopps is an elderly woman who recently discovered a lump in her right breast. Her primary care physician referred Mrs. Hopps to the Village Square Institute for further evaluation.

As you will learn later in this chapter, Nancy Hopps has a disorder that has affected one of the mammary organs of her reproductive system. She will be clinically evaluated for a possible cancerous tumor of the breast, and you will have the opportunity to interpret her chart note, the medical record dictated by her physician following Nancy's physical examination.

In this chapter you will learn common word elements (prefixes, combining forms, and suffixes) used to form medical terms related to both the male and female reproductive systems. Mastery of these terms, and the word parts from which they are constructed, will enable you to understand the health conditions and diagnostic procedures summarized in the patient chart notes presented throughout this chapter.

Let's begin our study of the male and female reproductive systems with a brief overview of their anatomy and physiology. Afterward, you will learn about diseases and disorders, diagnostic tests and procedures, and therapeutic methods for treating common reproductive health conditions.

Overview of Reproductive System Anatomy and Physiology

As the name implies, the reproductive system enables human beings to reproduce, ensuring the survival of the species. **Gonads** are the primary organs of reproduction. Male gonads, called the **testes**, produce sperm and the hormone *testosterone* (tĕs-TŎS-tĕ-rōn). The testes, also called *testicles*, are suspended in a sac called the **scrotum**, situated behind the **penis** (Figure 8.1). Testosterone stimulates development of the male sex organs and production of sperm.

Sperm is produced in the testes and transported through genital ducts: the **epididymis** (ĕp-ĭ-DĬD-ĭ-mĭs), **vas deferens** (also called the *ductus deferens*), and **urethra**. The seminal vesicles, bulbourethral (BŬL-bō-yū-RĒ-thrăl) gland, and prostate gland contribute fluids along the way to produce semen.

Female gonads, called the **ovaries**, produce **ova** (eggs) and secrete the hormones *estrogen* and *progesterone* (prō-JĔS-tĕr-ōn). These hormones regulate the reproductive cycle and development of the **breasts** (**mammary glands**) and other female sexual characteristics. Fertilization of the ovum (singular form of *ova*) usually occurs in the **uterine tubes** (also called **fallopian tubes**). If fertilization occurs, the ovum implants in the **uterus**, where the female reproductive system continues to nurture and protect the developing fetus during pregnancy. During childbirth, the baby is expelled from the **vagina** (Figure 8.2 on the next page).

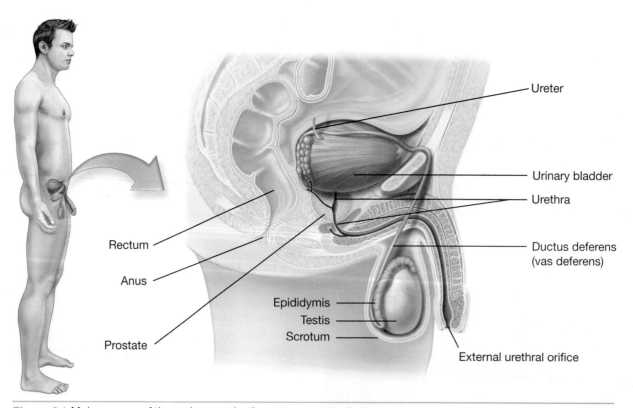

Figure 8.1 Major organs of the male reproductive system, sagittal view

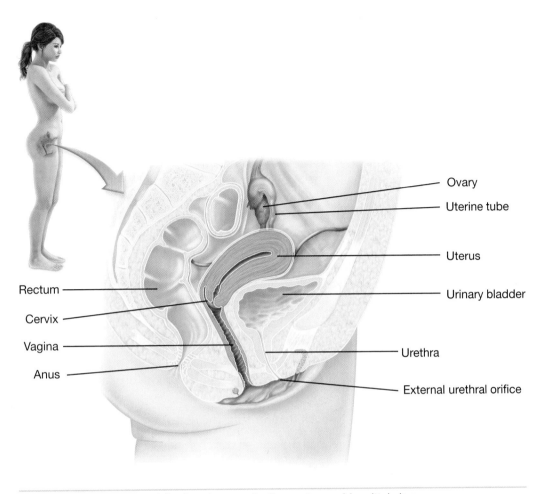

Figure 8.2 Major organs of the female reproductive system, midsagittal view

In summary, the primary functions of the male and female reproductive systems are to

- produce ova (eggs) and sperm;
- secrete hormones; and
- facilitate conception (fertilization) and pregnancy

The study of the male reproductive system is encompassed within the medical practice of **urology**, the study of the urinary tract. A **urologist** is a physician who specializes in the study, diagnosis, and treatment of diseases and disorders of the male reproductive system, as well as the male urinary tract. **Gynecology** is the study of the female reproductive system. A specialist in the study, diagnosis, and treatment of female reproductive system disorders is called a **gynecologist**.

Anatomy and Physiology Vocabulary

Now that you have been introduced to the major organs and basic functions of the male and female reproductive systems, following are brief definitions of the key terms presented in the anatomy and physiology overview.

Key Term	Definition
breasts	mammary glands
bulbourethral gland	small gland on either side of the prostate gland; secretes fluid that lubricates the penis during sexual intercourse
epididymis	small, oblong body that rests upon and beside the posterior surface of the testes; stores and transports sperm from the testes
gonads	primary organs of reproduction (testes in the male, ovaries in the female)
ovaries	female gonads
penis	male organ of reproduction and urination
prostate gland	gland that surrounds the neck of the bladder and the urethra in the male; aids in production and ejaculation of semen
scrotum	pouch that contains the testes
seminal vesicles	sac-like glands that lie behind the male bladder; hold fluid that mixes with sperm to create semen
sperm	fluid produced in the testes that consists of sperm cells
testes	male gonads
urethra	canal through which urine is discharged from the bladder to the outside of the body
uterine tubes	fallopian tubes
uterus	organ that contains and nourishes the developing fetus
vagina	tube that leads from the cervix, the neck-like passage at the lower end of the uterus, to the vulva (external genitals)
vas deferens	excretory duct of the testis; *ductus deferens*

E-Flash Card Activity: Anatomy and Physiology Vocabulary

Directions: After you have reviewed the anatomy and physiology vocabulary pertaining to the male and female reproductive systems, practice with the e-flash cards until you are comfortable with the spelling and definition of each term.

Identifying Major Organs of the Male Reproductive System

Directions: Label the diagram of the male reproductive system.

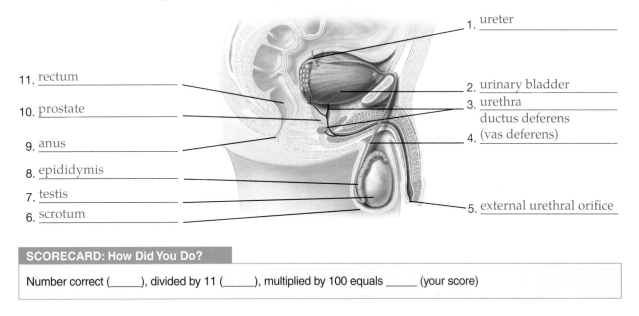

11. rectum

10. prostate

9. anus

8. epididymis

7. testis

6. scrotum

1. ureter

2. urinary bladder

3. urethra

4. ductus deferens (vas deferens)

5. external urethral orifice

SCORECARD: How Did You Do?

Number correct (_____), divided by 11 (_____), multiplied by 100 equals _____ (your score)

Identifying Major Organs of the Female Reproductive System

Directions: Label the diagram of the female reproductive system.

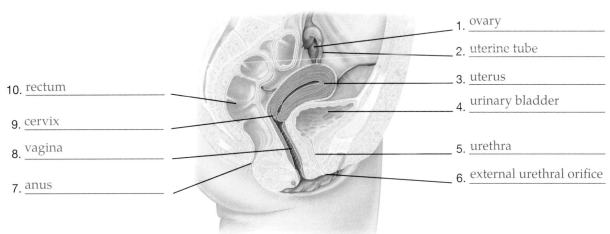

10. rectum

9. cervix

8. vagina

7. anus

1. ovary

2. uterine tube

3. uterus

4. urinary bladder

5. urethra

6. external urethral orifice

SCORECARD: How Did You Do?

Number correct (_____), divided by 10 (_____), multiplied by 100 equals _____ (your score)

Matching Anatomy and Physiology Vocabulary

Directions: Match the vocabulary term in Column A with its meaning in Column B.

Column A

K 1. gonads

N 2. testes

G 3. sperm

A 4. ovaries

O 5. breasts

B 6. uterine tubes

I 7. uterus

C 8. vagina

F 9. scrotum

M 10. epididymis

J 11. vas deferens

H 12. urethra

E 13. prostate gland

P 14. penis

D 15. seminal vesicles

L 16. bulbourethral gland

Column B

A. female gonads

B. fallopian tubes

C. tube that leads from the cervix, the neck-like passage at the lower end of the uterus, to the vulva (external genitals)

D. sac-like glands that lie behind the male bladder; hold fluid that mixes with sperm to create semen

E. gland that surrounds the neck of the bladder and the urethra in the male; aids in production and ejaculation of semen

F. pouch that contains the testes

G. fluid produced in the testes that consists of sperm cells

H. canal through which urine is discharged from the bladder to the outside of the body

I. organ that contains and nourishes the developing fetus

J. excretory duct of the testis; *ductus deferens*

K. primary organs of reproduction (testes in the male, ovaries in the female)

L. small gland on either side of the prostate gland; secretes fluid that lubricates the penis during sexual intercourse

M. small, oblong body that rests upon and beside the posterior surface of the testes; stores and transports sperm from the testes

N. male gonads

O. mammary glands

P. male organ of reproduction and urination

SCORECARD: How Did You Do?

Number correct (_____), divided by 16 (_____), multiplied by 100 equals _____ (your score)

Word Elements

In this section you will learn word elements—prefixes, combining forms, and suffixes—that are common to reproductive system terminology. By learning these word elements and understanding how they are combined to build medical terms, you will be able to analyze Mrs. Hopps's health condition (described in the Intern Experience at the beginning of this chapter) and identify a large number of terms associated with the reproductive systems.

E-Flash Card Activity: Word Elements

Directions: Review the word elements in the tables that follow. Then, practice with the e-flash cards until you are able to quickly recognize the different word parts (prefixes, combining forms, and suffixes) and their meanings. The e-flash cards are grouped together by prefixes, combining forms, and suffixes, followed by a cumulative review of all the word elements that you learned in this chapter.

Prefixes

Let's begin our study of medical word elements by looking at the prefixes listed in the table below. By now, you have mastered each of these prefixes and their meanings.

Prefix	Meaning
a-	not; without
dys-	painful; difficult
endo-	within
intra-	within
trans-	across

Combining Forms

Following are combining forms that appear in medical terms used to describe reproductive system anatomy and physiology, pathological conditions, diagnostic procedures, and therapeutic treatments. A few of these combining forms appear in medical terms used to describe other body systems.

Root Word/Combining Vowel	Meaning
cervic/o	cervix; neck
colp/o	vagina
cyst/o	sac containing fluid; bladder
gynec/o	woman; female
hyster/o	uterus
lapar/o	abdomen
mamm/o	breast
mast/o	breast
men/o	menstruation
metr/o, metri/o	uterus

(Continued)

Root Word/Combining Vowel	Meaning
oophor/o	ovary
orchid/o	testes
prostat/o	prostate gland
salping/o	uterine tube; fallopian tube
scrot/o	scrotum
testicul/o	testes
ur/o	urine; urinary tract
vagin/o	vagina
vas/o	vessel; duct

Suffixes

Following are suffixes commonly encountered in medical terms pertaining to the male and female reproductive systems. From your studies of other body systems, you are already familiar with most of these suffixes.

Suffix	Meaning
-al	pertaining to
-algia	pain
-ectomy	surgical removal; excision
-gram	record; image
-graphy	process of recording an image
-ic	pertaining to
-itis	inflammation
-logist	specialist in the study and treatment of
-logy	study of
-osis	abnormal condition
-pexy	surgical fixation
-plasty	surgical repair
-rrhagia	bursting forth (of blood)
-rrhaphy	suture
-rrhea	discharge; flow
-rrhexis	rupture
-scope	instrument used to observe
-scopy	process of observing

Matching Prefixes, Combining Forms, and Suffixes

Directions: In each exercise that follows, match the word element in Column A with its meaning in Column B. Some meanings may be used more than once.

Prefixes

Column A

B	1. trans-
D	2. dys-
C	3. a-
A	4. intra-
A	5. endo-

Column B

A. within
B. across
C. not; without
D. painful; difficult

Combining Forms

Column A

K	1. scrot/o
I	2. mast/o
D	3. colp/o
N	4. vas/o
E	5. hyster/o
O	6. oophor/o
C	7. cervic/o
G	8. testicul/o
I	9. mamm/o
L	10. prostat/o
F	11. cyst/o
D	12. vagin/o
J	13. men/o
M	14. ur/o
A	15. gynec/o
H	16. salping/o
E	17. metr/o, metri/o
G	18. orchid/o
B	19. lapar/o

Column B

A. woman; female
B. abdomen
C. cervix; neck
D. vagina
E. uterus
F. sac containing fluid; bladder
G. testes
H. uterine tube; fallopian tube
I. breast
J. menstruation
K. scrotum
L. prostate gland
M. urine; urinary tract
N. vessel; duct
O. ovary

Suffixes

Column A

H	1. -scope
A	2. -logist
E	3. -algia
B	4. -ic
D	5. -rrhaphy
B	6. -al
I	7. -ectomy
P	8. -rrhexis
M	9. -plasty
K	10. -gram
F	11. -scopy
L	12. -graphy
J	13. -logy
O	14. -rrhagia
N	15. -rrhea
Q	16. -osis
G	17. -itis
C	18. -pexy

Column B

A. specialist in the study and treatment of
B. pertaining to
C. surgical fixation
D. suture
E. pain
F. process of observing
G. inflammation
H. instrument used to observe
I. surgical removal; excision
J. study of
K. record; image
L. process of recording an image
M. surgical repair
N. discharge; flow
O. bursting forth (of blood)
P. rupture
Q. abnormal condition

SCORECARD: How Did You Do?

Number correct (_____), divided by 42 (_____), multiplied by 100 equals _____ (your score)

Breaking Down and Building Reproductive System Terms

Now that you have mastered common word parts used in medical terminology related to the reproductive systems, you have the ability to dissect and build a large number of terms that apply to reproductive anatomy and physiology, pathology, diagnostics, and treatments.

Term	Dissection	Word Part/Meaning	Term Meaning
Note: *For simplification, combining vowels have been omitted from the Word Part/Meaning column.*			
1. **amenorrhea** (ă-MĔN-ō-RĒ-ă)	a/men/o/rrhea	**a** = not; without **men** = menstruation **rrhea** = discharge; flow	without flow of menstruation
2. **cervical** (SĔR-vĭ-kăl)	cervic/al	**cervic** = cervix; neck **al** = pertaining to	pertaining to the cervix/neck
3. **colposcopy** (kŏl-PŎS-kō-pē)	colp/o/scopy	**colp** = vagina **scopy** = process of observing	process of observing the vagina
4. **dysmenorrhea** (dĭs-MĔN-ō-RĒ-ă)	dys/men/o/rrhea	**dys** = painful; difficult **men** = menstruation **rrhea** = discharge; flow	painful and difficult flow of menstruation
5. **endometriosis** (ĔN-dō-mē-trē-Ō-sĭs)	endo/metri/osis	**endo** = within **metr** = uterus **osis** = abnormal condition	abnormal condition within the uterus
6. **gynecology** (gī-nĕ-KŎL-ō-jē)	gynec/o/logy	**gynec** = woman; female **logy** = study of	study of the woman/female
7. **gynecologist** (gī-nĕ-KŎL-ō-jĭst)	gynec/o/logist	**gynec** = woman; female **logist** = specialist in the study of	specialist in the study of the woman/female
8. **hysterectomy** (HĬS-tĕr-ĔK-tō-mē)	hyster/ectomy	**hyster** = uterus **ectomy** = surgical removal; excision	excision of the uterus
9. **hysterosalpingogram** (HĬS-tĕr-ō-săl-PĬNG-gō-grăm)	hyster/o/salping/o/gram	**hyster** = uterus **salping** = uterine tube; fallopian tube **gram** = record; image	record/image of the uterus and uterine/fallopian tube
10. **hysterosalpingo-oophorectomy** (HĬS-tĕr-ō-săl-PING-gō ō-ŏ-for-ĔK-tō-mē)	hyster/o/salping/o oophor/ectomy	**hyster** = uterus **salping** = uterine tube; fallopian tube **oophor** = ovary **ectomy** = surgical removal; excision	excision of the uterus, uterine/fallopian tube, and ovary
11. **laparoscopy** (LĂP-ă-RŎS-kō-pē)	lapar/o/scopy	**lapar** = abdomen **scopy** = process of observing	process of observing the abdomen
12. **mammography** (mă-MŎG-ră-fē)	mamm/o/graphy	**mamm** = breast **graphy** = process of recording an image	process of recording an image of the breast
13. **mastectomy** (măs-TĔK-tō-mē)	mast/ectomy	**mast** = breast **ectomy** = surgical removal; excision	excision of the breast

Prefixes = Green   Root Words = **Red**   Suffixes = Blue

Term	Dissection	Word Part/Meaning	Term Meaning
14. **menorrhagia** (měn-ō-RĀ-jē-ă)	men/o/rrhagia	**men** = menstruation **rrhagia** = bursting forth (of blood)	bursting forth of menstruation
15. **menorrhea** (měn-ō-RĒ-ă)	men/o/rrhea	**men** = menstruation **rrhea** = discharge; flow	flow of menstruation
16. **oophorectomy** (ō-ŎF-ō-RĚK-tō-mē)	oophor/ectomy	**oophor** = ovary **ectomy** = surgical removal; excision	excision of the ovary
17. **orchidectomy** (or-kĭ-DĚK-tō-mē)	orchid/ectomy	**orchid** = testes **ectomy** = surgical removal; excision	excision of the testes
18. **prostatectomy** (PRŎS-tă-TĔK-tō-mē)	prostat/ectomy	**prostat** = prostate gland **ectomy** = surgical removal; excision	excision of the prostate gland
19. **prostatic** (prŏs-TĂT-ĭk)	prostat/ic	**prostat** = prostate gland **ic** = pertaining to	pertaining to the prostate gland
20. **prostatitis** (prŏs-tă-TĪ-tĭs)	prostat/itis	**prostat** = prostate gland **itis** = inflammation	inflammation of the prostate gland
21. **salpingitis** (săl-pĭn-JĪ-tĭs)	salping/itis	**salping** = uterine tube **itis** = inflammation	inflammation of the uterine/fallopian tube
22. **urologist** (ū-RŎL-ō-jĭst)	ur/o/logist	**ur** = urine; urinary tract **logist** = specialist in the study and treatment of	specialist in the study and treatment of the urinary tract
23. **urology** (ū-RŎL-ō-jē)	ur/o/logy	**ur** = urine; urinary tract **logy** = study of	study of the urine/urinary tract
24. **vaginitis** (VĂJ-ĭn-Ī-tĭs)	vagin/itis	**vagin** = vagina **itis** = inflammation	inflammation of the vagina
25. **vasectomy** (văs-ĔK-tō-mē)	vas/ectomy	**vas** = vessel; duct **ectomy** = surgical removal; excision	excision of a vessel/duct

Prefixes = Green   Root Words = Red   Suffixes = Blue

Using the pronunciation guide in the Breaking Down and Building chart, practice saying each medical term aloud. To hear the pronunciation of each term, go to the Pronounce It activity at the G-W companion website.

Audio Activity: Pronounce It

Directions: At the companion website, listen as each medical term listed below is pronounced. Practice pronouncing the terms until you are comfortable saying them aloud.

amenorrhea
(ă-MĔN-ō-RĒ-ă)

cervical
(SĔR-vĭ-kăl)

colposcopy
(kŏl-PŎS-kō-pē)

dysmenorrhea
(dĭs-MĔN-ō-RĒ-ă)

endometriosis
(ĔN-dō-mē-trē-Ō-sĭs)

gynecology
(gī-nĕ-KŎL-ō-jē)

gynecologist
(gī-nĕ-KŎL-ō-jĭst)

hysterectomy
(HĬS-tĕr-ĔK-tō-mē)

hysterosalpingogram
(HĬS-tĕr-ō-săl-PĬNG-gō-grăm)

hysterosalpingo-oophorectomy
(HĬS-tĕr-ō-săl-PING-gō ō-ŏ-for-ĔK-tō-mē)

laparoscopy
(LĂP-ă-RŎS-kō-pē)

mammography
(mă-MŎG-ră-fē)

mastectomy
(măs-TĔK-tō-mē)

menorrhagia
(mĕn-ō-RĀ-jē-ă)

menorrhea
(mĕn-ō-RĒ-ă)

oophorectomy
(ō-ŎF-ō-RĔK-tō-mē)

orchidectomy
(or-kĭ-DĔK-tō-mē)

prostatectomy
(PRŎS-tă-TĔK-tō-mē)

prostatic
(prŏs-TĂT-ĭk)

prostatitis
(prŏs-tă-TĪ-tĭs)

salpingitis
(săl-pĭn-JĪ-tĭs)

urologist
(ū-RŎL-ō-jĭst)

urology
(ū-RŎL-ō-jē)

vaginitis
(VĂJ-ĭn-Ī-tĭs)

vasectomy
(văs-ĔK-tō-mē)

Audio Activity: Spell It

Directions: Cover the medical terms in the Pronounce It activity with a sheet of paper. At the companion website, listen as the terms are read aloud. Correctly spell each term below.

1. amenorrhea
2. cervical
3. colposcopy
4. dysmenorrhea
5. endometriosis
6. gynecology
7. gynecologist
8. hysterectomy
9. hysterosalpingogram
10. hysterosalpingo-oophorectomy
11. laparoscopy
12. mammography
13. mastectomy
14. menorrhagia
15. menorrhea
16. oophorectomy
17. orchidectomy
18. prostatectomy
19. prostatic
20. prostatitis
21. salpingitis
22. urologist
23. urology
24. vaginitis
25. vasectomy

Break It Down

Directions: In the following exercise, dissect each medical term below into its word elements by placing a slash between each word part (prefix, root word, combining vowel, and suffix). Then define each term.

Example:
Medical Term: salpingitis
Dissection: salping/itis
Definition: inflammation of the uterine (fallopian) tube

Medical Term	Dissection
1. prostatitis	p r o s t a t/i t i s

Definition: inflammation of the prostate gland
_____

2. oophorectomy	o o p h o r/e c t o m y

Definition: excision of the ovary
_____

3. mammography	m a m m/o/g r a p h y

Definition: process of recording an image of the breast
_____

4. hysterosalpingo-oophorectomy	h y s t e r/o/s a l p i n g/o/- o o p h o r/e c t o m y

Definition: excision of the uterus, uterine/fallopian tube, and ovary
_____

5. endometriosis	e n d o/m e t r i/o s i s

Definition: abnormal condition within the uterus
_____

Medical Term	Dissection
6. dysmenorrhea	d y s / m e n / o / r r h e a

Definition: painful and difficult flow of menstruation

| 7. urologist | u r / o / l o g i s t |

Definition: specialist in the study and treatment of the urinary tract

| 8. salpingitis | s a l p i n g / i t i s |

Definition: inflammation of the uterine/fallopian tube

| 9. prostatectomy | p r o s t a t / e c t o m y |

Definition: excision of the prostate gland

| 10. urology | u r / o / l o g y |

Definition: study of the urine/urinary tract

| 11. gynecologist | g y n e c / o / l o g i s t |

Definition: specialist in the study of the woman/female

| 12. vasectomy | v a s / e c t o m y |

Definition: excision of a vessel/duct

| 13. amenorrhea | a / m e n / o / r r h e a |

Definition: without flow of menstruation

Medical Term	Dissection

14. vaginitis

v a g i n / i t i s

Definition: inflammation of the vagina

15. gynecology

g y n e c / o / l o g y

Definition: the study of the woman/female

16. menorrhagia

m e n / o / r r h a g i a

Definition: bursting forth of menstruation

17. hysterosalpingogram

h y s t e r / o / s a l p i n g / o / g r a m

Definition: record/image of the uterus and uterine/fallopian tube

18. hysterectomy

h y s t e r / e c t o m y

Definition: excision of the uterus

19. colposcopy

c o l p / o / s c o p y

Definition: process of observing the vagina

20. cervical

c e r v i c / a l

Definition: pertaining to the cervix/neck

Build It

Directions: In this exercise, build the medical terms that match the definitions provided by supplying the correct word elements.

P (Prefixes) = Green
RW (Root Words) = Red
S (Suffixes) = Blue
CV (Combining Vowel) = Purple

1. excision of a vessel/duct

vas	ectomy
RW	S

2. specialist in the study of the woman/female

gynec	o	logist
RW	CV	S

3. process of recording an image of the breast

mamm	o	graphy
RW	CV	S

4. record/image of the uterus and uterine/fallopian tube

hyster	o	salping	o	gram
RW	CV	RW	CV	S

5. abnormal condition within the uterus

endo	metri	osis
P	RW	S

6. without flow of menstruation

a	men	o	rrhea
P	RW	CV	S

7. inflammation of the uterine/fallopian tube

salping	itis
RW	S

8. process of observing the vagina

colp	o	scopy
RW	CV	S

9. process of observing the abdomen

lapar	o	scopy
RW	CV	S

10. excision of the breast

mast	ectomy
RW	S

11. painful and difficult flow of menstruation

dys	men	o	rrhea
P	RW	CV	S

12. specialist in the study and treatment of the urinary tract

ur	o	logist
RW	CV	S

13. flow of menstruation

men	o	rrhea
RW	CV	S

14. inflammation of the vagina

vagin	itis
RW	S

15. study of the woman/female

gynec	o	logy
RW	CV	S

16. pertaining to the cervix

cervic	al
RW	S

17. study of the urine/urinary tract

ur	o	logy
RW	CV	S

18. excision of the uterus

hyster	ectomy
RW	S

19. excision of the prostate gland

prostat	ectomy
RW	S

20. pertaining to the prostate

prostat	ic
RW	S

SCORECARD: How Did You Do?

Number correct (_____), divided by 20 (_____), multiplied by 100 equals _____ (your score)

Identify the Medical Word Part

Directions: For each medical word part shown below, indicate whether it is a prefix, root word, or suffix by circling the correct answer. Then write the meaning of the word part.

1. **metr**   Prefix   (Root Word)   Suffix

   Meaning: uterus _____

2. **graphy**   Prefix   Root Word   (Suffix)

   Meaning: process of recording an image _____

3. **dys**   (Prefix)   Root Word   Suffix

   Meaning: painful; difficult _____

4. **salping**   Prefix   (Root Word)   Suffix

   Meaning: uterine tube; fallopian tube _____

5. **cervic**   Prefix   (Root Word)   Suffix

   Meaning: cervix; neck _____

6. **oophor**   Prefix   (Root Word)   Suffix

   Meaning: ovary _____

7. **rrhagia**   Prefix   Root Word   (Suffix)

   Meaning: bursting forth (of blood) _____

8. **prostat**   Prefix   (Root Word)   Suffix

   Meaning: prostate gland _____

SCORECARD: How Did You Do?

Number correct (_____), divided by 8 (_____), multiplied by 100 equals _____ (your score)

Diseases and Disorders

Diseases and disorders of the male and female reproductive systems run the spectrum from the mild to the severe, and they have a number of different causes. In this section, we will briefly examine some common pathological conditions of these body systems.

Benign Prostatic Hypertrophy

Benign prostatic hypertrophy (prō-STĂT-ĭk hī-PĔR-trō-phē) (**BPH**) is a noncancerous enlargement of the prostate gland, or *prostate* (Figure 8.3). The prostate surrounds the urethra, a tube that carries urine from the bladder out of the body. As the prostate enlarges, it constricts (narrows) the urethra, impeding urine flow. Symptoms of BPH include *nocturia* (urinating often at night), *urinary retention* (inability to empty urine from the bladder), and *frequency* (urinating frequently). BPH occurs in many men as they age.

Breast Cancer

Breast cancer originates in the tissues of the breast (Figure 8.4 on the next page). It may be *invasive* or *noninvasive.* Breast cancer that is invasive has spread from the *lobule* (LŎB-yūl), or milk duct, to other tissue in the breast. Breast cancer that is noninvasive has not affected other tissue in the breast.

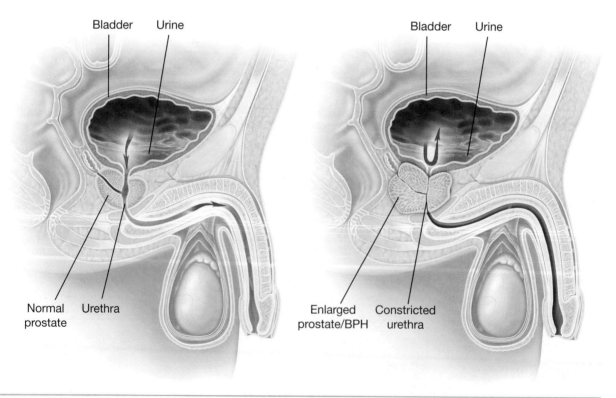

Figure 8.3 Benign prostatic hypertrophy is a noncancerous enlargement of the prostate gland.

Early-stage breast cancer usually does not cause symptoms. As the cancer grows, a woman may feel a painless lump in the breast or in the armpit. The lump is typically hard with uneven edges. There may be a change in the size, shape, or feel of the breast or nipple or a discharge from the nipple. Breast cancer is not limited to females. Men, too, can develop this type of cancer.

Different tests are used to diagnose breast cancer. A physician will perform a physical examination of both breasts, armpits, and the neck and chest area. **Mammography** (mă-MŎG-ră-fē) is used to screen for breast cancer. If a suspicious growth is detected in a mammogram, a breast ultrasound may be performed to determine whether the lump is solid (indicative of a tumor) or fluid-filled (characteristic of a cyst). Further testing may include a breast biopsy, computerized tomography (CT) scan, or magnetic resonance imaging (MRI) scan. These tests help the physician determine whether or not the cancer has spread. Use of a series of tests to establish the extent of cancerous growth—especially whether or not it has spread to other parts of the body—is called *staging*. Staging helps in guiding future treatment.

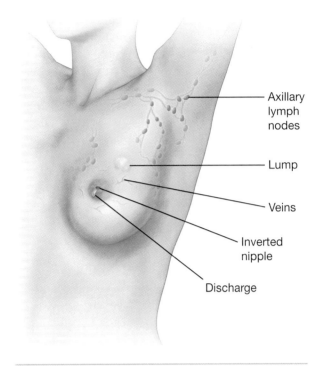

Figure 8.4 Breast cancer may originate anywhere within the tissues of the breast.

Chlamydia

Chlamydia is a common sexually transmitted disease (STD) caused by a bacterium (Figure 8.5). Sexually active individuals and those with multiple partners are at highest risk of contracting the disease.

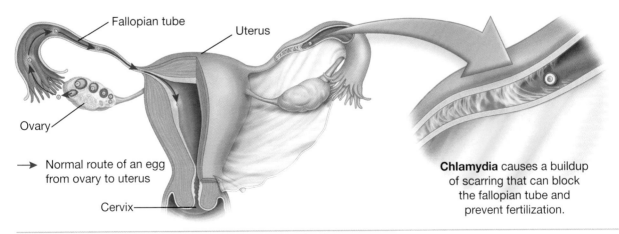

Figure 8.5 Untreated chlamydia can lead to fallopian tube damage.

Chlamydia infections in women may lead to **cervicitis** (sĕr-vĭ-SĪ-tĭs), inflammation of the cervix. Left untreated, it can result in fallopian tube damage. In men, chlamydia can lead to **urethritis** (yū-rĕ-THRĪ-tĭs), inflammation of the urethra. Male patients may experience a burning sensation during urination and/or a discharge from the penis or rectum. Some males also experience testicular tenderness. Chlamydia typically is treated with antibiotics.

Endometriosis

Endometriosis (ĕn-dō-MĒ-trē-Ō-sis) is a disorder in which the *endometrium* (ĕn-dō-MĒ-trē-ŭm), the tissue that lines the inside of the uterus, grows outside it (Figure 8.6). The displaced endometrium continues to function normally. It thickens, sloughs off, and bleeds with each menstrual cycle. But because the tissue is outside the uterus, it has no way to exit the body. It is trapped, causing irritation to surrounding body tissues and leading eventually to the formation of scar tissue and *adhesions* (abnormal tissue that binds organs together). The primary symptom of endometriosis is pelvic pain, often associated with the menstrual period. Painful intercourse, painful defecation, and infertility can be associated with this disease. The cause of endometriosis is unknown.

Gonorrhea

Gonorrhea is a curable sexually transmitted disease (STD). The bacterium that causes gonorrhea can infect the genital tract, mouth, or anus. In men, gonorrhea can cause pain with urination and a discharge from the penis. In women, it can cause bleeding between periods, pain with urination, and increased vaginal discharge. Gonorrhea does not always cause symptoms, so an infected person can unknowingly transmit the disease. Left untreated, the STD can lead to pelvic inflammatory disease (PID), which causes infertility or problems during pregnancy. Gonorrhea can pass from mother to baby during pregnancy. It is treated with antibiotics.

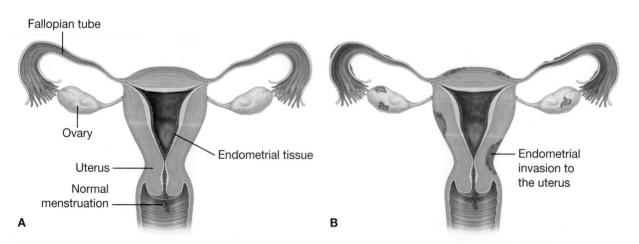

Figure 8.6 In endometriosis, the tissue that lines the inside of the uterus grows outside the uterus. The displaced tissue becomes trapped, causing irritation and eventually scar tissue and adhesions.

Genital Herpes

Genital herpes is a highly contagious sexually transmitted disease (STD) caused by the *herpes simplex virus* (*HSV*) (Figure 8.7). It is characterized by periodic outbreaks of painful, itchy, ulcer-like lesions of the genitals, skin, and mucus membranes. Some people infected with HSV are asymptomatic (without signs or symptoms). In fact, an infected person can still be contagious even if no sores are visible. Genital herpes cannot be cured, but it can be controlled with medication. Once a person has been infected, the virus lies dormant in the body and can reactivate several times a year. Use of condoms can help prevent transmission of the virus.

- Sexually transmitted virus

- Small, painful sores or blisters

- Usually heal in 1-3 weeks

- Can come back weeks, months, or years later

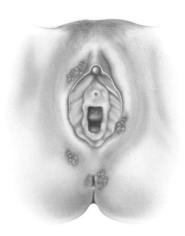

Figure 8.7 Genital herpes is a highly contagious, incurable sexually transmitted disease.

Pelvic Inflammatory Disease

Pelvic inflammatory disease (PID) is an infection of the female reproductive organs (Figure 8.8). Symptoms may include fever, chills, malaise (general feeling of unwellness), backache, tender abdomen, and a foul-smelling vaginal discharge. The initial infection is usually caused by an STD. PID occurs when the disease-causing microorganisms travel from the cervix to the upper genital tract. Untreated gonorrhea and chlamydia cause nearly all cases of PID. Antibiotic treatment is prescribed for PID.

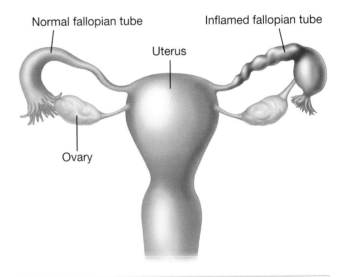

Normal fallopian tube

Inflamed fallopian tube

Uterus

Ovary

Figure 8.8 Pelvic inflammatory disease is an infection of the female reproductive organs. It is usually caused by a sexually transmitted disease.

Premenstrual Syndrome

Premenstrual syndrome (PMS) is a group of symptoms linked to the menstrual cycle. Its cause is unclear. PMS is characterized by a variety of symptoms, including tender breasts, mood swings, irritability, depression, fatigue, and food cravings. These problems tend to peak in women in their late 20s and early 30s. There are no specific physical or laboratory tests for the positive diagnosis of premenstrual syndrome.

Prostate Cancer

Prostate cancer originates in the prostate gland, a small, walnut-sized gland that surrounds the neck of the male bladder and urethra (Figure 8.9 on the next page). The prostate secretes an alkaline substance that

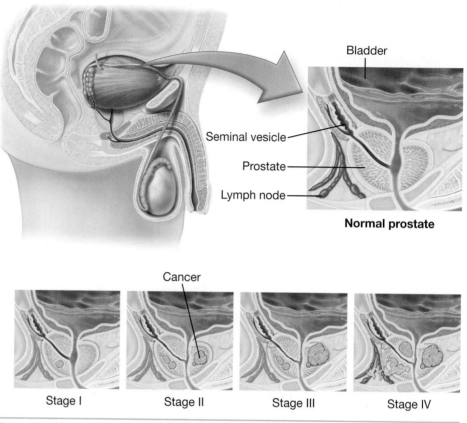

Bladder

Seminal vesicle

Prostate

Lymph node

Normal prostate

Cancer

Stage I

Stage II

Stage III

Stage IV

Figure 8.9 Stages of prostate cancer, from early to advanced stage. The cancer originates in the prostate gland, which surrounds the neck of the male bladder and urethra.

is a component of semen. Symptoms of prostate cancer are similar to those of benign prostatic hypertrophy (BPH): slow or weak urine stream, incontinence (leakage), feeling unable to fully empty the bladder, and nocturia. A biopsy may be performed if a rectal exam reveals that the prostate is enlarged or has a hard, uneven surface. During the biopsy, a sample of tissue is removed from the prostate and sent to a lab for analysis.

Syphilis

Syphilis (SĬF-ĭ-lĭs) is a sexually transmitted disease (STD) caused by a bacterium. It infects the genital area, lips, mouth, or anus by producing red, elevated areas on the skin that erode into small ulcers called *chancres* (SHĂNG-kĕrs). Syphilis is transmitted by direct sexual contact with an infected person. A pregnant woman infected with syphilis can pass the disease to her fetus. The disease is treated with antibiotics. Without treatment, syphilis can be life-threatening, severely damaging the heart, brain, or other vital organs.

Procedures and Treatments

In this section, you will learn about tests and procedures used to help diagnose pathological conditions of the male and female reproductive systems, as well as therapeutic methods commonly used to treat certain conditions.

Circumcision

Circumcision (sĕr-kŭm-SĬZH-ŭn) is the surgical removal of the foreskin, the skin that covers the tip of the penis (Figure 8.10). The procedure is performed soon after birth. There are medical benefits and risks to circumcision. Benefits include a lower risk of urinary tract infections (UTIs), penile cancer, and STDs. Risks include bleeding, pain, and infection after the procedure. Parents of a male newborn decide whether or not they want circumcision to be performed based on their religious, cultural, and personal beliefs.

Colposcopy

Colposcopy (kŏl-PŎS-kō-pē) is a diagnostic procedure used to examine the cervix, vagina, and vulva (external genitalia) (Figure 8.11 on the next page). It is performed using a *colposcope* (KŎL-pō-skōp), a surgical instrument that provides an enlarged view of the tissues in these areas. This enhanced view enables the physician to visually distinguish between normal and abnormal-appearing tissue and to take biopsies for pathological examination. Colposcopy is often performed if a pelvic exam or Pap test (discussed on the next page) revealed abnormalities. The main goal of colposcopy is to prevent cervical cancer by detecting precancerous lesions and treating them before they become cancerous.

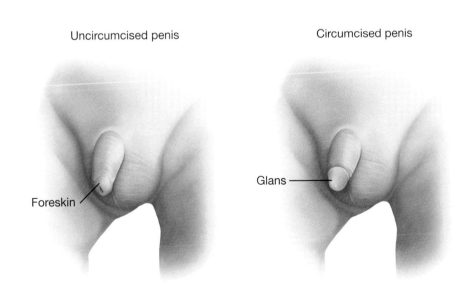

Uncircumcised penis

Circumcised penis

Glans

Foreskin

Figure 8.10 In circumcision, the foreskin of the penis is surgically removed shortly after birth.

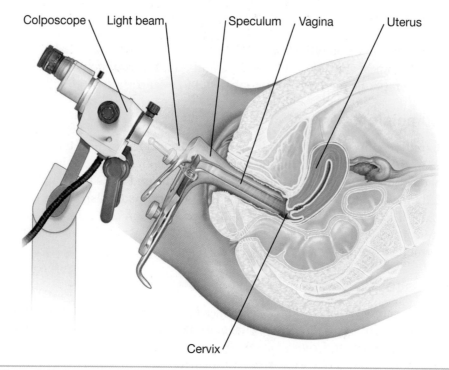

Colposcope   Light beam   Speculum   Vagina   Uterus

Cervix

Figure 8.11 Colposcopy is the diagnostic examination of the cervix, vagina, and vulva using a colposcope.

Digital Rectal Exam

A **digital rectal exam** is performed to evaluate the size and shape of the prostate gland. A physician inserts a finger into the rectum to *palpate* (lightly press with the fingers) the prostate through the wall of rectum. A digital rectal exam is used to screen for benign prostatic hypertrophy (BPH) and prostate cancer.

Dilation and Curettage

Dilation and curettage (kū-rĕ-TĂHZH), commonly referred to as a **D&C**, is the dilation (widening/opening) of the cervix and surgical removal of part of the lining of the uterus and/or contents of the uterus by curettage (scraping and scooping). Tissue removed during a D&C is sent to a laboratory for analysis. D&C may be performed as a diagnostic procedure or as a therapeutic gynecological procedure to treat a uterine condition. Symptoms that might indicate the need for a D&C are severe menstrual pain, abnormal uterine bleeding, postmenopausal bleeding, or an abnormal Pap test (discussed on the next page).

Laparoscopic Hysterectomy

Laparoscopic hysterectomy (LĂP-ă-rō-SKŎP-ĭk hĭs-tĕr-ĔK-tō-mē) is a minimally invasive surgical technique that allows the uterus to be removed without a large incision (Figure 8.12). The surgeon makes multiple, small incisions to insert instruments and uses a tiny camera to visualize the surgical site. The laparoscopic approach to hysterectomy is safer than open surgery because less tissue is cut, resulting in a lower risk of infection and faster healing time.

Pap Test

A **Pap test**, or **Pap smear**, is the microscopic examination of cells from the cervix (Figure 8.13). It is used as a screening tool for cervical cancer. During a Pap test, the physician inserts an instrument called a *speculum* into the vagina to open it slightly. Then cells are gently scraped from the opening of the cervix and sent to a lab for analysis.

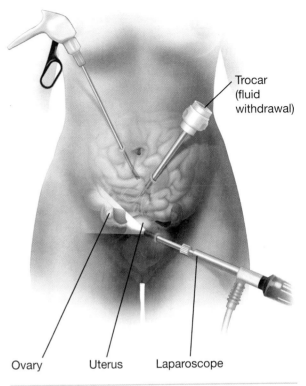

Trocar (fluid withdrawal)

Ovary   Uterus   Laparoscope

Figure 8.12 Laparoscopic hysterectomy is a safer alternative than open surgery for removal of the uterus.

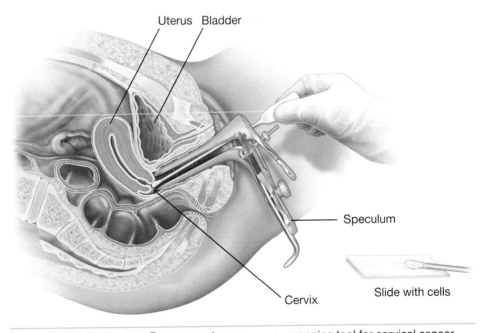

Uterus   Bladder

Speculum

Cervix

Slide with cells

Figure 8.13 A Pap test, or Pap smear, is a common screening tool for cervical cancer.

Transurethral Resection of the Prostate Gland

Transurethral (trăns-yū-RĒ-thrăl) **resection of the prostate (TURP)** is a type of prostate surgery done to relieve moderate to severe urinary symptoms caused by an enlarged prostate (Figure 8.14). As you learned earlier, another term for an enlarged prostate is *benign prostatic hypertrophy (BPH)*.

During the TURP procedure, an instrument called a *resectoscope* (rē-SĔK-tō-skōp) is inserted through the urethra to the prostate. Using the resectoscope, which functions as a both visual and surgical instrument, the physician removes the section of the prostate that is obstructing urine flow.

Vasectomy

A **vasectomy** is considered a permanent method of male contraception (Figure 8.15). During a vasectomy, the vas deferens from each testicle is clamped or cut, preventing the release of sperm. It is one of the most commonly used surgical sterilization procedures for men. A vasectomy only prevents pregnancy; it offers no protection against STDs.

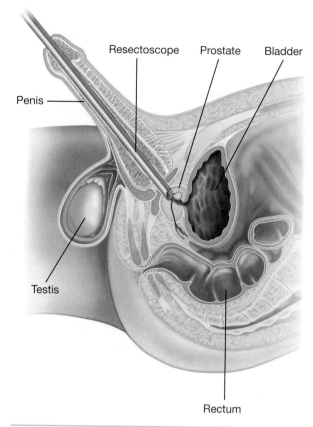

Figure 8.14 Transurethral resection of the prostate (TURP) is performed to relieve moderate to severe urinary symptoms caused by an enlarged prostate.

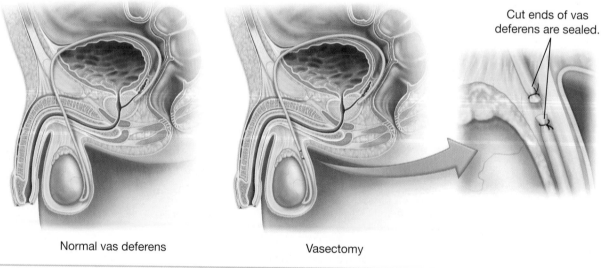

Normal vas deferens

Vasectomy

Cut ends of vas deferens are sealed.

Figure 8.15 Vasectomy is a permanent method of male contraception.

Tubal Ligation

Tubal ligation is a type of female contraception (birth control) that permanently prevents pregnancy (Figure 8.16). During tubal ligation, the uterine (fallopian) tubes are clamped, severed, or sealed. This procedure prevents eggs from reaching the uterus for fertilization and blocks sperm from traveling up the uterine tubes to the egg. A tubal ligation does not affect the menstrual cycle, nor does it offer protection from sexually transmitted diseases (STDs).

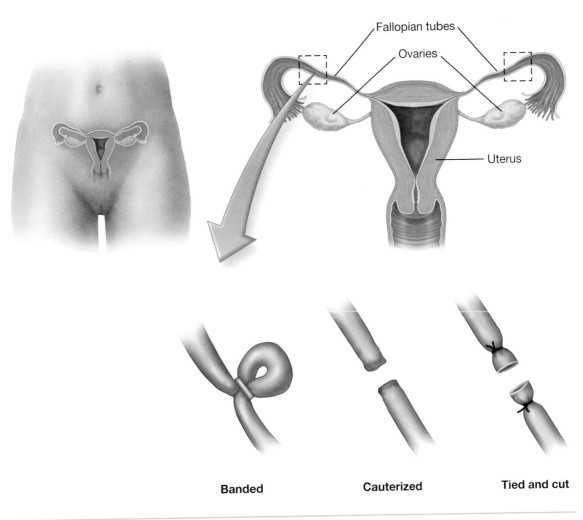

Fallopian tubes

Ovaries

Uterus

Banded   **Cauterized**   **Tied and cut**

Figure 8.16 Tubal ligation is a permanent method of female birth control.

Multiple Choice: Diseases and Disorders

Directions: Write the letter of the disease or disorder that matches each numbered definition below.

__C__ 1. Gonorrhea is
  a. found in women only.
  b. a benign tumor.
  c. passed to the fetus during pregnancy.
  d. a virus that lies dormant in the body and can reactivate several times a year.

__D__ 2. a sexually transmitted disease that produces chancres
  a. urethritis   c. endometriosis
  b. cervicitis   d. syphilis

__A__ 3. a common bacterial STD that can cause cervicitis in women and urethritis in men
  a. chlamydia
  b. genital herpes
  c. endometriosis
  d. benign prostatic hypertrophy

__A__ 4. an infection of the female reproductive organs
  a. pelvic inflammatory disease
  b. syphilis
  c. endometriosis
  d. chlamydia

__B__ 5. a highly contagious sexually transmitted disease caused by the herpes simplex virus (HSV)
  a. chlamydia   c. endometriosis
  b. genital herpes   d. gonorrhea

__B__ 6. a disorder in which the tissue lining the inside of the uterus grows outside the uterus
  a. chlamydia
  b. endometriosis
  c. genital herpes
  d. pelvic inflammatory disease

__B__ 7. a cancer that starts in the prostate gland
  a. genital herpes
  b. prostate cancer
  c. benign prostatic hypertrophy
  d. endometriosis

SCORECARD: How Did You Do?

Number correct (_____), divided by 7 (_____), multiplied by 100 equals _____ (your score)

Multiple Choice: Procedures and Treatments

Directions: Write the letter of the diagnostic procedure or therapeutic treatment that matches each numbered definition below.

__A__ 1. surgical removal of the foreskin
  a. circumcision
  b. transurethral resection of the prostate gland
  c. vasectomy
  d. tubal ligation

__C__ 2. surgery done to relieve moderate to severe urinary symptoms caused by an enlarged prostate
  a. prostectomy
  b. vasectomy
  c. transurethral resection of the prostate gland
  d. tubal ligation

__D__ 3. permanent method of male birth control
  a. transurethral resection of the prostate gland
  b. circumcision
  c. tubal ligation
  d. vasectomy

__A__ 4. microscopic examination of cells scraped from the cervix
  a. Pap test
  b. colposcopy
  c. dilation and curettage
  d. laparoscopic hysterectomy

B   5. dilation of the cervix and surgical removal of part of the lining of the uterus and uterine contents
    a. laparoscopic hysterectomy
    b. dilation and curettage
    c. Pap test
    d. colposcopy

D   6. diagnostic procedure for examining the cervix, vagina, and vulva
    a. Pap test
    b. dilation and curettage
    c. tubal ligation
    d. colposcopy

B   7. excision of the uterus
    a. circumcision
    b. laparoscopic hysterectomy
    c. vasectomy
    d. tubal ligation

A   8. permanent method of female birth control
    a. tubal ligation
    b. transurethral resection of the prostate gland
    c. vasectomy
    d. circumcision

SCORECARD: How Did You Do?

Number correct (_____), divided by 8 (_____), multiplied by 100 equals _____ (your score)

Identifying Abbreviations

Directions: Write the abbreviation for each medical term listed below.

Medical Term	Abbreviation
1. sexually transmitted disease	STD
2. herpes simplex virus	HSV
3. pelvic inflammatory disease	PID
4. benign prostatic hypertrophy	BPH
5. premenstrual syndrome	PMS
6. transurethral resection of the prostate gland	TURP
7. dilation and curettage	D&C

SCORECARD: How Did You Do?

Number correct (_____), divided by 7 (_____), multiplied by 100 equals _____ (your score)

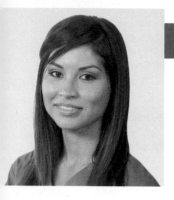

Analyzing the Intern Experience

In the Intern Experience described at the beginning of this chapter, we met Emily, an intern with the Village Square Institute. Emily was assigned to shadow Pam, a registered nurse (RN). Their first patient was Nancy Hopps, an elderly woman who recently discovered a lump in her right breast. Her primary care physician had referred Mrs. Hopps to the Village Square Institute for more in-depth clinical evaluation.

A doctor at the Institute examined Mrs. Hopps and obtained her personal and family health history. He then made a medical diagnosis and provided Mrs. Hopps with a treatment plan. Later, the doctor made a dictated recording of the patient's health information, which was subsequently transcribed into a chart note.

We will now learn more about Nancy Hopps's condition from a clinical perspective, interpreting the medical terms in his chart note as we analyze the scenario presented in the Intern Experience.

Audio Activity: Nancy Hopps's Chart Note

Directions: At the companion website, listen and read along as the physician dictates Nancy Hopps's chart note, shown below. Then do the exercise that appears after the chart note.

CHART NOTE

Patient Name: Hopps, Nancy
ID Number: HN 25780
Examination Date: January 12, 20xx

SUBJECTIVE
Mrs. Nancy Hopps is an 82-year-old female who is new to this practice. She was referred by her primary care physician after physical examination confirmed a lump in her right breast.

OBJECTIVE
Vital signs within normal limits, although **BP** is slightly elevated. Physical exam reveals a significant, easily **palpated** (lightly pressed with the palms and fingers) lump of the right breast that is somewhat hard with irregular borders.

ASSESSMENT
Possible breast **carcinoma**.

PLAN
Mammogram and a breast ultrasound will be performed in our office and sent to our radiology group for analysis.

Interpret Nancy Hopps's Chart Note

Directions: After listening to the dictated recording and reading the chart note on Nancy Hopps, provide the medical term that matches each definition below. You may encounter terms that were introduced in previous chapters.

Example: painful and difficult menstruation flow   *Answer:* dysmenorrhea

1. blood pressure

   BP

2. diagnostic procedure used to screen for breast cancer

   mammogram

3. examined by lightly pressing with the palms of the hands and the fingers

   palpated

4. cancerous tumor

   carcinoma

Working with Medical Records

In this activity, you will interpret the medical records (chart notes) of patients with reproductive system disorders. These examples illustrate typical medical records prepared in a real-world healthcare environment. To interpret these chart notes, you will apply your knowledge of word elements (prefixes, combining forms, and suffixes), diseases and disorders, and procedures and treatments related to the male and female reproductive systems.

Audio Activity: Juan Forsum's Chart Note

Directions: At the companion website, listen and read along as the physician dictates Juan Forsum's chart note, shown on the next page. Then do the exercise that appears after the chart note.

CHART NOTE

Patient Name: Forsum, Juan
ID Number: FJ 34896
Examination Date: April 4, 20xx

SUBJECTIVE
Juan returns to our office with continued problems of **nocturia**, urinary retention, and frequency. He returns due to increasing discomfort.

OBJECTIVE
The patient is a controlled diabetic with normal vital signs. Digital **rectal exam** revealed enlarged prostate.

ASSESSMENT
Benign prostatic hypertrophy

PLAN
Transurethral resection of the prostate (TURP)

Interpret Juan Forsum's Chart Note

Directions: After listening to the dictated recording and reading the chart note on Juan Forsum, provide the medical term that matches each definition below.

Example: inflammation of the prostate gland   *Answer:* prostatitis

1. noncancerous enlargement of the prostate gland

   benign prostatic hypertrophy

2. exam used to screen for BPH and prostate cancer

   rectal exam

3. type of prostate surgery performed to relieve moderate to severe urinary symptoms caused by an enlarged prostate

   transurethral resection of the prostate (TURP)

4. frequent urination at night

   nocturia

SCORECARD: How Did You Do?

Number correct (_____), divided by 4 (_____), multiplied by 100 equals _____ (your score)

Audio Activity: Richard Thomas's Chart Note

Directions: At the companion website, listen and read along as the physician dictates Richard Thomas's chart note, shown below. Then do the exercise that appears after the chart note.

CHART NOTE

Patient Name: Thomas, Richard
ID Number: RT 69024
Examination Date: August 29, 20xx

SUBJECTIVE
Patient complains of **scrotal** and genital pain. There is also discomfort during urination often associated with a **purulent** discharge.

OBJECTIVE
Richard is a sexually active 17-year-old male who, by his own admission, does not routinely use a condom. Physical exam reveals small, palpable lump on **lateral** aspect of the left **testis**.

ASSESSMENT
Evaluate for **gonorrhea**.

PLAN
Culture test for gonorrhea.

Assessment

Interpret Richard Thomas's Chart Note

Directions: After listening to the dictated recording and reading the chart note on Richard Thomas, provide the medical term that matches each definition below. You may encounter terms that were introduced in previous chapters.

Example: excision of a vessel or duct   *Answer*: vasectomy

1. pertaining to the side   lateral

2. curable sexually transmitted disease   gonorrhea

3. pertaining to pus   purulent

4. male gonad   testis

5. pertaining to the sac in which the testes are suspended   scrotal

SCORECARD: How Did You Do?

Number correct (_____), divided by 5 (_____), multiplied by 100 equals _____ (your score)

Chapter Review

Word Elements Summary

Prefixes

Prefix	Meaning
a-	not; without
dys-	painful; difficult
endo-	within
intra-	within
trans-	across

Combining Forms

Root Word/Combining Vowel	Meaning
cervic/o	cervix; neck
colp/o	vagina
cyst/o	sac containing fluid; bladder
gynec/o	woman; female
hyster/o	uterus
lapar/o	abdomen
mamm/o	breast
mast/o	breast
men/o	menstruation
metr/o, metri/o	uterus
oophor/o	ovary
orchid/o	testes
prostat/o	prostate gland
salping/o	uterine tube; fallopian tube
scrot/o	scrotum
testicul/o	testes
ur/o	urine; urinary tract
vagin/o	vagina
vas/o	vessel; duct

Suffixes

Suffix	Meaning
-al	pertaining to
-algia	pain
-ectomy	surgical removal; excision
-gram	record; image
-graphy	process of recording an image
-ic	pertaining to
-itis	inflammation
-logist	specialist in the study and treatment of
-logy	study of
-osis	abnormal condition
-pexy	surgical fixation
-plasty	surgical repair
-rrhagia	bursting forth (of blood)
-rrhaphy	suture
-rrhea	discharge; flow
-rrhexis	rupture
-scope	instrument used to observe
-scopy	process of observing

More Practice: Activities and Games

The activities on the following pages will help you reinforce your skills and check your mastery of the medical terminology that you learned in this chapter. Visit the companion website for More Practice games and activities.

Break It Down

Directions: In this exercise, dissect each medical term into its word elements by placing a slash between each word part (prefix, root word, combining vowel, and suffix). Then define each term.

Example:
Medical Term: oophorectomy
Dissection: oophor/ectomy
Definition: excision of the ovary

Medical Term	Dissection

1. prostatocystitis   p r o s t a t/o/c y s t/i t i s

Definition: inflammation of the sac of the prostate

2. metrosalpingography   m e t r o/s a l p i n g/o/g r a p h y

Definition: process of recording an image of the uterus and uterine/fallopian tube

3. mastalgia   m a s t/a l g i a

Definition: pain in the breast

4. intracervical   i n t r a/c e r v i c/a l

Definition: pertaining to within the cervix

5. orchidopexy   o r c h i d/o/p e x y

Definition: surgical fixation of the testes

6. mammoplasty   m a m m/o/p l a s t y

Definition: surgical repair of the breast

Medical Term	Dissection
7. laparoscope	l a p a r / o / s c o p e

Definition: instrument used to observe the abdomen

8. hysterorrhaphy	h y s t e r / o / r r h a p h y

Definition: suture of the uterus

9. colporrhexis	c o l p / o / r r h e x i s

Definition: rupture of the vagina

Audio Activity: Tyra McNamara's Chart Note

Directions: At the companion website, listen and read along as the physician dictates the following chart note on Tyra McNamara. Then do the exercise that appears after the chart note.

CHART NOTE

Patient Name: McNamara, Tyra
ID Number: MT 33412
Examination Date: July 28, 20xx

SUBJECTIVE
This newly married patient complains of painful intercourse, which is often associated with her **menstrual** period. She has random episodes of pain with urination and bowel movements.

OBJECTIVE
Patient had one child delivered vaginally. No history of **STDs** or cancer. **Dysmenorrhea** and **menorrhagia**.

ASSESSMENT
Probable **endometriosis**

PLAN
Patient prescribed hormonal contraceptives and ibuprofen to help reduce pelvic pain. Patient to return for follow-up.

Interpret Tyra McNamara's Chart Note

Directions: After listening to the dictated recording and reading the chart note on Tyra McNamara, provide the medical term that matches each definition below. You may encounter definitions and terms that were introduced in previous chapters.

Example: excision of the ovary   *Answer*: oophorectomy

1. pertaining to menstruation   menstrual

2. sexually transmitted diseases   STDs

3. painful menstration   dysmenorrhea

4. excessively heavy periods (bursting forth of menstruation)   menorrhagia

5. disorder in which the tissue that lines the inside of the uterus grows outside of it   endometriosis

Spelling

Directions: Circle the correctly spelled term in each row.

1.	dysmenarrhea	dysmenorrea	(dysmenorrhea)	dysmenerrhea
2.	(hysterorrhaphy)	hysteroraphy	hysterorraphy	hysterrorphy
3.	endometreosis	(endometriosis)	endommetriosis	endomietriosis
4.	menorrhagea	mennoragea	(menorrhagia)	menoragia
5.	orophorectomy	ooforectomy	oophoroctomy	(oophorectomy)
6.	(salpingitis)	salpinjitis	selpingitis	salpingittis
7.	urrology	(urology)	eurology	eurollogy
8.	orchidopeksy	orchydopexy	orchidopeksia	(orchidopexy)
9.	prostotectomy	prostytectomy	(prostatectomy)	prostetectomy
10.	(mastectomy)	masstectomy	mastechtomy	mastyctomy
11.	cervicol	cervicall	(cervical)	cervichal
12.	(gynecology)	guynecology	gyneccology	gynnecology

Dictionary Skills

Directions: Using a medical dictionary, such as *Taber's Cyclopedic Medical Dictionary*, look up the term **mastitis**.

For each medical term shown below, indicate whether the term appears on the same page as **mastitis**, before the page, or after the page. Use the following abbreviations in your answers:

O = on the same page   **B** = before the page   **A** = after the page

Write the definition of each term in the space provided.

Medical Term	O, B, A
	Answers in this column will vary.
1. mammography	

Definition: process of recording an image of the breast

2. mastoid _____

Definition: shaped like a breast

3. mastopexy _____

Definition: surgical fixation of the breast

4. mastalgia _____

Definition: pain in the breast

5. mastopathy _____

Definition: disease of the breast

6. mastology _____

Definition: the study of the breast

Chapter 9

The Respiratory System

pulmon / o / logy = the study of the lungs

Chapter Organization

- Intern Experience
- Overview of Respiratory System Anatomy and Physiology
- Word Elements
- Breaking Down and Building Respiratory System Terms
- Diseases and Disorders
- Procedures and Treatments
- Working with Medical Records
- Chapter Review

Chapter Objectives

After completing this chapter, you will be able to

1. label an anatomical diagram of the respiratory system;
2. dissect and define common medical terminology related to the respiratory system;
3. build terms used to describe respiratory system diseases and disorders, diagnostic procedures, and therapeutic treatments;
4. pronounce and spell common medical terminology related to the respiratory system;
5. understand that the processes of building and dissecting a medical term based on its prefix, word root, and suffix enable you to analyze an extremely large number of medical terms beyond those presented in this chapter;
6. interpret the meaning of abbreviations associated with the respiratory system; and
7. interpret medical records containing terminology and abbreviations related to the respiratory system.

You will see this icon at various points throughout this chapter. The icon indicates that you will find interactive activities and games on the Medical Terminology Companion Website. These activities and games will help you learn, practice, and expand your medical terminology knowledge and skills. Some of these activities are also available on the Medical Terminology Mobile Website.

Companion Website
www.g-wlearning.com/healthsciences

Mobile Site
www.m.g-wlearning.com/5800

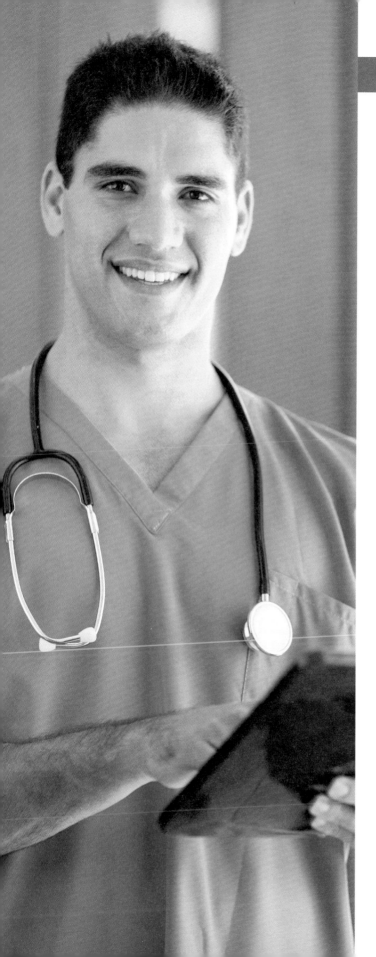

Intern Experience

Mark Lungus, an intern with the Oak Forest Urgent Care Center, has been assigned to shadow (observe and assist) Dr. Connor Wiley today. Mark and Dr. Wiley enter exam room 2, where they meet David, their first patient. David, a high school lacrosse player, was brought to the clinic after collapsing during a practice session.

David explains to Dr. Wiley that "it hurts to breathe" and he is "so tired." Lacrosse practice, rehearsals for the school play, and late nights spent studying and writing a research paper are wearing him down. Running late for lacrosse practice that afternoon, David had breathlessly dashed onto the field and lined up with his teammates. The coach had ordered them to run a series of grueling sprints and offense drills. At one point David's opponent pivoted and pushed off hard, slamming his lacrosse stick into David's chest. David could not catch his breath. The pain in his chest was so intense that he collapsed onto the grass, gasping for air. He could see the coach and the trainer rushing over to him.

David is suffering from an injury that has affected his respiratory system. To help you understand his health problem, this chapter will present word elements (combining forms, prefixes, and suffixes) that make up medical terms related to the respiratory system. As you learn these terms, you will recognize many common word elements from your study of body systems covered in previous chapters—particularly prefixes and suffixes, which are universal word elements.

We will begin our study of the respiratory system with a brief overview of its anatomy and physiology. Later in the chapter, you will learn about some common pathological conditions of the respiratory system, tests and procedures used to diagnose these conditions, and methods for treating them.

Overview of Respiratory System Anatomy and Physiology

Breathing is essential to life. You can live a few weeks without food and a few days without water, but only a few minutes without oxygen. The respiratory system carries oxygen into the body and excretes carbon dioxide. These processes occur in three steps:

- **ventilation**, which is normally accomplished by *inspiration* (drawing air into the lungs) and *expiration* (expelling air from the lungs);

- **exchange of gases**, which occurs in the lungs as (1) oxygen diffuses from the air sacs into the blood, and (2) carbon dioxide diffuses out of the blood as a waste product to be eliminated; and

- **transport** of oxygen from the lungs throughout the body and of carbon dioxide out of the body by the cardiovascular (circulatory) system.

Major Organs and Structures of the Respiratory System

The major organs of the respiratory system include the nose, **pharynx** (throat), **trachea** (windpipe), and **lungs** (Figure 9.1). The lungs are the primary organs of *respiration*, or breathing. Air flows into the nose, through the pharynx,

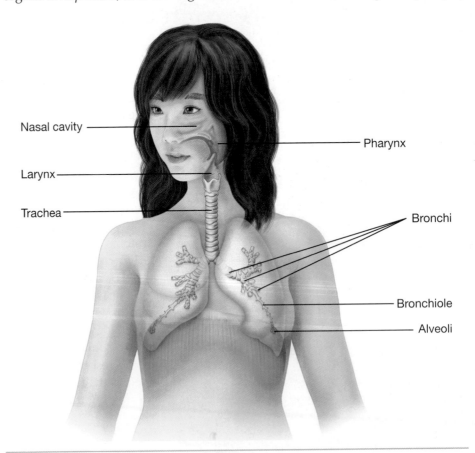

Figure 9.1 Major organs and structures of the respiratory system

and into the trachea. The trachea branches off into the **bronchi** (BRŎNG-kē), tubes that carry air directly into the lungs. (The singular form of *bronchi* is *bronchus*.) Your lungs are enveloped by the **pleura**, a thin membrane of tissue that also lines the chest cavity. The diameters of the bronchi grow increasingly smaller until the bronchi divide into tiny **bronchioles** ("little bronchi"). The bronchioles terminate at the **alveoli** (ăl-VĒ-ō-lē), where the oxygen from the air is exchanged for carbon dioxide, a waste product.

Functions of the Respiratory System

The human respiratory system serves three primary functions:

1. **Gas exchange** — Every cell in your body needs oxygen and produces carbon dioxide. Oxygen from the air enters the blood, and carbon dioxide leaves the blood as a waste product that is expelled by the lungs.
2. **Regulation of acid-base (pH) levels** — The respiratory system maintains a normal acid-base balance by continually adjusting the carbon dioxide levels in the blood.
3. **Protection** — The respiratory system protects the body against "foreign invaders" by filtering out airborne pollutants and some microorganisms.

Pulmonology is the medical specialty concerned with the study, diagnosis, and treatment of diseases and disorders of the respiratory system. A **pulmonologist** is a physician who specializes in the study, diagnosis, and treatment of respiratory system diseases and disorders.

Anatomy and Physiology Vocabulary

Now that you have been introduced to the basic structure and functions of the respiratory system, we will explore in more detail the key terms presented in the introduction.

Key Term	Definition
alveoli	tiny, grape-like sacs in which exchange of gases (oxygen and carbon) occurs
bronchi	tubes that carry air into the lungs
lungs	the primary organs of respiration (breathing)
pharynx	the throat
pleura	a thin, serous (watery) membrane that envelops each lung and also lines the chest cavity
pulmonologist	physician who specializes in the study and treatment of diseases and disorders of the respiratory system
pulmonology	the study of the respiratory system
trachea	windpipe

E-Flash Card Activity: Anatomy and Physiology Vocabulary

Directions: After you have reviewed the anatomy and physiology vocabulary related to the respiratory system, practice with the e-flash cards until you are comfortable with the spelling and definition of each term.

Identifying Major Organs and Structures of the Respiratory System

Directions: Label the diagram of the respiratory system.

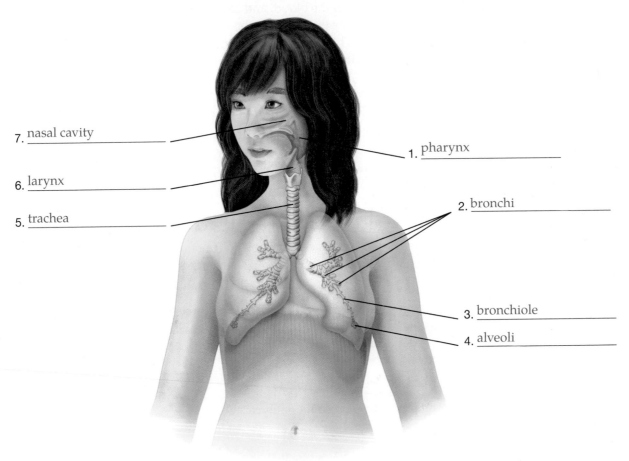

7. nasal cavity

6. larynx

5. trachea

1. pharynx

2. bronchi

3. bronchiole

4. alveoli

SCORECARD: How Did You Do?

Number correct (_____), divided by 7 (_____), multiplied by 100 equals _____ (your score)

Matching Anatomy and Physiology Vocabulary

Directions: Match the vocabulary term in Column A with its meaning in Column B.

Column A

<u>H</u> 1. pharynx

<u>G</u> 2. trachea

<u>D</u> 3. pleura

<u>B</u> 4. bronchi

<u>A</u> 5. alveoli

<u>E</u> 6. pulmonologist

<u>F</u> 7. pulmonology

<u>C</u> 8. lungs

Column B

A. tiny, grape-like sacs in which exchange of gases (oxygen and carbon) occurs

B. tubes that carry air into the lungs

C. the primary organs of respiration (breathing)

D. a thin, serous (watery) membrane that envelops each lung and also lines the chest cavity

E. physician who specializes in the study and treatment of diseases and disorders of the respiratory system

F. the study of the respiratory system

G. windpipe

H. the throat

SCORECARD: How Did You Do?

Number correct (_____), divided by 8 (_____), multiplied by 100 equals _____ (your score)

Word Elements

In this section you will learn word elements—prefixes, combining forms, and suffixes—that are common to the respiratory system. By learning these word elements and understanding how they are combined to build medical terms, you will be able to analyze David's health condition (described in the Intern Experience at the beginning of this chapter) and identify a large number of terms associated with the respiratory system.

E-Flash Card Activity: Word Elements

Directions: Review the word elements in the tables that follow. Then, practice with the e-flash cards until you are able to quickly recognize the different word parts (prefixes, combining forms, and suffixes) and their meanings. The e-flash cards are grouped together by prefixes, combining forms, and suffixes, followed by a cumulative review of all the word elements that you learned in this chapter.

Prefixes

Let's begin our study of word elements by looking at the prefixes listed in the table below. There is only one new prefix in this list; the others were introduced in previous chapters.

Prefix	Meaning
a-	not; without
an-	not; without
brady-	slow
dys-	painful; difficult
endo-	within
hyper-	above; above normal
hypo-	below; below normal
tachy-	fast

Combining Forms

Listed below are combining forms that appear in medical terms used to describe the respiratory system. Which of these combining forms have you already mastered?

Root Word/Combining Vowel	Meaning
bronch/o, bronchi/o	bronchial tube; bronchus
cyan/o	blue
embol/o	plug; embolus
hem/o	blood
lob/o	lobe (a defined portion of an organ or structure)
ox/o	oxygen
pharyng/o	pharynx; throat
pleur/o	pleura
pneum/o, pneumon/o	lung; air

(Continued)

Root Word/Combining Vowel	Meaning
pulmon/o	lung
rhin/o	nose
spir/o	breathe; breathing
sten/o	narrow; constricted
thorac/o	chest
trache/o	trachea; windpipe

Suffixes

Listed below are suffixes that appear in medical terms pertaining to the respiratory system. You are already familiar with most of these suffixes from your study of other body systems covered in previous chapters.

Suffix	Meaning
-al	pertaining to
-algia	pain
-centesis	surgical puncture to remove fluid
-ectasis	dilatation; dilation; expansion
-ectomy	surgical removal; excision
-gram	record; image
-ia	condition
-itis	inflammation
-logist	specialist in the study and treatment of
-logy	study of
-meter	measure
-osis	abnormal condition
-pnea	breathing
-scope	instrument used to observe
-thorax	chest; pleural cavity
-tomy	incision; cut into

Matching Prefixes, Combining Forms, and Suffixes

Directions: In each exercise below, match the word element in Column A with its meaning in Column B. Some meanings may be used more than once.

Prefixes

Column A		*Column B*
C	1. brady-	A. above; above normal
E	2. tachy-	B. not; without
B	3. a-	C. slow
F	4. hypo-	D. painful; difficult
G	5. endo-	E. fast
B	6. an-	F. below; below normal
D	7. dys-	G. within
A	8. hyper-	

Combining Forms

Column A		*Column B*
D	1. thorac/o	A. blue
M	2. pharyng/o	B. oxygen
I	3. pneumon/o	C. nose
N	4. lob/o	D. chest
K	5. trache/o	E. plug; embolus
J	6. bronchi/o	F. pleura
L	7. spir/o	G. blood
E	8. embol/o	H. lung
C	9. rhin/o	I. lung; air
B	10. ox/o	J. bronchial tube; bronchus
H	11. pulmon/o	K. trachea; windpipe
J	12. bronch/o	L. breathe; breathing
I	13. pneum/o	M. pharynx; throat
A	14. cyan/o	N. lobe
F	15. pleur/o	O. narrow; constricted
G	16. hem/o	
O	17. sten/o	

Suffixes

Column A

G	1.	-meter
E	2.	-ectomy
I	3.	-itis
C	4.	-al
M	5.	-tomy
H	6.	-pnea
B	7.	-centesis
P	8.	-osis
O	9.	-thorax
K	10.	-logist
F	11.	-ectasis
D	12.	-ia
N	13.	-algia
L	14.	-logy
J	15.	-scope
A	16.	-gram

Column B

A. record; image
B. surgical puncture to remove fluid
C. pertaining to
D. condition
E. surgical removal; excision
F. dilatation; dilation; expansion
G. measure
H. breathing
I. inflammation
J. instrument used to observe
K. specialist in the study and treatment of
L. study of
M. incision; cut into
N. pain
O. chest; pleural cavity
P. abnormal condition

SCORECARD: How Did You Do?

Number correct (_____), divided by 41 (_____), multiplied by 100 equals _____ (your score)

Breaking Down and Building Respiratory System Terms

Now that you have mastered the prefixes, combining forms, and suffixes for medical terminology pertaining to the respiratory system, you have the ability to dissect and build a large number of terms related to this body system.

On the next page is a list of medical terms commonly used in pulmonology, the medical specialty concerning the study, diagnosis, and treatment of the respiratory system. For each term, a dissection has been provided, along with the meaning of each word element and the definition of the term as a whole.

Term	Dissection	Word Part/Meaning	Term Meaning
Note: *For simplification, combining vowels have been omitted from the Word Part/Meaning column.*			
1. **apnea** (ĂP-nē-ă)	a/pnea	**a** = not; without **pnea** = breathing	without breathing
2. **anoxia** (ăn-ŎK-sē-ă)	an/ox/ia	**an** = not; without **ox** = oxygen **ia** = condition	condition of without oxygen
3. **bradypnea** (brăd-ĭp-NĒ-ă)	brady/pnea	**brady** = slow **pnea** = breathing	slow breathing
4. **bronchiectasis** (BRŎNG-kē-ĕk-TĀ-sĭs)	bronchi/ectasis	**bronchi** = bronchial tube; bronchus **ectasis** = dilatation; dilation; expansion	dilatation of the bronchus
5. **bronchitis** (brŏng-KĪ-tĭs)	bronch/itis	**bronch** = bronchial tube; bronchus **itis** = inflammation	inflammation of the bronchus
6. **bronchogram** (BRŎNG-kō-grăm)	bronch/o/gram	**bronch** = bronchial tube; bronchus **gram** = record; image	record or image of the bronchus
7. **bronchopneumonia** (BRŎNG-kō-nū-MŌ-nē-ă)	bronch/o/pneumon/ia	**bronch** = bronchial tube; bronchus **pneumon** = lung; air **ia** = condition	condition of the bronchus and lung
8. **bronchoscope** (BRŎNG-kō-skōp)	bronch/o/scope	**bronch** = bronchial tube; bronchus **scope** = instrument used to observe	instrument used to observe the bronchus
9. **dyspnea** (DĬSP-nē-ă)	dys/pnea	**dys** = painful; difficult **pnea** = breathing	painful or difficult breathing
10. **hemothorax** (hē-mō-THOR-ăks)	hem/o/thorax	**hem** = blood **thorax** = chest; pleural cavity	blood in the pleural cavity
11. **hyperpnea** (hī-PĔRP-nē-ă)	hyper/pnea	**hyper** = above; above normal **pnea** = breathing	above-normal breathing
12. **hypopnea** (hī-PŎP-nē-ă)	hypo/pnea	**hypo** = below normal **pnea** = breathing	below-normal breathing

Prefixes = Green   Root Words = Red   Suffixes = Blue

Term	Dissection	Word Part/Meaning	Term Meaning
13. **pharyngitis** (făr-ĭn-JĪ-tĭs)	pharyng/itis	**pharyng** = throat **itis** = inflammation	inflammation of the throat
14. **pneumothorax** (nū-mō-THOR-ăks)	pneum/o/thorax	**pneum** = lung; air **thorax** = chest; pleural cavity	air in the pleural cavity
15. **pneumonia** (nū-MŌ-nē-ă)	pneumon/ia	**pneumon** = lung; air **ia** = condition	condition of the lung
16. **pneumonocentesis** (NŪ-mō-nō-sĕn-TĒ-sĭs)	pneumon/o/centesis	**pneumon** = lung; air **centesis** = surgical puncture to remove fluid	surgical puncture to remove fluid in the lung
17. **pulmonologist** (pŭl-mŏn-ŎL-ō-jĭst)	pulmon/o/logist	**pulmon** = lung **logist** = specialist in the study and treatment of	specialist in the study and treatment of the lungs
18. **pulmonology** (pŭl-mŏn-ŎL-ō-jē)	pulmon/o/logy	**pulmon** = lung **logy** = study of	study of the lungs
19. **rhinitis** (rī-NĪ-tĭs)	rhin/itis	**rhin** = nose **itis** = inflammation	inflammation of the nose
20. **spirometer** (spī-RŎM-ĕt-ĕr)	spir/o/meter	**spir** = breathe; breathing **meter** = measure	measure of breathing
21. **tachypnea** (tăk-ĭp-NĒ-ă)	tachy/pnea	**tachy** = fast **pnea** = breathing	fast breathing
22. **tracheal** (TRĀ-kē-ăl)	trache/al	**trache** = trachea **al** = pertaining to	pertaining to the trachea
23. **tracheitis** (trā-kē-Ī-tĭs)	trache/itis	**trache** = trachea **itis** = inflammation	inflammation of the trachea
24. **tracheostenosis** (TRĀ-kē-ō-stĕn-Ō-sĭs)	trache/o/sten/osis	**trache** = trachea **sten** = narrow; constricted **osis** = abnormal condition	abnormal condition of a narrow/constricted trachea
25. **tracheotomy** (trā-kē-ŎT-ō-mē)	trache/o/tomy	**trache** = trachea **tomy** = incision; cut into	incision to the trachea

Prefixes = Green   Root Words = Red   Suffixes = Blue

Using the pronunciation guide in the Breaking Down and Building chart, practice saying each medical term aloud. To hear the pronunciation of each term, go to the Pronounce It activity at the G-W companion website.

Audio Activity: Pronounce It

Directions: At the companion website, listen as each medical term listed below is pronounced. Practice pronouncing the terms until you are comfortable saying them aloud.

apnea
(ĂP-nē-ă)

anoxia
(ăn-ŎK-sē-ă)

bradypnea
(brăd-ĭp-NĒ-ă)

bronchiectasis
(BRŎNG-kē-ĕk-TĀ-sĭs)

bronchitis
(brŏng-KĪ-tĭs)

bronchogram
(BRŎNG-kō-grăm)

bronchopneumonia
(BRŎNG-kō-nū-MŌ-nē-ă)

bronchoscope
(BRŎNG-kō-skōp)

dyspnea
(DĬSP-nē-ă)

hemothorax
(hē-mō-THOR-ăks)

hyperpnea
(hī-PĔRP-nē-ă)

hypopnea
(hī-PŎP-nē-ă)

pharyngitis
(făr-ĭn-JĪ-tĭs)

pneumothorax
(nū-mō-THOR-ăks)

pneumonia
(nū-MŌ-nē-ă)

pneumonocentesis
(NŪ-mō-nō-sĕn-TĒ-sĭs)

pulmonologist
(pŭl-mŏn-ŎL-ō-jĭst)

pulmonology
(pŭl-mŏn-ŎL-ō-jē)

rhinitis
(rī-NĪ-tĭs)

spirometer
(spī-RŎM-ĕt-ĕr)

tachypnea
(tăk-ĭp-NĒ-ă)

tracheal
(TRĀ-kē-ăl)

tracheitis
(trā-kē-Ī-tĭs)

tracheostenosis
(TRĀ-kē-ō-stĕn-Ō-sĭs)

tracheotomy
(trā-kē-ŎT-ō-mē)

Audio Activity: Spell It

Directions: Cover the medical terms in the Pronounce It activity with a sheet of paper. At the companion website, listen as the terms are read aloud. Correctly spell each term below.

1. apnea
2. anoxia
3. bradypnea
4. bronchiectasis
5. bronchitis
6. bronchogram
7. bronchopneumonia
8. bronchoscope
9. dyspnea
10. hemothorax
11. hyperpnea
12. hypopnea
13. pharyngitis
14. pneumothorax
15. pneumonia
16. pneumonocentesis
17. pulmonologist
18. pulmonology
19. rhinitis
20. spirometer
21. tachypnea
22. tracheal
23. tracheitis
24. tracheostenosis
25. tracheotomy

Break It Down

Directions: Dissect each medical term below into its word elements by placing a slash between each word part (prefix, root word, combining vowel, and suffix). Then define each term.

Example:
Medical Term: pulmonologist
Dissection: pulmon/o/logist
Definition: specialist in the study and treatment of the lungs

Medical Term	Dissection
1. rhinitis	r h i n / i t i s

Definition: inflammation of the nose

2. pharyngitis	p h a r y n g / i t i s

Definition: inflammation of the throat

3. hemothorax	h e m / o / t h o r a x

Definition: blood in the pleural cavity

4. pulmonology	p u l m o n / o / l o g y

Definition: study of the lungs

5. apnea	a / p n e a

Definition: without breathing

Medical Term	Dissection

6. tachypnea

t a c h y / p n e a

Definition: fast breathing

7. pneumonocentesis

p n e u m o n / o / c e n t e s i s

Definition: surgical puncture to remove fluid in the lung

8. bronchitis

b r o n c h / i t i s

Definition: inflammation of the bronchus

9. tracheotomy

t r a c h e / o / t o m y

Definition: incision to the trachea

10. anoxia

a n / o x / i a

Definition: condition of without oxygen

11. dyspnea

d y s / p n e a

Definition: painful or difficult breathing

12. pneumothorax

p n e u m / o / t h o r a x

Definition: air in the pleural cavity

13. tracheostenosis

t r a c h e / o / s t e n / o s i s

Definition: abnormal condition of a narrow/constricted trachea

Medical Term	Dissection
14. bronchiectasis	b r o n c h i / e c t a s i s

Definition: dilatation of the bronchus

15. spirometer	s p i r / o / m e t e r

Definition: measure of breathing

16. tracheal	t r a c h e / a l

Definition: pertaining to the trachea

17. bradypnea	b r a d y / p n e a

Definition: slow breathing

18. bronchogram	b r o n c h / o / g r a m

Definition: record or image of the bronchus

19. tracheitis	t r a c h e / i t i s

Definition: inflammation of the trachea

20. pneumonia	p n e u m o n / i a

Definition: condition of the lung

SCORECARD: How Did You Do?

Number correct (_____), divided by 20 (_____), multiplied by 100 equals _____ (your score)

Build It

Directions: Build the medical term that matches each definition below by supplying the correct word elements.

P (Prefixes) = Green
RW (Root Words) = Red
S (Suffixes) = Blue
CV (Combining Vowel) = Purple

1. air in the pleural cavity

pneum	o	thorax
RW	CV	S

2. above-normal breathing

hyper	pnea
P	S

3. below-normal breathing

hypo	pnea
P	S

4. blood in the pleural cavity

hem	o	thorax
RW	CV	RW

5. condition of the lung

pneumon	ia
RW	S

6. condition of the bronchus and lung

bronch	o	pneumon	ia
RW	CV	RW	S

7. slow breathing

brady	pnea
RW	S

8. dilatation of the bronchus

bronchi	ectasis
RW	S

9. fast breathing

tachy	pnea
P	S

10. incision to the trachea

trache	o	tomy
RW	CV	S

11. inflammation of the bronchus

bronch	itis
RW	S

12. inflammation of the nose

rhin	itis
RW	S

13. inflammation of the throat

pharyng	itis
RW	S

14. inflammation of the trachea

trache	itis
RW	S

15. instrument used to observe the bronchus

bronch	o	scope
RW	CV	S

16. measure of breathing

spir	o	meter
RW	CV	S

17. surgical puncture to remove fluid in the lung

pneum	o	centesis
RW	CV	S

18. record or image of the bronchus

bronch	o	gram
RW	CV	S

19. specialist in the study and treatment of the lungs

pulmon	o	logist
RW	CV	S

20. without breathing

a	pnea
P	S

SCORECARD: How Did You Do?

Number correct (_____), divided by 20 (_____), multiplied by 100 equals _____ (your score)

Diseases and Disorders

Diseases and disorders of the respiratory system run the spectrum from the mild to the severe, and they have a number of different causes. In this section, we will briefly explore some common respiratory pathological conditions.

Asthma

As you learned in chapter 5, **asthma** is a disorder caused by inflammation of the bronchi (airways) in the lungs (Figure 9.2). When an asthma attack occurs, the muscles surrounding the bronchi constrict (narrow), and the lining (mucous membranes) of the bronchi swell. Both the constriction and swelling reduce the amount of air that can pass through the lungs. The result is wheezing, shortness of breath, coughing, and tightness in the chest. The etiology (cause) of asthma is unknown.

In people who are sensitive to environmental *allergens* (allergy-causing substances), inhalation can trigger asthma symptoms. Examples of common asthma-inducing allergens are dust, pet hair or dander, pollen, and mold. Even emotional stress can trigger an asthma attack. The duration of an asthma attack may be a few minutes or a few days.

Treatments for asthma include limiting exposure to irritants that can trigger an asthma attack and using prescription medications such as bronchodilators, anti-inflammatory drugs, and inhaled steroids. An asthma attack that severely restricts airflow is life threatening and requires immediate medical intervention.

Pneumonia

Pneumonia is an inflammation in one or both lungs often caused by a bacterium or virus (Figure 9.3). Exudate (ĔKS-yū-dāt), fluid such as pus or cellular debris that leaks from blood vessels, clogs the air spaces of the lungs, preventing gas exchange. Symptoms of pneumonia include persistent cough, shortness of breath, chest pain, and fever with chills and sweating.

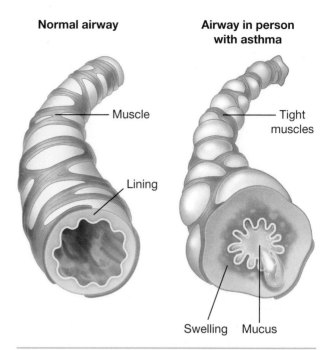

Normal airway

Airway in person with asthma

Muscle — Tight muscles — Lining — Swelling — Mucus

Figure 9.2 During an asthma attack, the muscles surrounding the bronchi constrict, and the bronchial lining swells.

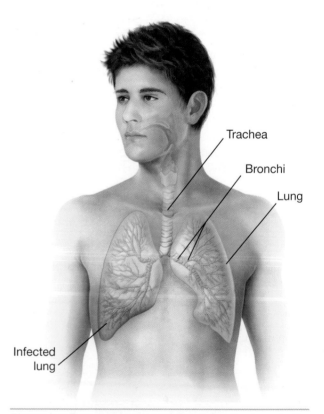

Trachea — Bronchi — Lung — Infected lung

Figure 9.3 Pneumonia is an inflammation in one or both lungs caused by an infection.

Pneumothorax

A **pneumothorax** is a collapsed lung. It occurs when air escapes from the lung and collects in the pleural space, the small area between the lungs and thoracic cavity (Figure 9.4). This accumulation of air puts pressure on the lungs, preventing them from expanding. Symptoms of pneumothorax include shortness of breath and sharp pain in the chest upon deep breathing or coughing. The condition is caused by a penetrating chest injury, such as a gunshot or knife wound or a rib fracture that punctures the lung.

Bronchitis

Bronchitis is an inflammation of the lining of the bronchial tubes, which deliver air to and from the lungs (Figure 9.5). Bronchitis may be either *acute* (appearing suddenly and worsening quickly) or *chronic* (developing gradually and worsening over an extended period of time).

Acute bronchitis is a condition that can develop from a respiratory infection or the common cold. *Chronic bronchitis* is a more serious condition resulting from long-term irritation or inflammation of the bronchial tubes. Symptoms include fatigue, fever, chills, and a productive cough of *sputum*, mucus or fluid coughed up from the lungs. The sputum may be clear, white, or yellowish-green in color. Chronic bronchitis is one of the conditions included in the disease called chronic obstructive pulmonary disease (COPD), discussed on the next page.

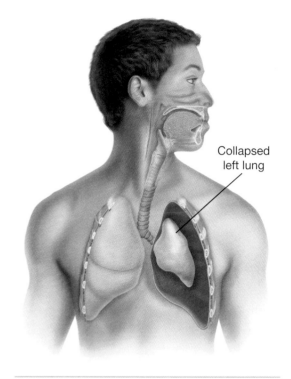

Collapsed left lung

Figure 9.4 A pneumothorax is a collapsed lung.

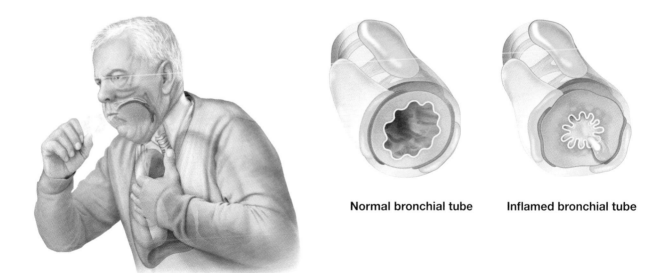

Normal bronchial tube   Inflamed bronchial tube

Figure 9.5 Bronchitis is an inflammation of the lining of the bronchial tubes.

Chronic Obstructive Pulmonary Disease

Chronic obstructive pulmonary disease (COPD) is a progressive disease marked by difficulty breathing (Figure 9.6). It is caused by damage to the lungs over many years and is often, but not always, associated with smoking. Tobacco smoke irritates the bronchi and destroys the elastic fibers in the lungs, making it harder to breathe.

COPD is often a combination of two diseases: chronic bronchitis and emphysema. In **chronic bronchitis**, the bronchial tubes become inflamed and secrete excessive mucus. Bronchial inflammation and excessive mucous secretions can narrow or block the bronchial tubes, making breathing difficult.

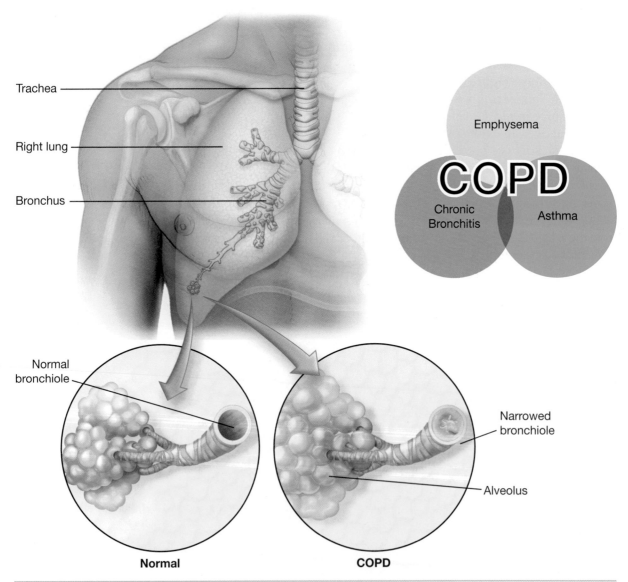

Figure 9.6 COPD is often a combination of emphysema and chronic bronchitis. Although asthma is also marked by constricted bronchial airflow and inflammation, it is recognized as a distinct disease.

Chronic bronchitis is characterized by a long-term cough with mucus production. In **emphysema** (ĕm-fĭ-SĒ-mă), the walls of the alveoli (tiny air sacs in the lungs) have become damaged and lost their elasticity. Less air gets into and out of the lungs, causing **dyspnea** (DĬSP-nē-ă), or difficulty breathing, and lethargy. Because lung damage is irreversible, COPD worsens over time.

Croup

Croup (krūp) is difficulty breathing and a "barking" cough due to inflammation around the larynx (vocal cords) and trachea (Figure 9.7). It is common in infants and children. The cough reflex forces air through the swollen, constricted airway, causing the vocal cords to vibrate with a harsh sound, similar to that of a barking seal. To diagnose croup, the physician listens through a stethoscope for a crackling or rattling sound during inspiration (breathing in) or expiration (breathing out). A rattle or crackle, medically described as *rales*, may be either a loud, low-pitched sound or a very short, high-pitched sound from the lungs.

Upper Respiratory Infection

An **upper respiratory infection (URI)** is any type of infection of the head and chest that is caused by a virus. It can affect the nose, throat, sinuses, and ears. It also can affect the eustachian tube (which connects the middle ear and throat), the trachea, larynx, or bronchial tube.

A URI typically is referred to as the "common cold." It produces a collection of symptoms such as a cough, sore throat, headache, slight fever, ear congestion, and fatigue.

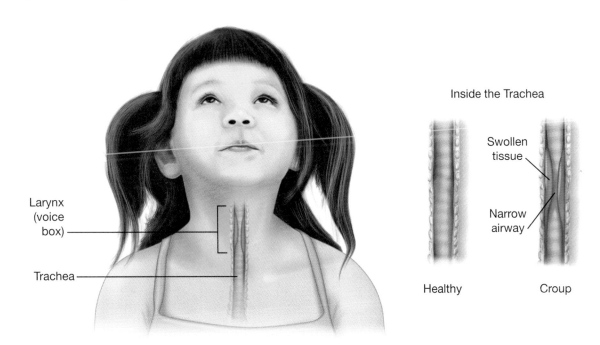

Figure 9.7 Croup is marked by difficulty breathing and a "barking" cough due to inflammation around the larynx and trachea. The disease is common in infants and children.

Obstructive Sleep Apnea

Obstructive sleep apnea (commonly called "sleep apnea") is a condition in which airflow pauses or decreases during sleep due to narrowing or blockage of the airway. As a result, a person with obstructive sleep apnea often snores loudly. A pause in breathing is called an *apnea episode*. The reduced oxygen intake that occurs with sleep apnea causes the person to feel sleepy or drowsy throughout the day.

Pleural Effusion

A **pleural effusion** (ĕ-FYŪ-zhŭn) is an excessive accumulation of fluid between the pleurae, the layers of tissue that envelop the lungs and line the thoracic (chest) cavity (Figure 9.8).

During the act of respiration the lungs expand, the ribs move out, and the diaphragm moves down. Your body naturally produces pleural fluid in small amounts to lubricate the tissue that surrounds the lungs and lines the thoracic cavity. This slippery fluid allows the two surfaces to slide easily against each other. An excessive amount of fluid impairs the ability of the lungs to expand and move, making breathing difficult and painful.

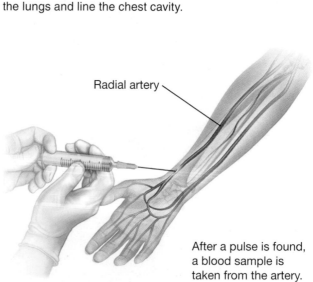

Ribs

Pleural space

Pleural effusion

Figure 9.8 Pleural effusion is an excessive accumulation of fluid between the pleurae, the layers of tissue that surround the lungs and line the chest cavity.

Procedures and Treatments

We will now take a brief look at some diagnostic tests and procedures and therapeutic treatments common to the respiratory system.

Arterial Blood Gas

An **arterial blood gas (ABG) test** measures the levels of oxygen and carbon dioxide in the blood and determines the acidity (pH) of the blood (Figure 9.9). A blood sample typically is collected from the radial artery in the wrist. An ABG test evaluates how well the lungs move oxygen into the blood and remove carbon dioxide from the blood.

Radial artery

After a pulse is found, a blood sample is taken from the artery.

Figure 9.9 An arterial blood gas (ABG) test is used to measure oxygen and carbon dioxide levels in the blood. It also helps determine the acidity (pH) of the blood.

Cardiopulmonary Resuscitation

Cardiopulmonary resuscitation (CPR) is a life-saving technique used when cardiac arrest has occurred (breathing or heartbeat has stopped). When the heart stops, lack of oxygenated blood can cause brain damage in as little as four minutes. The American Heart Association recommends that CPR begin with chest compressions until emergency support arrives. CPR can keep oxygenated blood flowing to the brain and other vital organs until medical professionals can attempt to restore a normal heart rhythm.

Chest X-Ray

A **chest X-ray (CXR)** is a radiographic image of the structure of the thoracic cavity and its organs (Figure 9.10). A chest X-ray is typically taken in the posteroanterior (PA) and lateral positions to obtain detailed anatomical images. These images are analyzed to determine the presence of conditions such as pneumonia, lung disease, pleural effusion, or lung tumor.

Continuous Positive Airway Pressure

Continuous positive airway pressure (CPAP) is a treatment in which a machine is used to deliver a constant flow of mild air pressure through the airways (Figure 9.11). It helps patients with breathing problems maintain adequate levels of arterial oxygen.

CPAP is used to treat conditions such as sleep apnea and respiratory distress syndrome in newborns. The continuous flow of mild air pressure helps keep the alveoli open at the end of exhalation, boosting oxygenation and decreasing the amount of effort needed to breathe. In patients with sleep apnea, CPAP is typically administered through a mask placed over the patient's nose or both the nose and the mouth.

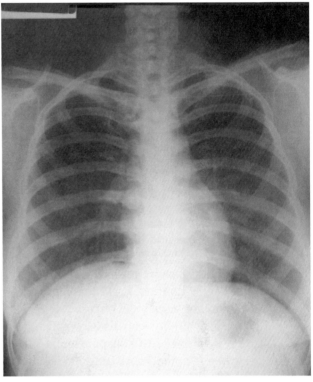

Santibhavank P/Shutterstock.com

Figure 9.10 A chest X-ray is a radiographic image of the structure of the thoracic cavity and its organs.

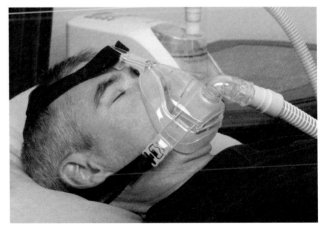

Brian Chase/Shutterstock.com

Figure 9.11 CPAP is a common treatment for sleep apnea.

Pulmonary Function Test

A **pulmonary function test (PFT)** is any of a group of tests that measures lung function (Figure 9.12). The patient breathes into an instrument called a *spirometer* (spī-RŎM-ĕt-ĕr), which determines lung capacity by measuring the volume of air taken in by the lungs during inhalation and released during exhalation. The spirometer records the rate at which air is taken in and expelled by the lungs. PFTs are used to evaluate a broad range of lung diseases, such as asthma, chronic bronchitis, and emphysema.

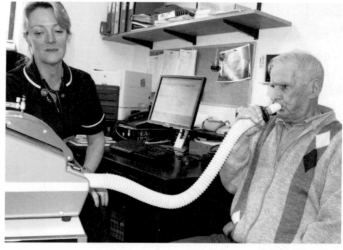

Life in View / Science Source

Figure 9.12 During a pulmonary function test, the patient breathes into a spirometer, which measures lung function.

Sputum Culture and Sensitivity

A **sputum culture and sensitivity (C&S)** involves two separate lab tests. In a *culture test*, microorganisms from a sample of a patient's sputum (mucus or fluid from the lungs) are placed in a culture medium and grown. Once a pathogen has been identified, a *sensitivity* test is done to determine what medicine (typically an antibiotic) will effectively treat a pulmonary infection.

In a manual sensitivity test, disks containing various antibiotics are placed on a culture plate along with a suspension of the isolated bacteria. If the infection is bacterial, the antibiotics that are most effective in treating the infection will inhibit bacterial growth near the disks.

Tuberculin Skin Test

The **tuberculin skin test**, or **TB skin test**, is used to determine whether or not a patient has been exposed to tuberculosis (TB), a highly contagious bacterial disease of the lungs (Figure 9.13). The TB skin test is also called the *PPD skin test* or the *Mantoux* (MÄN-tū) *test*. A sample of the TB bacillus (a purified protein derivative extracted from the disease-causing bacterium), abbreviated *PPD*, is injected intradermally (beneath the epidermis, or outer layer of skin). The skin test is interpreted 48 to 72 hours after the injection to detect exposure to TB.

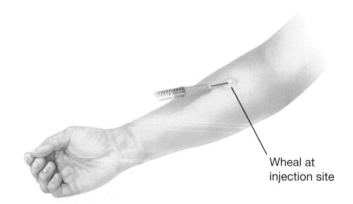

Wheal at injection site

Figure 9.13 The tuberculin (TB) test helps determine whether or not a person has been exposed to the bacterium that causes tuberculosis.

Thoracentesis

Thoracentesis (THOR-ă-sĕn-TĒ-sĭs) is a procedure in which excess fluid is removed from the pleural space, the area between the lungs and the chest wall (Figure 9.14). In certain respiratory disorders and diseases, abnormal fluid buildup in the pleural space puts pressure on the lungs, making breathing difficult.

As you learned earlier in this chapter, excessive buildup of pleural fluid is called a *pleural effusion*. In thoracentesis, a thin needle or plastic tube is inserted into the pleural space to extract excess fluid, allowing the patient to breathe more easily. The fluid is often sent to a pathologist for analysis.

Ventilation/Perfusion Scan

A **ventilation/perfusion scan (VPS)** is also called a **lung scan** or **V/Q scan**. It is a diagnostic nuclear medicine test that measures airflow and blood flow in the lungs. It is used to help diagnose a variety of conditions such as pulmonary embolism, pleural effusion, and pulmonary edema.

During a ventilation/perfusion scan, the patient inhales radioactive gas, which is detected by a machine and converted into an image that reveals details about the patient's lung ventilation (airflow) and lung perfusion (blood flow).

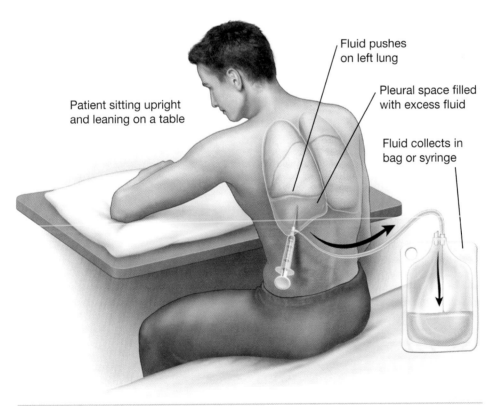

Figure 9.14 Thoracentesis is a procedure for removing fluid buildup in the pleural space, the area between the lungs and chest wall.

Multiple Choice: Diseases and Disorders

Directions: Write the letter of the disease or disorder that matches each numbered definition below.

_D_ 1. a combination of two diseases: chronic bronchitis and emphysema
   a. croup
   b. pleural effusion
   c. pneumothorax
   d. chronic obstructive pulmonary disease

_B_ 2. inflammation of the lining of the bronchial tubes
   a. pneumonia   c. pleural effusion
   b. bronchitis   d. asthma

_C_ 3. collapsed lung
   a. pleural effusion
   b. pneumonia
   c. pneumothorax
   d. chronic obstructive pulmonary disease

_A_ 4. inflammation around the larynx and trachea
   a. croup   c. bronchitis
   b. pneumonia   d. pleural effusion

_D_ 5. disorder caused by inflammation of the bronchi (airways of the lungs)
   a. pneumonia   c. pleural effusion
   b. pneumothorax   d. asthma

_A_ 6. infection of the head and chest caused by a virus
   a. upper respiratory infection
   b. pleural effusion
   c. pneumothorax
   d. chronic obstructive pulmonary disease

_C_ 7. excessive accumulation of fluid between the pleura, the layers of tissue that envelop the lungs and line the chest cavity
   a. pneumonia   c. pleural effusion
   b. bronchitis   d. asthma

_C_ 8. condition in which airflow pauses or decreases during sleep due to narrowing or blockage of the airway
   a. pneumothorax
   b. pneumonia
   c. obstructive sleep apnea
   d. chronic obstructive pulmonary disease

_C_ 9. inflammation of the lungs commonly caused by infection from a bacterium or virus
   a. upper respiratory infection
   b. pleural effusion
   c. pneumonia
   d. chronic obstructive pulmonary disease

SCORECARD: How Did You Do?

Number correct (_____), divided by 9 (_____), multiplied by 100 equals _____ (your score)

Multiple Choice: Procedures and Treatments

Directions: Write the letter of the diagnostic procedure or therapeutic treatment that matches each numbered definition below.

_B_ 1. test used to determine if a patient has been exposed to tuberculosis
   a. pulmonary function test
   b. tuberculin skin test
   c. thoracentesis
   d. sputum culture and sensitivity

_A_ 2. any of a group of tests that measures lung function
   a. pulmonary function test
   b. tuberculin skin test
   c. thoracentesis
   d. sputum culture and sensitivity

_A_ 3. procedure in which excess fluid is removed from the pleural space
   a. thoracentesis
   b. chest X-ray
   c. sputum culture and sensitivity
   d. arterial blood gas test

_D_ 4. test that measures blood levels of oxygen and carbon dioxide as well as the acidity of the blood
   a. pulmonary function test
   b. tuberculin skin test
   c. thoracentesis
   d. arterial blood gas test

_B_ 5. treatment in which a machine is used to deliver a constant flow of mild air pressure through the airways
  a. thoracentesis
  b. constant positive airway pressure
  c. ventilation/perfusion scan
  d. cardiopulmonary resuscitation

_D_ 6. test that identifies which bacterium, virus, or fungus is causing a pulmonary illness and helps determine the most effective antibiotic treatment
  a. pulmonary function test
  b. tuberculin skin test
  c. thoracentesis
  d. sputum culture and sensitivity

_D_ 7. life-saving technique involving the use of chest compressions following cardiac arrest
  a. thoracentesis
  b. constant positive airway pressure
  c. ventilation/perfusion scan
  d. cardiopulmonary resuscitation

SCORECARD: How Did You Do?

Number correct (_____), divided by 7 (_____), multiplied by 100 equals _____ (your score)

Identify Abbreviations

Directions: Write the abbreviation for each medical term listed below.

Medical Term	Abbreviation
1. tuberculosis	TB
2. arterial blood gas	ABG
3. culture and sensitivity	C&S
4. upper respiratory infection	URI
5. pulmonary function test	PFT
6. chest X-ray	CXR
7. continuous positive airway pressure	CPAP
8. ventilation/perfusion scan	VPS
9. cardiopulmonary resuscitation	CPR
10. chronic obstructive pulmonary disease	COPD

SCORECARD: How Did You Do?

Number correct (_____), divided by 10 (_____), multiplied by 100 equals _____ (your score)

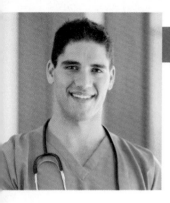

Analyzing the Intern Experience

In the Intern Experience described at the beginning of this chapter, we met Mark, a medical intern with the Oak Forest Urgent Care Center. Mark observed and assisted Dr. Connor Wiley as he examined and talked with David, a high school lacrosse player who came to the clinic because of chest pain and difficulty breathing.

After examining David and obtaining his personal and family health history, Dr. Wiley made a medical diagnosis and provided David with a treatment plan. Later, the physician made a dictated recording of the patient's health information, which was subsequently transcribed into a chart note.

We will now learn more about David's condition from a clinical perspective, interpreting the medical terms in his chart note as we analyze the scenario presented in the Intern Experience.

 ### Audio Activity: David Marino's Chart Note

Directions: At the companion website, listen and read along as the physician dictates David Marino's chart note, shown below. Then do the exercise that appears after the chart note.

CHART NOTE

Patient Name: Marino, David
ID Number: DMM1782
Examination Date: September 7, 20xx

SUBJECTIVE
David is a 17-year-old high school student who complains of shortness of breath and sudden chest pain during lacrosse practice.

OBJECTIVE
Patient presents with pronounced **dyspnea** and elevated pulse and **BP**. Temperature is 101. The **pharynx** is clear. The right lung shows decreased breath sounds with air exchange. **Chest X-ray** reveals a collapsed lower lobe of the right lung.

ASSESSMENT
Pneumothorax due to blunt force rib fracture.

PLAN
Inserted chest tube to reinflate lung. Patient is stable and will be transferred by ambulance to General Hospital.

Interpret David Marino's Chart Note

Directions: After listening to the dictated recording and reading the chart note on David Marino, provide the medical term that matches each definition below. You may encounter terms that were introduced in previous chapters.

Example: dilatation of the bronchus   *Answer:* bronchiectasis

1. collapsed lung   pneumothorax

2. the throat   pharynx

3. difficulty breathing   dyspnea

4. radiographic image of the structure and
   organs of the thoracic cavity   chest X-ray

5. blood pressure   BP

SCORECARD: How Did You Do?

Number correct (_____), divided by 5 (_____), multiplied by 100 equals _____ (your score)

Working with Medical Records

In this activity, you will interpret the medical records (chart notes) of patients with respiratory system disorders. These examples illustrate typical medical records prepared in a real-world healthcare environment. To interpret these chart notes, you will apply your knowledge of word elements (prefixes, combining forms, and suffixes), diseases and disorders, and procedures and treatments related to the respiratory system.

Audio Activity: Emma LaCross's Chart Note

Directions: At the companion website, listen and read along as the physician dictates the following chart note on Emma LaCross. Then do the exercise that appears after the chart note.

CHART NOTE

Patient Name: LaCross, Emma
ID Number: YPU2975
Examination Date: June 10, 20xx

SUBJECTIVE
This 2-year-old female presents with a sore throat and cough that started last night and, according to the mother, "sounded quite croupy." The patient's temperature was not taken.

OBJECTIVE
Patient is alert, well hydrated, afebrile (without fever), and in no acute distress. Both **tympanic** (pertaining to the eardrum) membranes are clear. Throat is mildly injected (filled with fluid). No **exudate** or enlarged tonsils. Neck is supple without **adenopathy**. Lungs are clear with no wheezing or **rales**. Heart is without murmur (abnormal or extra sound heard during a heartbeat).

ASSESSMENT
Croup

PLAN
Mother will use a vaporizer, elevate the child's head when resting, and push fluids. Prescribed Robitussin® DM at bedtime only. Patient should return in 2–4 days if no improvement. Discussed with the mother the normal course of croup and suggested she return or visit an urgent care facility if the condition worsens.

Assessment

Interpret Emma LaCross's Chart Note

Directions: After listening to the dictated recording and reading the chart note on Emma LaCross, provide the medical term that matches each definition below. You may encounter terms that were introduced in previous chapters.

Example: inflammation of the trachea   *Answer:* tracheitis

1. crackling or rattling sound heard in the lungs   rales

2. inflammation around the larynx and trachea   croup

3. disease of the glands   adenopathy

4. pertaining to the eardrum   tympanic

5. fluid that leaks from blood vessels and clogs the air spaces of the lungs   exudate

SCORECARD: How Did You Do?

Number correct (_____), divided by 5 (_____), multiplied by 100 equals _____ (your score)

Audio Activity: Azaria Taylor's Chart Note

Directions: At the companion website, listen and read along as the physician dictates the following chart note on Azaria Taylor. Then do the exercise that appears after the chart note.

CHART NOTE

Patient Name: Taylor, Azaria
ID Number: GLW0331
Examination Date: April 22, 20xx

SUBJECTIVE
This is a 9-year-old female who returns with about 10 days of nasal congestion, cough, and running a fever of 101–103°.

OBJECTIVE
Patient is cooperative but subdued with mild, audible nasal congestion. Throat is clear and neck supple without adenopathy. Coarse **rales** heard in the left lung bases, both posteriorly and laterally. No wheezes or grunting. **CXR** results show consolidation (density) in the left middle lobe and infiltrate (fluid accumulation) in the left lower lobe.

ASSESSMENT
Left middle and lower lobe **pneumonia**.

PLAN
Augmentin® (antibiotic drug), 250 mg chewable, one t.i.d. (3 times a day) x 10 days. Patient should drink fluids for fever control. Recheck in 10 days. Repeat chest X-ray in 4 weeks to verify clearing.

Assessment

Interpret Azaria Taylor's Chart Note

Directions: After listening to the dictated recording and reading the chart note on Azaria Taylor, provide the medical term that matches each definition below.

Example: pain in the chest   *Answer:* thoracalgia

1. crackling or rattling sound heard in lungs   rales

2. chest X-ray   CXR

3. inflammation of the lungs usually caused by a bacterial or viral infection   pneumonia

SCORECARD: How Did You Do?

Number correct (_____), divided by 3 (_____), multiplied by 100 equals _____ (your score)

Chapter Review

Word Elements Summary

Prefixes

Prefix	Meaning
a-	not; without
an-	not; without
brady-	slow
dys-	painful; difficult
endo-	within
hyper-	above; above normal
hypo-	below; below normal
tachy-	fast

Combining Forms

Root Word/Combining Vowel	Meaning
bronch/o, bronchi/o	bronchial tube; bronchus
cyan/o	blue
embol/o	plug; embolus
hem/o	blood
lob/o	lobe (a defined portion of an organ or structure)
ox/o	oxygen
pharyng/o	pharynx; throat
pleur/o	pleura
pneum/o, pneumon/o	lung; air
pulmon/o	lung
rhin/o	nose
spir/o	breathe; breathing
sten/o	narrow; constricted
thorac/o	chest
trache/o	trachea; windpipe

Suffixes

Suffix	Meaning
-al	pertaining to
-algia	pain
-centesis	surgical puncture to remove fluid
-ectasis	dilatation; dilation; expansion
-ectomy	surgical removal; excision
-gram	record; image
-ia	condition
-itis	inflammation
-logist	specialist in the study and treatment of
-logy	study of
-meter	measure
-osis	abnormal condition
-pnea	breathing
-scope	instrument used to observe
-thorax	chest; pleural cavity
-tomy	incision; cut into

More Practice: Activities and Games

The activities on the following pages will help you reinforce your skills and check your mastery of the medical terminology that you learned in this chapter. Visit the companion website for More Practice games and activities.

Audio Activity: Daniel Elliot's Chart Note

Directions: At the companion website, listen and read along as the physician dictates the following chart note on Daniel Elliot. Then do the exercise that appears after the chart note.

CHART NOTE

Patient Name: Elliott, Daniel
ID Number: FRU9764
Examination Date: January 30, 20xx

SUBJECTIVE
This is a 54-year-old male with **emphysema**, **dyspnea**, and increasing weakness. For the last 2 months he has had recurring nocturnal (occurring at night) dyspnea up to 3 times a night but denies problems of orthopnea (difficult breathing when lying flat). He states that he uses an albuterol inhaler for **asthma**, which seems to relieve the symptoms. He is barrel-chested with a productive cough of white **sputum**. Patient is a nonsmoker. **Afebrile** (without fever) with no chills or lower-extremity **edema**.

OBJECTIVE
Mr. Elliott is a thin, gaunt gentleman appearing older than his stated age. BP is 148/64. Pulse is 92. Respirations are 30. Heart is regular in rhythm. Lungs display good air movement with diffuse expiratory (pertaining to exhaling or breathing out) wheezing and prolongation of the expiratory phase. **CXR** reveals flattened diaphragm, increased AP (anteroposterior) diameter and box-car lung shapes consistent with severe emphysema. **Pulmonary function test** before and after albuterol treatment shows severe obstructive changes with no improvement following treatment.

ASSESSMENT
Patient has shortness of breath secondary to **COPD** exacerbation (symptoms made worse by another disease).

PLAN
Refer patient to **pulmonary** medicine specialist.

Assessment

Interpret Daniel Elliot's Chart Note

Directions: After listening to the dictated recording and reading the chart note on Daniel Elliot, provide the medical term that matches each definition below. You may encounter terms that were introduced in previous chapters.

Example: condition of the bronchus and lung   *Answer:* bronchopneumonia

1. disorder caused by inflammation of the bronchi (airways) of the lungs

   asthma

2. pertaining to the lungs

   pulmonary

3. mucus or fluid coughed up from the lungs

   sputum

4. painful or difficult breathing

   dyspnea

5. chest X-ray

   CXR

(Continued on next page)

6. form of COPD in which the walls of the alveoli (tiny air sacs in the lungs) have become damaged and lost their elasticity

emphysema

7. swelling

edema

8. any of a group of tests that measures lung function

pulmonary function test

9. progressive lung disease marked by difficulty breathing; caused by damage to the lungs over a period of years

COPD

10. without fever

afebrile

Break It Down

Directions: In this exercise, dissect each medical term below into its word elements by placing a slash between each word part (prefix, root word, combining vowel, and suffix). Then define each term.

Example:
Medical Term: hyperpnea
Dissection: hyper/pnea
Definition: above-normal breathing

Medical Term

Dissection

1. hyperoxia

h y p e r /o x /i a

Definition: condition of above-normal oxygen

2. bronchiectasis

b r o n c h i /e c t a s i s

Definition: dilation of the bronchial tube/bronchus

3. thoracalgia

t h o r a c /a l g i a

Definition: chest pain

Medical Term	Dissection
4. cyanosis	c y a n/o s i s

Definition: abnormal condition of blue

5. endotracheal	e n d o/t r a c h e/a l

Definition: pertaining to within the trachea/windpipe

6. thoracentesis	t h o r a/c e n t e s i s

Definition: surgical puncture to remove fluid from the chest

7. lobotomy	l o b/o/t o m y

Definition: incision to a lobe

8. thoracotomy	t h o r a c/o/t o m y

Definition: incision to the chest

9. tachypnea	t a c h y/p n e a

Definition: fast breathing

10. bronchostenosis	b r o n c h/o/s t e n/o s i s

Definition: abnormal condition of a narrow/constricted bronchus

11. spirometer	s p i r/o/m e t e r

Definition: measure of breathing

Identify the Medical Word Part

Directions: For each medical word part shown below, indicate whether it is a prefix, root word, or suffix by circling the correct answer. Then write the meaning of the word part.

1. **hypo**　　　　　(Prefix)　　　　Root Word　　　Suffix

   Meaning: below; below normal

2. **centesis**　　　Prefix　　　Root Word　　　(Suffix)

   Meaning: surgical puncture to remove fluid

3. **pleur**　　　　Prefix　　　(Root Word)　　　Suffix

   Meaning: pleura

4. **pulmon**　　　Prefix　　　(Root Word)　　　Suffix

   Meaning: lung

5. **tachy**　　　　(Prefix)　　　Root Word　　　Suffix

   Meaning: fast

6. **thorax**　　　Prefix　　　Root Word　　　(Suffix)

   Meaning: chest; pleural cavity

7. **pnea**　　　　Prefix　　　Root Word　　　(Suffix)

   Meaning: breathing

8. **bronch**　　　Prefix　　　(Root Word)　　　Suffix

   Meaning: bronchial tube/bronchus

Chapter 10
The Cardiovascular System

cardi / o / logy: the study of the heart

Chapter Organization

- Intern Experience
- Overview of Cardiovascular System Anatomy and Physiology
- Word Elements
- Breaking Down and Building Cardiovascular System Terms
- Diseases and Disorders
- Procedures and Treatments
- Analyzing the Intern Experience
- Working with Medical Records
- Chapter Review

Chapter Objectives

After completing this chapter, you will be able to

1. label an anatomical diagram of the cardiovascular system;
2. dissect and define common medical terminology related to the cardiovascular system;
3. build terms used to describe cardiovascular system diseases and disorders, diagnostic procedures, and therapeutic treatments;
4. pronounce and spell common medical terminology related to the cardiovascular system;
5. understand that the processes of building and dissecting a medical term based on its prefix, word root, and suffix enable you to analyze an extremely large number of medical terms beyond those presented in this chapter;
6. interpret the meaning of abbreviations associated with the cardiovascular system; and
7. interpret medical records containing terminology and abbreviations related to the cardiovascular system.

You will see this icon at various points throughout this chapter. The icon indicates that you will find interactive activities and games on the Medical Terminology Companion Website. These activities and games will help you learn, practice, and expand your medical terminology knowledge and skills. Some of these activities are also available on the Medical Terminology Mobile Website.

Companion Website
www.g-wlearning.com/healthsciences

Mobile Site
www.m.g-wlearning.com/5800

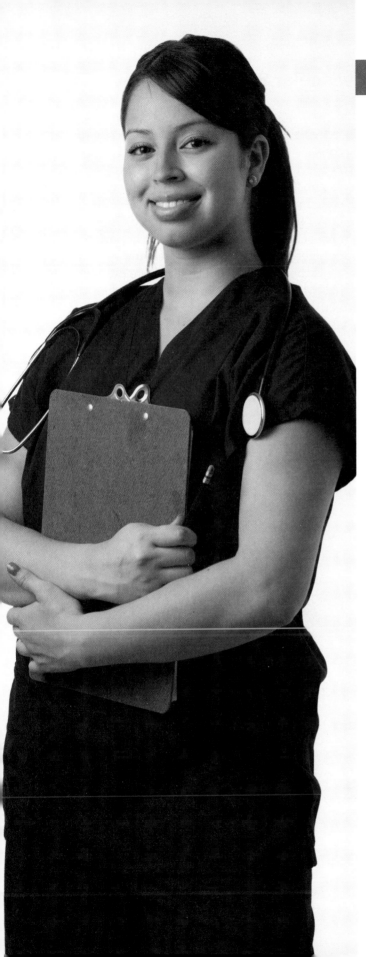

Intern Experience

Layla Stern, an intern with Guardian Urgent Care Center, enters exam room 1, where a middle-aged man is lying on the examination table. He is pale and sweating profusely. A young woman who appears to be in her twenties is hovering near the man, and she is clearly distressed. When Layla begins the triage interview, she learns that Peggy, the young woman, had begged her father, Jim Flowers, to let her go to Citadel Stadium to see her favorite singer. Since Peggy's birthday was approaching, he agreed to take her and her best friend, Mira, to the concert. As they neared the stadium, Peggy was so excited that she didn't notice her father massaging his chest and left arm. When he missed the turn into the parking lot, Peggy yelled and then suddenly noticed that her father was "very pale and sweating a lot." Alarmed, she told him to pull the car over to the side of the road. She helped her father shift into the passenger seat and then drove him to the urgent care center only a few blocks from the stadium.

As you will learn later in this chapter, Jim Flowers has a health condition that has affected his heart, the organ that pumps blood throughout the body. You will have the opportunity to analyze and interpret Jim's patient chart note, the medical record dictated by his physician after the physical examination that Jim received.

In this chapter you will learn common word elements (prefixes, combining forms, and suffixes) used to form medical terms pertaining to the cardiovascular system. Mastery of these terms, and the word parts from which they are constructed, will enable you to understand the health conditions, diagnostic procedures, and therapeutic treatments summarized in the patient chart notes presented throughout this chapter.

Let's begin our study of the cardiovascular system with a brief overview of its anatomy and physiology.

Overview of Cardiovascular System Anatomy and Physiology

The **cardiovascular** (KĂR-dē-ō-VĂS-kyū-lăr) system, or **circulatory** (SĔR-kyŭ-lă-TOR-ē) **system**, consists of the heart and blood vessels (Figure 10.1). This is a huge transportation network. Think of it as a major highway system that transports substances necessary for our survival yet also removes waste that is generated along the way. The cardiovascular system allows continuous movement of blood through the heart and blood vessels. This highway system is composed of a dense network of many different types of blood vessels that work together to transport oxygen and nutrients throughout the body and remove carbon dioxide and other waste products.

Arteries are blood vessels that carry blood away from the heart. They distribute oxygen and nutrients to cells, tissues, and organs throughout the body. Arterioles are very small arterial branches that connect arteries to capillaries. **Capillaries** (KĂP-ĭ-lăr-ēz) are tiny vessels in which the exchange of oxygen, nutrients, and waste products occurs. **Veins** are the blood vessels that carry blood toward the heart. They transport carbon dioxide and other waste products away from the cells, tissues, and organs. **Venules** (VĔN-yulz) are very small veins that connect capillaries to larger veins.

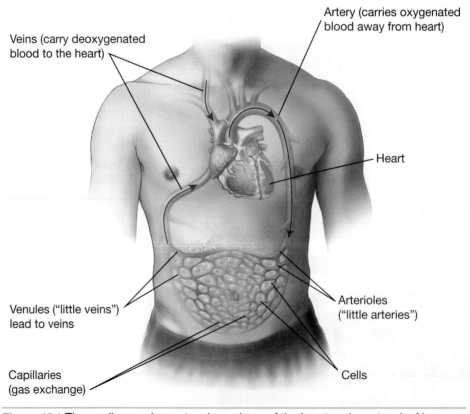

Figure 10.1 The cardiovascular system is made up of the heart and a network of large and progressively smaller blood vessels.

While the arteries, veins, and capillaries make up the dense transportation network of the cardiovascular system, the **heart** functions as the muscular force behind this system. The heart pumps the blood that contains oxygen and nutrients, which our bodies need to survive. Blood also picks up waste products from the cells and delivers them to organs that can eliminate them from the body, such as the lungs, kidneys, and intestines. Dysfunction within the cardiovascular system produces, at best, serious health issues; total failure results in death.

Cardiology (kär-dē-ŎL-ō-jē) is the medical specialty concerned with the study of the heart. A **cardiologist** (kär-dē-ŎL-ō-jĭst) is a physician who specializes in the study, diagnosis, and treatment of diseases and disorders of the heart—and, by extension, the cardiovascular system.

Anatomy and Physiology Vocabulary

Now that you have been introduced to the basic structure and functions of the cardiovascular system, we will explore in a bit more detail the key terms presented in the introduction.

Key Term	Definition
arteries	vessels that carry blood away from the heart and distribute oxygen and nutrients to cells, tissues, and organs
arterioles	very small arterial branches that connect arteries to capillaries
capillaries	tiny vessels in which the exchange of oxygen, nutrients, and waste products occurs
cardiovascular system	the body system that consists of the heart and blood vessels; *circulatory system*
circulatory system	another term for *cardiovascular system*
heart	muscular organ that pumps blood throughout the body
veins	vessels that carry blood toward the heart and remove carbon dioxide and other waste products from cells, tissues, and organs
venules	very small veins that connect capillaries to larger veins

E-Flash Card Activity: Anatomy and Physiology Vocabulary

Directions: After you have reviewed the anatomy and physiology vocabulary related to the cardiovascular system, practice with the e-flash cards until you are comfortable with the spelling and definition of each term.

Identifying Major Organs and Structures of the Cardiovascular System

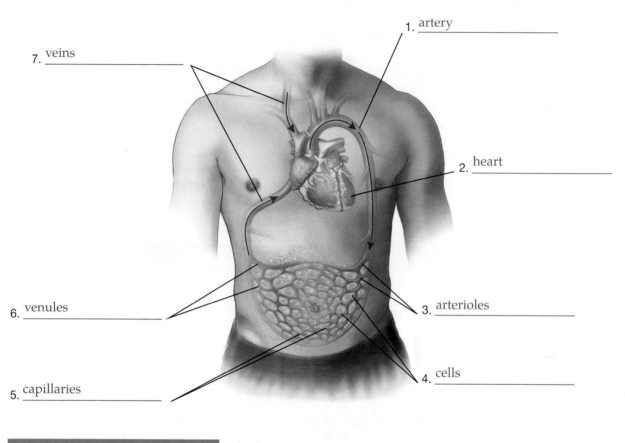

1. artery _____

7. veins _____

2. heart _____

6. venules _____

3. arterioles _____

4. cells _____

5. capillaries _____

Matching Anatomy and Physiology Vocabulary

Directions: Match the vocabulary term in Column A with its meaning in Column B.

Column A

_F_ 1. veins

_H_ 2. arteries

_C_ 3. cardiovascular system

_E_ 4. capillaries

_D_ 5. circulatory system

_A_ 6. heart

_B_ 7. venules

_G_ 8. arterioles

Column B

A. muscular organ that pumps blood throughout the body

B. very small veins that connect capillaries to larger veins

C. the body system that consists of the heart and blood vessels; *circulatory system*

D. another term for *cardiovascular system*

E. tiny vessels in which the exchange of oxygen, nutrients, and waste products occurs

F. vessels that carry blood toward the heart and transport carbon dioxide and other waste products away from the cells, tissues, and organs

G. very small arterial branches that connect arteries to capillaries

H. vessels that carry blood away from the heart and distribute oxygen and nutrients to cells, tissues, and organs

SCORECARD: How Did You Do?

Number correct (_____), divided by 8 (_____), multiplied by 100 equals _____ (your score)

Word Elements

In this section you will learn word elements—prefixes, combining forms, and suffixes—that are common to the cardiovascular system. By learning these word elements and understanding how they are combined to build medical terms, you will be able to analyze Jim's health condition (described in the Intern Experience at the beginning of this chapter) and identify a large number of terms associated with the cardiovascular system.

E-Flash Card Activity: Word Elements

Directions: Review the word elements in the tables that follow. Then, practice with the e-flash cards until you are able to quickly recognize the different word parts (prefixes, combining forms, and suffixes) and their meanings. The e-flash cards are grouped together by prefixes, combining forms, and suffixes, followed by a cumulative review of all the word elements that you learned in this chapter.

Prefixes

Let's begin our study of cardiovascular system word elements by looking at the prefixes listed in the table below. By now, you are familiar with all of these prefixes.

Prefix	Meaning
a-	not; without
brady-	slow
dys-	painful; difficult
hyper-	above; above normal
hypo-	below; below normal
intra-	within
peri-	around
tachy-	fast

Combining Forms

Listed below are combining forms commonly used in medical terms related to the cardiovascular system.

Root Word/Combining Vowel	Meaning
angi/o	blood vessel
arteri/o	artery
ather/o	fatty substance
cardi/o	heart
coron/o	heart
cyan/o	blue
electr/o	electrical activity
hem/o, hemat/o	blood
isch/o	to keep back
my/o	muscle
phleb/o	vein
pulmon/o	lung
sten/o	narrow; constricted
tens/o	pressure; tension
thromb/o	clot
vas/o	vessel; duct
ven/o, ven/i	vein

Suffixes

Listed below are suffixes that appear in medical terms pertaining to the cardiovascular system. From your study of body systems covered in previous chapters, you are already familiar with most of these suffixes.

Suffix	Meaning
-ac	pertaining to
-al	pertaining to
-ary	pertaining to
-ation	process; condition; state of being or having
-emia	blood condition
-gram	record; image
-ia	condition
-ion	process
-itis	inflammation
-logist	specialist in the study and treatment of
-logy	study of
-megaly	large; enlargement
-oma	tumor; mass
-osis	abnormal condition
-ous	pertaining to
-pathy	disease
-penia	deficiency; abnormal reduction
-plasty	surgical repair
-pnea	breathing
-rrhage	bursting forth (of blood)
-rrhexis	rupture
-sclerosis	hardening
-stasis	stop; stand still
-tic	pertaining to
-tomy	incision; cut into
-trophy	development

Matching Prefixes, Combining Forms, and Suffixes

Directions: In each exercise that follows, match the word element in Column A with its meaning in Column B. Some meanings may be used more than once.

Prefixes

Column A

D	1.	dys-
G	2.	intra-
F	3.	tachy-
A	4.	brady-
C	5.	a-
H	6.	peri-
B	7.	hyper-
E	8.	hypo-

Column B

A. slow
B. above; above normal
C. not; without
D. painful; difficult
E. below; below normal
F. fast
G. within
H. around

Combining Forms

Column A

D	1.	isch/o
J	2.	sten/o
L	3.	pulmon/o
N	4.	vas/o
I	5.	thromb/o
B	6.	phleb/o
K	7.	hem/o
B	8.	ven/o
G	9.	angi/o
F	10.	electr/o
A	11.	arteri/o
E	12.	my/o
H	13.	coron/o
H	14.	cardi/o
M	15.	tens/o
C	16.	cyan/o
O	17.	ather/o
B	18.	ven/i
K	19.	hemat/o

Column B

A. artery
B. vein
C. blue
D. to keep back
E. muscle
F. electrical activity
G. blood vessel
H. heart
I. clot
J. narrow; constricted
K. blood
L. lung
M. pressure; tension
N. vessel; duct
O. fatty substance

Suffixes

Column A

P	1. -sclerosis
D	2. -ia
E	3. -itis
B	4. -logist
G	5. -logy
I	6. -megaly
F	7. -oma
O	8. -emia
A	9. -ous
A	10. -ac
A	11. -al
R	12. -gram
L	13. -plasty
A	14. -ary
H	15. -osis
N	16. -rrhexis
S	17. -pnea
Q	18. -ation
M	19. -rrhage
C	20. -trophy
J	21. -pathy
K	22. -penia
U	23. -ion
T	24. -stasis
A	25. -tic
V	26. -tomy

Column B

A. pertaining to
B. specialist in the study and treatment of
C. development
D. condition
E. inflammation
F. tumor; mass
G. study of
H. abnormal condition
I. large; enlargement
J. disease
K. deficiency; abnormal reduction
L. surgical repair
M. bursting forth (of blood)
N. rupture
O. blood condition
P. hardening
Q. process; condition; state of being or having
R. record; image
S. breathing
T. stop; stand still
U. process
V. incision; cut into

SCORECARD: How Did You Do?

Number correct (_____), divided by 53 (_____), multiplied by 100 equals _____ (your score)

Breaking Down and Building Cardiovascular System Terms

Now that you have mastered the prefixes, combining forms, and suffixes for medical terminology pertaining to the cardiovascular system, you have the ability to dissect and build a large number of terms related to this body system.

Below is a list of medical terms commonly used in cardiology, the medical specialty concerning the study, diagnosis, and treatment of diseases and disorders of the cardiovascular system. For each term, a dissection has been provided, along with the meaning of each word element and the definition of the term as a whole.

Term	Dissection	Word Part/Meaning	Term Meaning
Note: *For simplification, combining vowels have been omitted from the Word Part/Meaning column.*			
1. **angioplasty** (ĂN-jē-ō-PLĂS-tē)	angi/o/plasty	**angi** = blood vessel **plasty** = surgical repair	surgical repair of a blood vessel
2. **arteriosclerosis** (är-TĒ-rē-ō-sklĕ-RŌ-sĭs)	arteri/o/sclerosis	**arteri** = artery **sclerosis** = hardening	hardening of the artery
3. **atherosclerosis** (ĂTH-ĕr-ō-sklĕ-RŌ-sĭs)	ather/o/sclerosis	**ather** = fatty substance **sclerosis** = hardening	hardening of a fatty substance
4. **bradycardia*** (BRĀD-ē-KĂR-dē-ă)	brady/card/ia	**brady** = slow **cardi** = heart **ia** = condition	condition of a slow heart
5. **cardiac** (KĂR-dē-ăk)	cardi/ac	**cardi** = heart **ac** = pertaining to	pertaining to the heart
6. **cardiologist** (kär-dē-ŎL-ō-jĭst)	cardi/o/logist	**cardi** = heart **logist** = specialist in the study and treatment of	specialist in the study and treatment of the heart
7. **cardiology** (kär-dē-ŎL-ō-jē)	cardi/o/logy	**cardi** = heart **logy** = study of	study of the heart
8. **cardiomegaly** (KĂR-dē-ō-MĔG-ă-lē)	cardi/o/megaly	**cardi** = heart **megaly** = large; enlargement	enlargement of the heart
9. **cardiomyopathy** (KĂR-dē-ō-mī-ŎP-ă-thē)	cardi/o/my/o/pathy	**cardi** = heart **my** = muscle **pathy** = disease	disease of the heart muscle
10. **cardiopulmonary** (KĂR-dē-ō-PŬL-mō-nĕr-ē)	cardi/o/pulmon/ary	**cardi** = heart **pulmon** = lung **ary** = pertaining to	pertaining to the heart and lung
11. **coronary** (KOR-ō-nār-ē)	coron/ary	**coron** = heart **ary** = pertaining to	pertaining to the heart
12. **electrocardiogram** (ĕ-LĔK-trō-KĂR-dē-ō-gram)	electr/o/cardi/o/gram	**electr** = electrical activity **cardi** = heart **gram** = record; image	record of the electrical activity of the heart

Prefixes = Green   Root Words = Red   Suffixes = Blue

Term	Dissection	Word Part/Meaning	Term Meaning
13. **hemorrhage** (HĔM-ĕ-rĭj)	hem/o/rrhage	**hem** = blood **rrhage** = bursting forth (of blood)	bursting forth of blood
14. **hemostasis** (HĒ-mō-STĀ-sĭs)	hem/o/stasis	**hem** = blood **stasis** = stop; stand still	stop blood (flow)
15. **hypertension** (hī-pĕr-TĔN-shŭn)	hyper/tens/ion	**hyper** = above; above normal **tens** = pressure; tension **ion** = process	process of above-normal pressure/tension
16. **hypertrophy** (hī-PĔR-trŏ-fē)	hyper/trophy	**hyper** = above; above normal **trophy** = development	above-normal development
17. **hypotension** (hī-pō-TĔN-shun)	hypo/tens/ion	**hypo** = below; below normal **tens** = pressure; tension **ion** = process	process of below-normal pressure/tension
18. **myocardial** (mī-ō-KĀR-dē-ăl)	my/o/cardi/al	**my** = muscle **cardi** = heart **al** = pertaining to	pertaining to the heart muscle
19. **pericarditis*** (PĔR-ĭ-kär-DĪ-tĭs)	peri/card/itis	**peri** = around **card** = heart **itis** = inflammation	inflammation around the heart
20. **phlebitis** (flĕ-BĪ-tĭs)	phleb/itis	**phleb** = vein **itis** = inflammation	inflammation of a vein
21. **stenotic** (stĕ-NŎT-ĭk)	sten/o/tic	**sten** = narrow; constricted **tic** = pertaining to	pertaining to (being) narrow/constricted
22. **tachycardia*** (tăk-ē-KĀR-dē-ă)	tachy/card/ia	**tachy** = fast **card** = heart **ia** = condition	condition of a fast heart
23. **thrombophlebitis** (THRŎM-bō-flĕ-BĪ-tĭs)	thromb/o/phleb/itis	**thromb** = clot **phleb** = vein **itis** = inflammation	inflammation of a clot in a vein
24. **thrombosis** (thrŏm-BŌ-sĭs)	thromb/osis	**thromb** = clot **osis** = abnormal condition	abnormal condition of a clot
25. **venous** (VĒ-nŭs)	ven/ous	**ven** = vein **ous** = pertaining to	pertaining to the vein

Prefixes = Green   Root Words = Red   Suffixes = Blue

*Note that in the terms *bradycardia*, *pericarditis*, and *tachycardia*, the letter i is dropped from the root word before the suffix is attached.

Using the pronunciation guide in the Breaking Down and Building chart, practice saying each medical term aloud. To hear the pronunciation of each term, go to the Pronounce It activity at the G-W companion website.

Audio Activity: Pronounce It

Directions: At the companion website, listen as each medical term listed below is pronounced. Practice pronouncing the terms until you are comfortable saying them aloud.

angioplasty
(ĂN-jē-ō-PLĂS-tē)

arteriosclerosis
(är-TĒ-rē-ō-sklĕ-RŌ-sĭs)

atherosclerosis
(ĂTH-ĕr-ō-sklĕ-RŌ-sĭs)

bradycardia
(BRĀD-ē-KÄR-dē-ă)

cardiac
(KÄR-dē-ăk)

cardiologist
(kär-dē-ŎL-ō-jĭst)

cardiology
(kär-dē-ŎL-ō-jē)

cardiomegaly
(KÄR-dē-ō-MĔG-ă-lē)

cardiomyopathy
(KÄR-dē-ō-mī-ŎP-ă-thē)

cardiopulmonary
(KÄR-dē-ō-PŬL-mō-nĕr-ē)

coronary
(KOR-ō-nār-ē)

electrocardiogram
(ĕ-LĔK-trō-KÄR-dē-ō-gram)

hemorrhage
(HĔM-ĕ-rĭj)

hemostasis
(HĒ-mō-STĀ-sĭs)

hypertension
(hī-pĕr-TĔN-shŭn)

hypertrophy
(hī-PĔR-trŏ-fē)

hypotension
(hī-pō-TĔN-shun)

myocardial
(mī-ō-KÄR-dē-ăl)

pericarditis
(PĔR-ĭ-kär-DĪ-tĭs)

phlebitis
(flĕ-BĪ-tĭs)

stenotic
(stĕ-NŎT-ĭk)

tachycardia
(tăk-ē-KÄR-dē-ă)

thrombophlebitis
(THRŎM-bō-flĕ-BĪ-tĭs)

thrombosis
(thrŏm-BŌ-sĭs)

venous
(VĒ-nŭs)

Audio Activity: Spell It

Directions: Cover the medical terms in the Pronounce It activity with a sheet of paper. At the companion website, listen as the terms are read aloud. Correctly spell each term below.

1. angioplasty
2. arteriosclerosis
3. atherosclerosis
4. bradycardia
5. cardiac
6. cardiologist
7. cardiology
8. cardiomegaly
9. cardiomyopathy
10. cardiopulmonary
11. coronary
12. electrocardiogram
13. hemorrhage
14. hemostasis
15. hypertension
16. hypertrophy
17. hypotension
18. myocardial
19. pericarditis
20. phlebitis
21. stenotic
22. tachycardia
23. thrombophlebitis
24. thrombosis
25. venous

Break It Down

Directions: In the exercise that follows, dissect each medical term into its word elements by placing a slash between each word part (prefix, root word, combining vowel, and suffix). Then define each term.

Example:

Medical Term: cardiologist

Dissection: cardi/o/logist

Definition: specialist in the study and treatment of the heart

Medical Term	Dissection

1. venous — v e n/o u s

Definition: pertaining to the vein

2. cardiac — c a r d i/a c

Definition: pertaining to the heart

3. angioplasty — a n g i/o/p l a s t y

Definition: surgical repair of a blood vessel

4. hypertension — h y p e r/t e n s/i o n

Definition: process of above-normal pressure/tension

5. cardiopulmonary — c a r d i/o/p u l m o n/a r y

Definition: pertaining to the heart and lung

6. pericarditis — p e r i/c a r d/i t i s

Definition: inflammation around the heart

Medical Term	Dissection

7. stenotic

s t e n / o / t i c

Definition: pertaining to (being) narrow/constricted

8. arteriosclerosis

a r t e r i / o / s c l e r o s i s

Definition: hardening of the artery

9. cardiology

c a r d i / o / l o g y

Definition: study of the heart

10. hemostasis

h e m / o / s t a s i s

Definition: stop blood (flow)

11. hypotension

h y p o / t e n s / i o n

Definition: process of below-normal pressure/tension

12. thrombosis

t h r o m b / o s i s

Definition: abnormal condition of a clot

13. myocardial

m y / o / c a r d i / a l

Definition: pertaining to the heart muscle

14. electrocardiogram

e l e c t r / o / c a r d i / o / g r a m

Definition: record of the electrical activity of the heart

Medical Term	Dissection
15. atherosclerosis	a t h e r / o / s c l e r o s i s

Definition: hardening of a fatty substance

| 16. bradycardia | b r a d y / c a r d / i a |

Definition: condition of a slow heart

| 17. phlebitis | p h l e b / i t i s |

Definition: inflammation of a vein

| 18. tachycardia | t a c h y / c a r d / i a |

Definition: condition of a fast heart

| 19. coronary | c o r o n / a r y |

Definition: pertaining to the heart

| 20. thrombophlebitis | t h r o m b / o / p h l e b / i t i s |

Definition: inflammation of a clot in a vein

SCORECARD: How Did You Do?

Number correct (_____), divided by 20 (_____), multiplied by 100 equals _____ (your score)

Build It

Directions: In the following exercise, build the medical term that matches each definition by supplying the correct word elements.

P (Prefixes) = Green
RW (Root Words) = Red
S (Suffixes) = Blue
CV (Combining Vowel) = Purple

1. abnormal condition of a clot

thromb	osis
RW	S

2. above-normal development

hyper	trophy
P	S

3. condition of a fast heart

tachy	card	ia
P	RW	S

4. condition of a slow heart

brady	card	ia
P	RW	S

5. disease of the heart muscle

cardi	o	my	o	pathy
RW	CV	RW	CV	S

6. bursting forth (of blood)

hem	o	rrhage
RW	CV	S

7. hardening of a fatty substance

ather	o	sclerosis
RW	CV	S

8. hardening of the artery

arteri	o	sclerosis
RW	CV	S

9. inflammation of a clot in a vein

thromb	o	phleb	itis
RW	CV	RW	S

10. enlargement of the heart

$$\underset{\text{RW}}{\text{cardi}} \quad \underset{\text{CV}}{\text{o}} \quad \underset{\text{S}}{\text{megaly}}$$

11. process of above-normal pressure/tension

$$\underset{\text{P}}{\text{hyper}} \quad \underset{\text{RW}}{\text{tens}} \quad \underset{\text{S}}{\text{ion}}$$

12. pertaining to (being) narrow/constricted

$$\underset{\text{RW}}{\text{sten}} \quad \underset{\text{CV}}{\text{o}} \quad \underset{\text{S}}{\text{tic}}$$

13. pertaining to the heart

$$\underset{\text{RW}}{\text{coron}} \quad \underset{\text{S}}{\text{ary}}$$

14. pertaining to the heart and lung

$$\underset{\text{RW}}{\text{cardi}} \quad \underset{\text{CV}}{\text{o}} \quad \underset{\text{RW}}{\text{pulmon}} \quad \underset{\text{S}}{\text{ary}}$$

15. pertaining to the vein

$$\underset{\text{RW}}{\text{ven}} \quad \underset{\text{S}}{\text{ous}}$$

16. record of the electrical activity of the heart

$$\underset{\text{RW}}{\text{electr}} \quad \underset{\text{CV}}{\text{o}} \quad \underset{\text{RW}}{\text{cardi}} \quad \underset{\text{CV}}{\text{o}} \quad \underset{\text{S}}{\text{gram}}$$

17. stop blood (flow)

$$\underset{\text{RW}}{\text{hem}} \quad \underset{\text{CV}}{\text{o}} \quad \underset{\text{S}}{\text{stasis}}$$

18. study of the heart

$$\underset{\text{RW}}{\text{cardi}} \quad \underset{\text{CV}}{\text{o}} \quad \underset{\text{S}}{\text{logy}}$$

19. surgical repair of a blood vessel

$$\underset{\text{RW}}{\text{angi}} \quad \underset{\text{CV}}{\text{o}} \quad \underset{\text{S}}{\text{plasty}}$$

SCORECARD: How Did You Do?

Number correct (_____), divided by 19 (_____), multiplied by 100 equals _____ (your score)

Diseases and Disorders

From the mild to the severe, diseases and disorders of the cardiovascular system have a variety of causes, some of which are rooted in genetics; others, in lifestyle habits. In this section, we will briefly explore some common pathological conditions of the cardiovascular system and their etiologies (causes).

Aneurysm

An **aneurysm** (ĂN-yū-rĭzm) is the *dilatation* (widening) and thinning of an artery due to a weakness in the arterial wall (Figures 10.2 and 10.3). Each time the heart beats, the thin, weakened wall of the artery balloons outward. Damage to the arterial wall may be congenital (present at birth) or the result of arteriosclerosis (discussed in the next entry). The continuous, repetitive force of each heartbeat can cause the thin blood vessel to rupture. If the aneurysm is located in a critical artery such as in the brain or aorta (large, main artery of the body), sudden death can result.

Arteriosclerosis

Arteriosclerosis (är-TĒ-rē-ō-sklĕ-RŌ-sĭs) is commonly called "hardening of the arteries." As we age, our arteries naturally thicken, grow narrower, and lose their elasticity. Blood vessels affected by arteriosclerosis become less flexible and unable to accommodate increases in blood volume. This limited flexibility can lead to *hypertension* (high blood pressure) and clots that obstruct blood flow.

Atherosclerosis

Atherosclerosis (ĂTH-ĕr-ō-sklĕ-RŌ-sĭs), the most common form of arteriosclerosis, is a chronic (long-term) disease in which the arteries that supply blood to the heart muscle become *stenotic* (narrowed) from fatty deposits called *plaque* (Figure 10.4 on the next page). The fatty plaque builds up along the internal wall of the artery, slowing blood flow and depriving the heart of oxygenated blood, a condition called *ischemia* (ĭs-KĒ-mē-ă).

Ischemia causes cell death and damage to surrounding tissues. Myocardial ischemia, which affects the heart muscle, produces a condition called **angina pectoris** (ĂN-jĭ-nă PĔK-tō-rĭs), more commonly known as severe chest pain. The term *angina pectoris* is often shortened to *angina*.

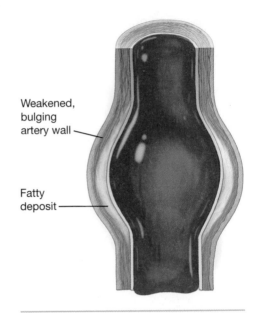

Weakened, bulging artery wall

Fatty deposit

Figure 10.2 An aneurysm is the widening and thinning of an artery due to weakness in the arterial wall. It can be the result of accumulation of fatty deposits in the artery wall.

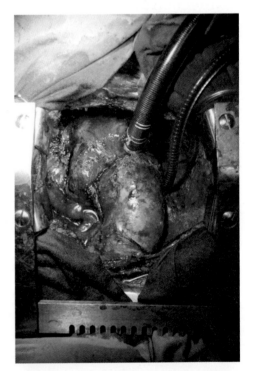

kalewa/Shutterstock.com

Figure 10.3 An aneurysm in one of the large arteries of the heart, shown during "open" surgical repair.

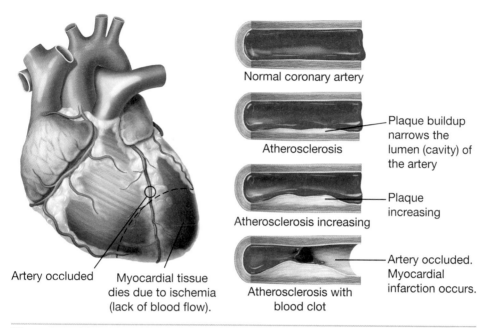

Normal coronary artery

Atherosclerosis

Plaque buildup narrows the lumen (cavity) of the artery

Atherosclerosis increasing

Plaque increasing

Atherosclerosis with blood clot

Artery occluded. Myocardial infarction occurs.

Artery occluded

Myocardial tissue dies due to ischemia (lack of blood flow).

Figure 10.4 Atherosclerosis is marked by stenosis (narrowing) of the arteries that supply blood to the heart muscle. Stenosis is caused by buildup of fatty deposits in the arteries.

Congestive Heart Failure

Congestive heart failure (CHF) occurs when the heart muscle cannot pump enough oxygenated and nutrient-rich blood throughout the body (Figure 10.5). When the heart muscle becomes less effective, blood may back up within other areas of the body, causing fluid buildup in organs, tissues, and extremities. The patient may experience weakness, dyspnea (difficulty breathing), and edema (swelling).

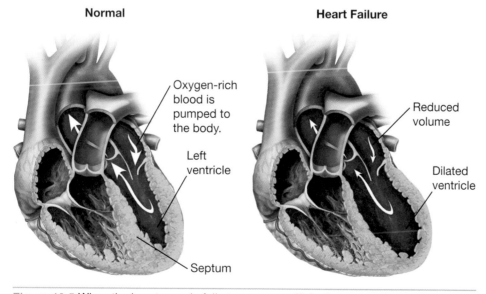

Normal

Heart Failure

Oxygen-rich blood is pumped to the body.

Left ventricle

Septum

Reduced volume

Dilated ventricle

Figure 10.5 When the heart muscle fails to pump a sufficient amount of oxygen throughout the body, the result is congestive heart failure.

The reduction of blood flow to the heart is called *coronary artery disease* (CAD). As time progresses, conditions such as *stenosis* (narrowed arteries of the heart), coronary artery disease, or hypertension may weaken the heart, making it too stiff to pump efficiently. To compensate for this inefficiency, the heart undergoes *hypertrophy* (hī-PĔR-trŏ-fē), or enlargement. More specifically, the thickness of the heart muscle increases. Cardiac hypertrophy temporarily improves blood flow but leads to irregular heartbeat, fluid congestion in the lungs, and retention of fluid in other areas of the body.

Myocardial Infarction

An *infarct* (ĬN-färkt) is an area of tissue that has died due to a lack of oxygenated blood. A **myocardial infarction (MI)**, commonly called a *heart attack*, occurs when the heart muscle is deprived of oxygen (Figure 10.6).

Just like the rest of the body, the heart is supplied with oxygen and nutrients through the arteries. When a coronary artery is occluded (blocked) by a blood clot, for example, the heart is deprived of oxygen, resulting in death of a portion of the muscle (infarction). Heart tissue that dies during an MI does not regenerate, permanently affecting the heart's blood-pumping efficiency.

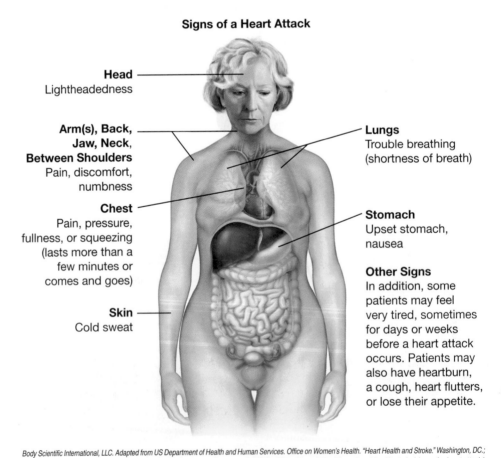

Signs of a Heart Attack

Head
Lightheadedness

Arm(s), Back, Jaw, Neck, Between Shoulders
Pain, discomfort, numbness

Chest
Pain, pressure, fullness, or squeezing (lasts more than a few minutes or comes and goes)

Skin
Cold sweat

Lungs
Trouble breathing (shortness of breath)

Stomach
Upset stomach, nausea

Other Signs
In addition, some patients may feel very tired, sometimes for days or weeks before a heart attack occurs. Patients may also have heartburn, a cough, heart flutters, or lose their appetite.

Body Scientific International, LLC. Adapted from US Department of Health and Human Services. Office on Women's Health. "Heart Health and Stroke." Washington, DC.; available at http://womenshealth.gov/heart-health-stroke/signs-of-a-heart-attack/.

Figure 10.6 Common signs of myocardial infarction, or heart attack.

Varicose Veins

Varicose (VĂR-ĭ-kōs) **veins** are veins that have lost their elasticity (Figures 10.7 and 10.8). As a result, they appear *edematous* (ĕ-DĔM-ă-tŭs) (swollen) and tortuous (having many twists and turns). This appearance is due to the failure of valves within the veins to prevent the backflow of blood. Incompetent valves cause the blood to pool and the veins to swell. A varicose vein disorder can involve both deep veins and superficial (close to the surface) veins. Superficial varicose veins are called "spider veins" and often cause cosmetic embarrassment.

Procedures and Treatments

In this section, you will learn about tests and procedures used to help diagnose pathological conditions of the cardiovascular system, as well as therapeutic methods commonly used to treat certain conditions.

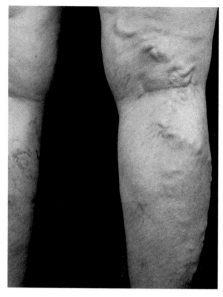

Dr. Barry Slaven/Visuals Unlimited Inc.

Figure 10.7 A patient with varicose veins in the legs, a common site of occurrence

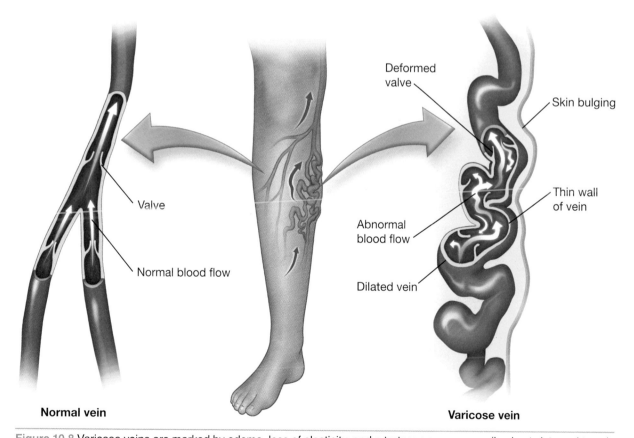

Figure 10.8 Varicose veins are marked by edema, loss of elasticity, and a tortuous appearance (having twists and turns).

Cardiac Catheterization

Cardiac catheterization (KĂTH-ĕ-tĕr-ĭ-ZĀ-shŭn) is a procedure in which a catheter (narrow, flexible tube) is inserted into a vein or artery leading to the heart (Figure 10.9). The catheter insertion usually originates in the groin. Frequently, the catheter is inserted in the femoral artery yet may be introduced through the arm. A contrast agent is then injected through the catheter to "image" the heart, measure cardiac pressures, and withdraw blood samples for analysis (Figure 10.10).

Cardiopulmonary Resuscitation

Cardiopulmonary resuscitation, or **CPR**, is an emergency-response procedure used in an effort to resuscitate a patient who has had a myocardial infarction (heart attack). First responders apply chest compressions or, if available, use an *automated external defibrillator* (AED). This machine delivers an electrical charge to the heart (*defibrillation*) that can restore normal heart rhythm.

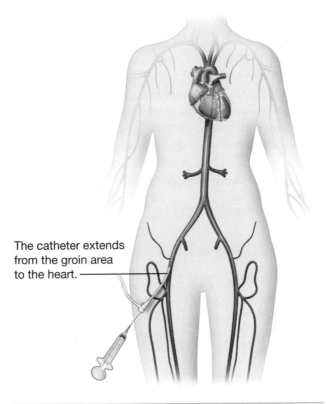

The catheter extends from the groin area to the heart.

Figure 10.9 Cardiac catheterization is a procedure in which images are taken of the heart, cardiac pressures are measured, and blood is withdrawn for laboratory analysis.

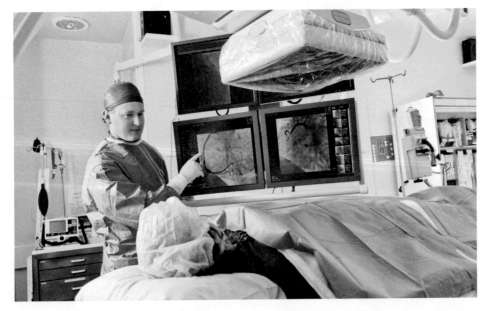

epstock/Shutterstock.com

Figure 10.10 A catheterization lab, or "cath" lab, in a modern hospital

Doppler Sonography

Doppler sonography is a technique used to measure blood flow and blood pressure by "bouncing" ultrasound (high-frequency sound waves) off red blood cells as they circulate through the body. Unlike standard sonography procedures, which cannot show blood flow, Doppler sonography shows images of body organs and tissues as well as blood flow.

During Doppler sonography, sound waves are directed toward the heart to detect and record cardiac anomalies (Figure 10.11). This imaging technique creates moving images of heart muscle contraction, heart valve movement, and blood flow. Doppler sonography is not only limited to the heart but also is used extensively to evaluate venous and arterial blood flow in other areas of the body.

Electrocardiogram

An **electrocardiogram (ECG)** is a diagnostic procedure used to record the electrical activity of the heart (Figure 10.12). ECG aids in diagnosing dysfunction of, or damage to, cardiac tissue.

If a patient has intermittent yet persistent chest pain or *arrhythmia* (painful or irregular heart contractions), a cardiologist may instruct a patient to wear a device called a *Holter monitor*. Because heart irregularities are difficult to capture on a single ECG, the Holter monitor is worn by the patient for about 24 hours. The patient keeps track of all daily activities in a diary. Then the cardiologist compares this data to the electrical activity of the heart recorded by the Holter monitor. This comparison provides the cardiologist with further insight to help identify the etiology (cause) of the heart dysfunction or damage.

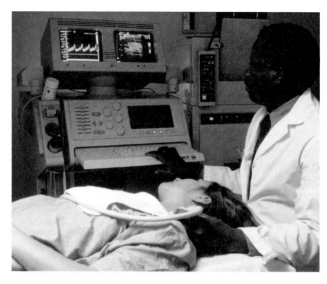

Ouellette Theroux/Publiphoto/Science Source

Figure 10.11 In Doppler sonography, blood flow and blood pressure are measured by "bouncing" ultrasound (high-frequency sound waves) off red blood cells as they travel through the body.

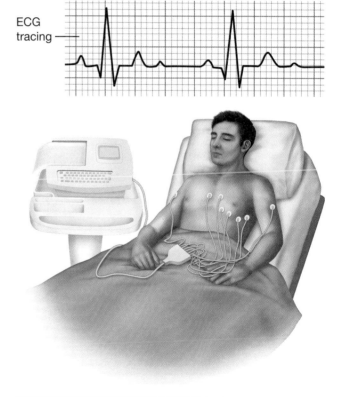

ECG tracing

Figure 10.12 Electrocardiogram, or ECG, is a common procedure for identifying cardiac dysfunction or damage.

Pacemaker

An irregular rate or rhythm of the heart is called *arrhythmia*. *Bradycardia*, for example, is a type of arrhythmia in which the heart beats too slowly. *Tachycardia* is a form of arrhythmia in which the heart beats too fast.

Cardiac arrhythmia may be treated with the insertion of a **pacemaker** (Figures 10.13, 10.14, and 10.15). A pacemaker is a device that corrects arrhythmia by stimulating contraction of the heart muscle with mild electrical impulses.

In more severe cases of cardiac arrhythmia, or when a patient has suffered a heart attack or is at high risk of having one, an electronic device called an **implantable cardioverter defibrillator (ICD)** is surgically placed inside the chest cavity. The ICD has wires with electrodes that are attached to the heart. The high-energy electrical impulses delivered by the ICD will shock the heart if a life-threatening arrhythmia occurs or the heart stops beating.

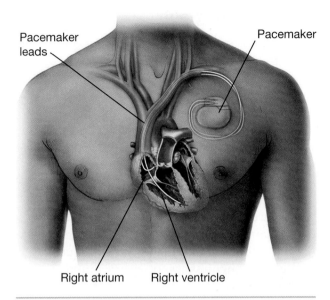

Figure 10.13 A pacemaker, which helps maintain normal heart rhythm, typically has two leads: one that enters the right atrium (right upper chamber of the heart) and one that enters the right ventricle (lower right chamber of the heart). The pacemaker works by making contractions in these chambers occur "in sync" (together at the same rate).

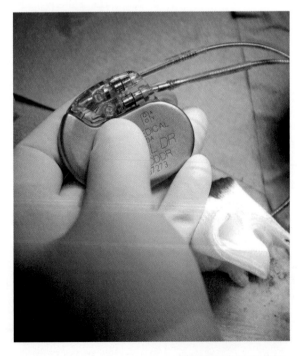

Figure 10.14 A surgeon holds a pacemaker that is about to be implanted in a patient's chest.

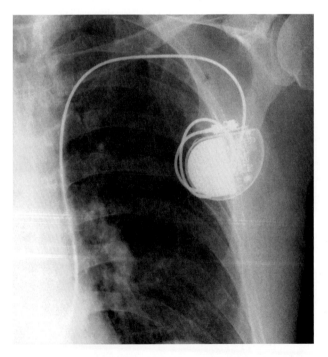

Figure 10.15 An X-ray image of a pacemaker in a patient's chest cavity.

Multiple Choice: Diseases and Disorders

Directions: Write the letter of the disease or disorder that matches each numbered definition.

B   1. disease in which the arteries thicken, narrow, and lose their elasticity
   a. aneurysm
   b. arteriosclerosis
   c. congestive heart failure
   d. varicose veins

C   2. event in which the heart muscle is deprived of oxygen
   a. atherosclerosis
   b. aneurysm
   c. myocardial infarction
   d. congestive heart failure

A   3. disease in which the heart muscle cannot pump enough oxygenated blood
   a. congestive heart failure
   b. atherosclerosis
   c. aneurysm
   d. myocardial infarction

B   4. dilatation and thinning of an artery due to weakness in the arterial wall
   a. atherosclerosis
   b. aneurysm
   c. myocardial infarction
   d. congestive heart failure

D   5. veins that have lost their elasticity and appear swollen and tortuous
   a. atherosclerotic veins
   b. arteriosclerotic veins
   c. stenotic veins
   d. varicose veins

C   6. chronic disease in which the arteries that supply blood to the heart muscle become narrowed from fatty deposits
   a. aneurysm
   b. myocardial infarction
   c. atherosclerosis
   d. varicose veins

SCORECARD: How Did You Do?

Number correct (_____), divided by 6 (_____), multiplied by 100 equals _____ (your score)

Multiple Choice: Procedures and Treatments

Directions: Write the letter of the diagnostic procedure or therapeutic treatment that matches each numbered definition.

A   1. diagnostic procedure used to record the electrical activity of the heart
   a. electrocardiogram
   b. Doppler sonography
   c. cardiopulmonary resuscitation
   d. cardiac catheterization

B   2. procedure in which high-frequency sound waves are used to measure blood flow and blood pressure
   a. cardiopulmonary resuscitation
   b. Doppler sonography
   c. cardiac catheterization
   d. electrocardiogram

A   3. device that delivers mild electrical impulses to the heart to correct arrhythmia
   a. pacemaker
   b. Doppler sonography
   c. electrocardiogram
   d. cardiac catheterization

B   4 procedure in which a narrow, flexible tube is inserted into a vein or artery leading to the heart
   a. Doppler sonography
   b. cardiac catheterization
   c. pacemaker
   d. electrocardiogram

(Continued on next page)

<u>C</u> 5. emergency-response procedure used to try to revive a patient who has suffered a heart attack
   a. cardiac catheterization
   b. Doppler sonography
   c. cardiopulmonary resuscitation
   d. electrocardiogram

<u>B</u> 6. device surgically placed within the chest cavity to shock the heart when a dangerous arrhythmia occurs or the heart stops beating
   a. cardiac catheter
   b. implantable cardioverter defibrillator
   c. pacemaker
   d. cardiopulmonary resuscitator

SCORECARD: How Did You Do?

Number correct (_____), divided by 6 (_____), multiplied by 100 equals _____ (your score)

Assessment

Identifying Abbreviations

Directions: Write the abbreviation for each medical term listed below.

Medical Term	Abbreviation
1. myocardial infarction	MI
2. congestive heart failure	CHF
3. implantable cardioverter defibrillator	ICD
4. electrocardiogram	ECG
5. cardiopulmonary resuscitation	CPR
6. coronary artery disease	CAD
7. automated external defibrillator	AED

SCORECARD: How Did You Do?

Number correct (_____), divided by 7 (_____), multiplied by 100 equals _____ (your score)

Analyzing the Intern Experience

In the Intern Experience described at the beginning of this chapter, we met Layla, a medical intern with the Guardian Urgent Care Center. Layla shadowed (observed and assisted) the doctor as he examined and talked with Jim Flowers, a middle-aged man who came to the immediate-care center because of cardiac symptoms, including chest pain and profuse sweating.

After examining Mr. Flowers and obtaining his personal and family health history, the physician made a pending medical diagnosis of congestive heart failure and ordered a cardiac catheterization procedure. Later, the physician made a dictated recording of the patient's health information, which was subsequently transcribed into a chart note.

We will now learn more about Jim Flowers' condition from a clinical perspective, interpreting the medical terms in his chart note as we analyze the scenario presented in the Intern Experience.

Audio Activity: Jim Flowers' Chart Note

Directions: At the companion website, listen and read along as the physician dictates Jim Flowers' chart note, shown below. Then do the exercise that appears after the chart note.

CHART NOTE

Patient Name: Flowers, Jim
ID Number: 95432
Examination Date: February 18, 20xx

SUBJECTIVE
Jim is a 55-year-old male who presents to the Guardian Urgent Care Clinic after an episode of intense chest pain and tingling and numbness of his left arm that occurred while driving his daughter to a concert. The pain was relieved by placing a nitroglycerin tablet under his tongue. Because of concerns from both his daughter and wife, he is here today for a follow-up.

OBJECTIVE
BP is 110/84, respirations 20, pulse is 90/min and regular. Temperature normal. His chest X-ray reveals a **pacemaker** on the left, **cardiomegaly**, and increased markings suggestive of **congestive heart failure**. The **ECG** reveals normal rate and rhythm.

ASSESSMENT
1. **Angina pectoris**.
2. Cardiomegaly.
3. Possible **CHF**.

PLAN
Admit patient to County Hospital for **cardiac catheterization**.

Interpret Jim Flowers' Chart Note

Directions: After listening to the dictated recording and reading the chart note on Jim Flowers, provide the medical term that matches each definition below.

Example: inflammation of a vein   *Answer:* phlebitis

1. disease in which the heart muscle cannot pump enough oxygenated and nutrient-rich blood throughout the body

    congestive heart failure

2. procedure in which a narrow, flexible tube is inserted into a vein or artery leading to the heart

    cardiac catheterization

3. severe chest pain caused by myocardial ischemia (disruption of blood flow to the heart muscle caused by obstruction of a blood vessel)

    angina pectoris

4. diagnostic procedure used to record the electrical activity of the heart

    ECG

5. enlargement of the heart

    cardiomegaly

6. device that delivers mild electrical impulses to the heart to correct arrhythmia

    pacemaker

7. abbreviation for *congestive heart failure*

    CHF

SCORECARD: How Did You Do?

Number correct (_____), divided by 7 (_____), multiplied by 100 equals _____ (your score)

Working with Medical Records

In this activity, you will interpret the medical records (chart notes) of patients with cardiovascular system disorders. These examples illustrate typical medical records prepared in a real-world healthcare environment. To interpret these chart notes, you will apply your knowledge of word elements (prefixes, combining forms, and suffixes), diseases and disorders, and procedures and treatments related to the cardiovascular system.

Audio Activity: Carrie Geiger's Chart Note

Directions: At the companion website, listen and read along as the physician dictates the following chart note on Carrie Geiger. Then do the exercise that appears after the chart note. You may encounter terms that were introduced in previous chapters.

CHART NOTE

Patient Name: Geiger, Carrie
ID Number: 67854
Examination Date: April 4, 20xx

SUBJECTIVE
Carrie is a 24-year-old female who presents with swelling, redness, and tenderness of the right **posterior** extremity, present for the past 72 hours and becoming more uncomfortable and swollen. She has some pain with walking. It is worse after being on her feet all day. She recalls no direct trauma to the area. She is on birth control pills. Nonsmoker.

OBJECTIVE
She has localized **erythema**, induration (areas of hardened tissue), tenderness, and **edema** along the right lower extremity. **Varicose veins** noted distally and proximally.

ASSESSMENT
Chronic **venous** insufficiency with superficial **thrombophlebitis**. No deep vein venous **thrombosis**.

PLAN
Ibuprofen 60 mg BID with food (take a 60-mg tablet of ibuprofen twice a day). Apply warm compresses to the affected area for 30–60 minutes TID (three times a day). Elevate leg as needed. Will recheck in 2–3 weeks or sooner if no improvement.

Assessment

Interpret Carrie Geiger's Chart Note

Directions: After listening to the dictated recording and reading the chart note on Carrie Geiger, provide the medical term that matches each definition below. You may encounter terms that were introduced in previous chapters.

Example: enlargement of the heart   *Answer:* cardiomegaly

1. pertaining to the veins   venous
2. abnormal condition of a clot   thrombosis
3. veins that appear swollen and tortuous due to loss of elasticity   varicose veins
4. inflammation of a clot in a vein   thrombophlebitis
5. redness of the skin   erythema
6. swelling   edema
7. pertaining to the back (of the body)   posterior

SCORECARD: How Did You Do?

Number correct (_____), divided by 7 (_____), multiplied by 100 equals _____ (your score)

Audio Activity: Richard Thomas's Chart Note

Directions: At the companion website, listen and read along as the physician dictates the following chart note on Richard Thomas. Then do the exercise that appears after the chart note.

CHART NOTE

Patient Name: Thomas, Richard
ID Number: 61842
Examination Date: July 19, 20xx

SUBJECTIVE
This 71-year-old male has a history of multiple episodes of **epistaxis** (nosebleeds). No history of nose trauma. **Hemorrhage** comes on spontaneously, usually at night or in the early morning. He may go a couple of months with one and then gets one every day for a few weeks. They start at rest and occasionally with exertion. He has been able to stop the bleeding by applying direct pressure to the nose. He has no other bleeding problems. He is currently taking antihypertensive (pertaining to preventing or controlling high blood pressure) medications.

OBJECTIVE
Blood pressure is 176/80; pulse 80. There is no active bleeding at this time. A small, dried blood clot is noted in the left nostril, which may be the bleeding site.

ASSESSMENT
1. **Hypertension**
2. Recurrent epistaxis

PLAN
Patient was given Procardia XL® sublingually (pertaining to under the tongue), with blood pressure dropping to 140/75. Vaseline® jelly was applied to the left nostril anteriorly. Patient was instructed in treatment of nosebleeds if they recur. Patient instructed to take Procardia XL once daily. Follow up for blood pressure check in 2 weeks.

Assessment

Interpret Richard Thomas's Chart Note

Directions: After listening to the dictated recording and reading the chart note on Richard Thomas, provide the medical term that matches each definition below.

Example: inflammation around the heart   *Answer:* pericarditis

1. bursting forth (excessive discharge) of blood   hemorrhage

2. process of above-normal pressure   hypertension

3. nosebleeds   epistaxis

SCORECARD: How Did You Do?

Number correct (_____), divided by 3 (_____), multiplied by 100 equals _____ (your score)

Chapter Review

Word Elements Summary

Prefixes

Prefix	Meaning
a-	not; without
brady-	slow
dys-	painful; difficult
hyper-	above; above normal
hypo-	below; below normal
intra-	within
peri-	around
tachy-	fast

Combining Forms

Root Word/Combining Vowel	Meaning
angi/o	blood vessel
arteri/o	artery
ather/o	fatty substance
cardi/o	heart
coron/o	heart
cyan/o	blue
electr/o	electrical activity
hem/o, hemat/o	blood
isch/o	to keep back
my/o	muscle
phleb/o	vein
pulmon/o	lung
sten/o	narrow; constricted
tens/o	pressure; tension
thromb/o	clot
vas/o	vessel; duct
ven/o, ven/i	vein

Suffixes

Suffix	Meaning
-ac	pertaining to
-al	pertaining to
-ary	pertaining to
-ation	process; condition; state of being or having
-emia	blood condition
-gram	record; image
-ia	condition
-ion	process
-itis	inflammation
-logist	specialist in the study and treatment of
-logy	study of
-megaly	large; enlargement
-oma	tumor; mass
-osis	abnormal condition
-ous	pertaining to
-pathy	disease
-penia	deficiency; abnormal reduction
-plasty	surgical repair
-pnea	breathing
-rrhage	bursting forth (of blood)
-rrhexis	rupture
-sclerosis	hardening
-stasis	stop; stand still
-tic	pertaining to
-tomy	incision; cut into
-trophy	development

More Practice: Activities and Games

The activities on the following pages will help you reinforce your skills and check your mastery of the medical terminology that you learned in this chapter. Visit the companion website for More Practice games and activities.

Break It Down

Directions: Dissect each medical term below into its word elements by placing a slash between each word part (prefix, root word, combining vowel, and suffix). Then define each term.

Example:
Medical Term: arteriosclerosis
Dissection: arteri/o/sclerosis
Definition: hardening of the arteries

Medical Term	**Dissection**
1. cardiorrhexis	c a r d i /o/ r r h e x i s

Definition: rupture of the heart

| 2. hematoma | h e m a t /o m a |

Definition: tumor of the blood

| 3. phlebography | p h l e b /o/ g r a p h y |

Definition: process of recording an image of a vein

| 4. ischemia | i s c h /e m i a |

Definition: condition of keeping back blood

| 5. hemangioma | h e m /a n g i /o m a |

Definition: tumor of the blood and blood vessel

Medical Term	Dissection

6. phlebotomy   p h l e b / o / t o m y

Definition: incision to a vein (to withdraw blood)
_____

7. arteriorrhexis   a r t e r i / o / r r h e x i s

Definition: rupture of an artery
_____

8. thrombostasis   t h r o m b / o / s t a s i s

Definition: the stopping of a clot
_____

9. pericardial   p e r i / c a r d i / a l

Definition: pertaining to the area around the heart
_____

10. stenocardia   s t e n / o / c a r d / i a

Definition: condition of a narrow/constricted heart
_____

11. thromboangiitis   t h r o m b / o / a n g i / i t i s

Definition: inflammation of a clot in a blood vessel
_____

12. angioma   a n g i / o m a

Definition: tumor in a blood vessel
_____

Audio Activity: Samuel Gibson's Chart Note

Directions: At the companion website, listen and read along as the physician dictates the following chart note on Samuel Gibson. Then do the exercise that appears after the chart note.

CHART NOTE

Patient Name: Gibson, Samuel
ID Number: 25448
Date of Service: March 1, 2014

SUBJECTIVE
Mr. Gibson is an obese 64-year-old male who is slightly **dyspneic** (pertaining to difficulty breathing) with a history of **hypertension** who yesterday experienced chest discomfort. The patient describes persistent pain across the upper chest with associated severe **dyspnea**. This occurred while walking his dog. Chest discomfort resolved after resting on a bench. The patient awoke today to chest pain and seeks advice.

OBJECTIVE
Blood pressure is 144/91 with a pulse of 80. Respiratory rate is 16/min. Heart is regular in rate and rhythm. **Cardiac** risk factors include hypertension, obesity, and a positive family history of **CAD**. **Electrocardiogram** is normal.

ASSESSMENT
1. Unstable **angina pectoris**
2. Hypertension

PLAN
Admit patient to County Hospital to exclude **myocardial infarction** and to initiate therapy with beta blockers (drugs used to reduce hypertension), aspirin, and heparin (blood thinner). The patient will also undergo **cardiac catheterization**.

Assessment

Interpret Samuel Gibson's Chart Note

Directions: After listening to the dictated recording and reading the chart note on Samuel Gibson, provide the medical term that matches each definition below. You may encounter terms that were introduced in previous chapters.

Example: disease of the heart muscle   *Answer:* cardiomyopathy

1. difficulty breathing   dyspnea

2. above-normal blood pressure   hypertension

3. the reduction of blood flow to the heart; coronary artery disease   CAD

(Continued)

4. record of the electrical activity of the heart   electrocardiogram

5. procedure in which a narrow, flexible tube is inserted into a vein or artery leading to the heart   cardiac catheterization

6. severe chest pain   angina pectoris

7. pertaining to the heart   cardiac

8. event in which the heart muscle is deprived of oxygen   myocardial infarction

9. pertaining to difficulty breathing   dyspneic

10. blood pressure   BP

Spelling

Directions: Circle the correctly spelled term in each row.

1.	cardiamegaly	chardiomegaly	(cardiomegaly)	cardioalmegaly
2.	(hemostasis)	hemastasis	haemastasis	hemmastasis
3.	periocarditis	peracarditis	pericharditis	(pericarditis)
4.	myacardial	(myocardial)	myocardeal	myochardial
5.	(hypertrophy)	hypertrophe	hyperotrophy	hypertroephy
6.	bradicardia	bradichardia	(bradycardia)	bradychardia
7.	cardiamyopathy	cardeomyopathy	cardialmyopathy	(cardiomyopathy)
8.	(angioplasty)	angialplasty	angeoplasty	anginoplasty
9.	phlobitis	phleabitis	(phlebitis)	phlebytis
10.	tachychardia	(tachycardia)	tachycardea	tachychardea
11.	thromboesis	(thrombosis)	thrombosys	thrombolsis
12.	(venous)	veinous	venious	veneous

Identify the Medical Word Part

Directions: For each medical word part shown below, indicate whether it is a prefix, root word, or suffix by circling the correct answer. Then write the meaning of the word part.

1. **cardi**   Prefix   (Root Word)   Suffix

   Meaning: heart _____

2. **ather**   Prefix   (Root Word)   Suffix

   Meaning: fatty substance _____

3. **emia**   Prefix   Root Word   (Suffix)

   Meaning: blood condition _____

4. **tachy**   (Prefix)   Root Word   Suffix

   Meaning: fast _____

5. **ation**   Prefix   Root Word   (Suffix)

   Meaning: process; condition; state of being or having _____

6. **rrhage**   Prefix   Root Word   (Suffix)

   Meaning: bursting forth (of blood) _____

7. **steno**   Prefix   (Root Word)   Suffix

   Meaning: narrow/constricted _____

8. **thromb**   Prefix   (Root Word)   Suffix

   Meaning: clot _____

9. **tens**   Prefix   (Root Word)   Suffix

   Meaning: pressure; tension _____

10. **pulmon**   Prefix   (Root Word)   Suffix

    Meaning: lung _____

Cumulative Review

Chapters 8–10: Reproductive System, Respiratory System, and Cardiovascular System

Directions: Check your mastery of common word elements used in medical terminology related to the male and female reproductive systems, respiratory system, and cardiovascular system. Write the definition of each prefix, combining form, and suffix listed below. For more cumulative review practice, visit the companion website.

Prefixes

a-	not; without
an-	not; without
brady-	slow
dys-	painful; difficult
endo-	within
hyper-	above; above normal
hypo-	below; below normal
intra-	within
peri-	around
tachy-	fast
trans-	across

Combining Forms

angi/o	blood vessel
arteri/o	artery
ather/o	fatty substance
bronch/o, bronchi/o	bronchial tube; bronchus
cardi/o	heart
coron/o	heart
cyan/o	blue
cervic/o	cervix; neck

colp/o	vagina
cyst/o	bladder; sac containing fluid
electr/o	electrical activity
embol/o	plug; embolus
gynec/o	woman; female
hem/o, hemat/o	blood
hyster/o	uterus
isch/o	to keep back
lapar/o	abdomen
lob/o	lobe (a defined portion of an organ or structure)
mamm/o	breast
mast/o	breast
men/o	menstruation
metr/o, metri/o	uterus
my/o	muscle
oophor/o	ovary
orchid/o	testes
ox/o	oxygen
pharyng/o	pharynx; throat
phleb/o	vein
pleur/o	pleura
pneum/o	lung; air
pneumon/o	lung; air
prostat/o	prostate gland
pulmon/o	lung
rhin/o	nose
salping/o	uterine tube; fallopian tube
scrot/o	scrotum

spir/o	breathe; breathing
sten/o	narrow; constricted
tens/o	pressure; tension
testicul/o	testes
thorac/o	chest
thromb/o	clot
trache/o	trachea; windpipe
ur/o	urine; urinary tract
vagin/o	vagina
vas/o	vessel; duct
ven/o, ven/i	vein

Suffixes

-ac	pertaining to
-al	pertaining to
-algia	pain
-ary	pertaining to
-ation	process; condition; state of being or having
-centesis	surgical puncture to remove fluid
-ectasis	dilatation; dilation; expansion
-ectomy	surgical removal; excision
-emia	blood condition
-gram	record; image
-graphy	process of recording an image
-ia	condition
-ic	pertaining to
-ion	process
-itis	inflammation

-logist	specialist in the study and treatment of
-logy	study of
-megaly	large; enlargement
-meter	measure
-oma	tumor; mass
-osis	abnormal condition
-ous	pertaining to
-pathy	disease
-penia	deficiency; abnormal reduction
-pexy	surgical fixation
-plasty	surgical repair
-pnea	breathing
-rrhage	bursting forth (of blood)
-rrhagia	bursting forth (of blood)
-rrhaphy	suture
-rrhea	discharge; flow
-rrhexis	rupture
-sclerosis	hardening
-scope	instrument used to observe
-scopy	process of observing
-stasis	stop; stand still
-thorax	chest; pleural cavity
-tic	pertaining to
-tomy	incision; cut into
-trophy	development

Chapter 11

The Endocrine System

endo / crin / o / logy = the study of secretions within

Chapter Organization

- Intern Experience
- Overview of Endocrine System Anatomy and Physiology
- Word Elements
- Breaking Down and Building Endocrine System Terms
- Diseases and Disorders
- Tests and Procedures
- Analyzing the Intern Experience
- Working with Medical Records
- Chapter Review

Chapter Objectives

After completing this chapter, you will be able to

1. label an anatomical diagram of the endocrine system;
2. dissect and define common medical terminology related to the endocrine system;
3. build terms used to describe endocrine system diseases and disorders and diagnostic procedures;
4. pronounce and spell common medical terminology related to the endocrine system;
5. understand that the processes of building and dissecting a medical term based on its prefix, word root, and suffix enable you to analyze an extremely large number of medical terms beyond those presented in this chapter;
6. interpret the meaning of abbreviations associated with the endocrine system; and
7. interpret medical records containing terminology and abbreviations related to the endocrine system.

You will see this icon [↗] at various points throughout this chapter. The icon indicates that you will find interactive activities and games on the Medical Terminology Companion Website. These activities and games will help you learn, practice, and expand your medical terminology knowledge and skills. Some of these activities are also available on the Medical Terminology Mobile Website.

Companion Website
www.g-wlearning.com/healthsciences

Mobile Site
www.m.g-wlearning.com/5800

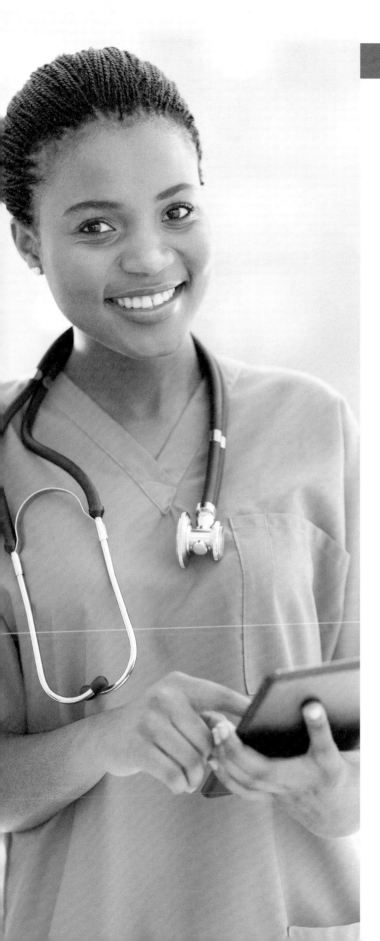

Liza Stephens has just finished the "textbook learning" part of a medical assistant degree program, and she is eager to put her knowledge and skills to work. Liza has been assigned by the school to serve an internship with the Stringfield Medical Associates, an internal medicine practice. She is reporting to Jeff Blishmer, an LPN (licensed practical nurse) who assists Dr. Pitcher.

Today Liza meets Mrs. Kathryn Noah, a 78-year-old patient with poor ambulation (walking). Liza assists her into a wheelchair and pushes the chair into an exam room. Liza listens as Mrs. Noah tells the nurse that she has a fever and feelings of numbness and tingling in her left big toe. Jeff, the nurse, notes that the toe is bluish in color, accompanied by a foul-smelling discharge. After recording these details in Mrs. Noah's medical record, Jeff uses his laptop to electronically signal to the physician that the patient is ready to be seen.

As you will learn later in this chapter, Mrs. Noah is suffering from a condition that has affected her endocrine system. To help you understand her health problem, this chapter will present word elements (combining forms, prefixes, and suffixes) that make up medical terms related to the endocrine system. As you learn these terms, you will recognize many common word elements from your study of body systems covered in previous chapters—particularly prefixes and suffixes, which are universal word elements.

We will begin our study of the endocrine system with a brief overview of its anatomy and physiology. Later in the chapter you will learn about some common endocrinological (ĔN-dō-krĭ-nō-LŎJ-ĭk-ăl) conditions and tests for diagnosing them.

Overview of Endocrine System Anatomy and Physiology

The **endocrine system** is composed of glands that are widely distributed throughout the body (Figure 11.1). The term *endocrine* means "to secrete within." Endocrine glands secrete chemicals called **hormones** directly within the bloodstream, which transports them to organs, glands, and tissues that need those hormones to function properly. Endocrine glands play a vital role in maintaining homeostasis, a state of equilibrium within the body.

The endocrine system communicates with the nervous system to regulate bodily functions. While the nervous system responds rapidly to changes in both the internal environment (body) and in the external environment (outside world), the endocrine system responds in a more measured fashion through hormonal secretions that effect longer-lasting physiological change.

Hormones are powerful chemical substances that travel through the bloodstream to targeted organs or glands. Excessive hormonal secretion (*hypersecretion*) or too little secretion (*hyposecretion*) disrupts the body's homeostatic state, causing the target gland or organ to malfunction. Endocrine disorders and diseases affect metabolism and other vital bodily functions, such as brain development, bone health, cardiovascular function, and digestion.

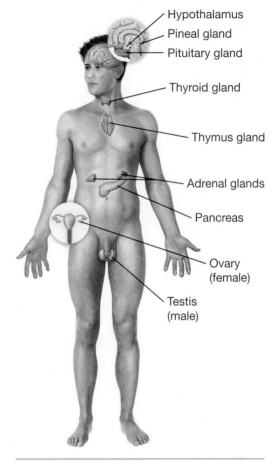

Hypothalamus
Pineal gland
Pituitary gland
Thyroid gland
Thymus gland
Adrenal glands
Pancreas
Ovary (female)
Testis (male)

Figure 11.1 The endocrine system is made up of glands that are distributed throughout the body.

Major Functions of the Endocrine System

The endocrine system regulates processes that occur slowly and effect long-lasting change within the body. These processes include

- growth and development of cells and tissues;
- metabolism (the process by which the body obtains energy from food);
- reproductive development and function; and
- mood.

Endocrinology (ĔN-dō-krĭ-NŎL-ō-jē) is the branch of medicine involving the study, diagnosis, and treatment of diseases and disorders of the endocrine glands. An **endocrinologist** (ĔN-dō-krĭ-NŎL-ō-jĭst) is a physician who specializes in treating diseases and disorders of the endocrine system.

Anatomy and Physiology Vocabulary

Now that you have been introduced to the basic structure and functions of the endocrine system, we will explore in more detail the key terms presented in the introduction.

Key Term	Definition
adrenal gland	triangle-shaped gland that sits atop each kidney; releases hormones that control metabolism, water and sodium levels, blood sugar levels, reproductive function, and response to stress
endocrine system	body system consisting of glands and hormones that maintain homeostasis (state of equilibrium)
endocrinologist	specialist in the study, diagnosis, and treatment of endocrine system diseases and disorders
endocrinology	the study of the endocrine system
homeostasis	a state of physiological equilibrium within the body
hormones	chemical substances that travel in the bloodstream to targeted glands or organs and are critical to homeostasis (normal body function)
hypothalamus	the part of the anterior brain that regulates body temperature, hunger, thirst, sleep, and emotions
ovaries	female reproductive glands
pancreas	gland behind the stomach that regulates insulin and glucose production and secretes digestive enzymes
parathyroid glands	four glands situated behind the thyroid gland; help metabolize calcium and phosphorus
pineal gland	small, pine-cone-shaped structure in the brain that secretes melatonin, a hormone that regulates sleep
pituitary gland	small, gray, rounded body attached to the base of the brain; secretes hormones that regulate growth, reproduction, and various metabolic activities
testes	male reproductive glands
thymus gland	gland located above the heart; important in the development of immunity in newborns
thyroid gland	gland in the base of the neck, located in front of and on both sides of the upper part of the trachea (windpipe) and the lower part of the larynx (throat); plays a vital role in metabolism and other life-sustaining functions

E-Flash Card Activity: Anatomy and Physiology Vocabulary

Directions: After you have reviewed the anatomy and physiology vocabulary related to the endocrine system, practice with the e-flash cards until you are comfortable with the spelling and definition of each term.

Identifying Major Glands of the Endocrine System

Directions: Label the anatomical diagram of the endocrine system.

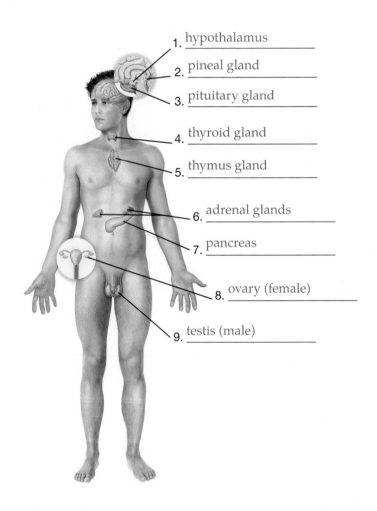

1. hypothalamus _____
2. pineal gland _____
3. pituitary gland _____
4. thyroid gland _____
5. thymus gland _____
6. adrenal glands _____
7. pancreas _____
8. ovary (female) _____
9. testis (male) _____

SCORECARD: How Did You Do?

Number correct (_____), divided by 9 (_____), multiplied by 100 equals _____ (your score)

Matching Anatomy and Physiology Vocabulary

Directions: Match the vocabulary term in Column A with its meaning in Column B.

Column A

- D 1. homeostasis
- K 2. hypothalamus
- E 3. adrenal gland
- G 4. pineal gland
- H 5. ovaries
- I 6. endocrinologist
- O 7. hormones
- N 8. parathyroid glands
- B 9. testes
- C 10. thyroid gland
- L 11. endocrinology
- M 12. pancreas
- A 13. pituitary gland
- F 14. endocrine system
- J 15. thymus gland

Column B

A. small, gray, rounded body attached to the base of the brain; secretes hormones that regulate growth, reproduction, and various metabolic activities

B. male reproductive glands

C. gland in the base of the neck, located in front of and on both sides of the upper part of the trachea (windpipe) and the lower part of the larynx (throat); plays a vital role in metabolism and other life-sustaining functions

D. a state of physiological equilibrium within the body

E. triangle-shaped gland that sits atop each kidney; releases hormones that control metabolism, water and sodium levels, blood sugar levels, reproductive function, and response to stress

F. body system consisting of glands and hormones that maintain homeostasis (state of equilibrium) in the body

G. small, pine-cone-shaped structure in the brain that secretes melatonin, a hormone that regulates sleep

H. female reproductive glands

I. specialist in the study, diagnosis, and treatment of endocrine system diseases and disorders

J. gland located above the heart; important in the development of immunity in newborns

K. the part of the anterior brain that regulates body temperature, hunger, thirst, sleep, and emotions

L. the study of the endocrine system

M. large gland behind the stomach that regulates insulin and glucose production and secretes digestive enzymes

N. four glands situated behind the thyroid gland; involved in the metabolism of calcium and phosphorus

O. chemical substances that travel in the bloodstream to targeted glands or organs and are critical to homeostasis (normal body function)

SCORECARD: How Did You Do?

Number correct (_____), divided by 15 (_____), multiplied by 100 equals _____ (your score)

Word Elements

In this section you will learn word elements—prefixes, combining forms, and suffixes—that are common to the endocrine system. By learning these word elements and understanding how they are combined to build medical terms, you will be able to analyze Mrs. Noah's health condition (described in the Intern Experience at the beginning of this chapter) and identify a large number of terms associated with the endocrine system.

 ## E-Flash Card Activity: Word Elements

Directions: Review the word elements in the tables that follow. Then, practice with the e-flash cards until you are able to quickly recognize the different word parts (prefixes, combining forms, and suffixes) and their meanings. The e-flash cards are grouped together by prefixes, combining forms, and suffixes, followed by a cumulative review of all the word elements that you learned in this chapter.

Prefixes

Let's begin our study of endocrine system word elements by looking at the prefixes listed in the table below. At this point in your studies, you have mastered all of these prefixes.

Prefix	Meaning
endo-	within
hyper-	above; above normal
hypo-	below; below normal
para-	beside; near
poly-	many; much

Combining Forms

The following combining forms appear in medical terms used to describe the endocrine system. Which of these have you already mastered?

Root Word/Combining Vowel	Meaning
acr/o	extremity
aden/o	gland
adren/o, adrenal/o	adrenal gland
carcin/o	cancer

(Continued)

Root Word/Combining Vowel	Meaning
crin/o	to secrete
dips/o	thirst
gluc/o	glucose; sugar
glyc/o	glucose; sugar
glycos/o	glucose; sugar
thym/o	thymus gland
thyr/o, thyroid/o	thyroid gland
ur/o	urine; urinary tract

Suffixes

Listed below are suffixes that appear in medical terms related to the endocrine system. From your study of body systems covered in previous chapters, you are already familiar with most of these suffixes.

Suffix	Meaning
-al	pertaining to
-e	noun suffix with no meaning
-ectomy	surgical removal; excision
-emia	blood condition
-ia	condition
-ic	pertaining to
-ism	condition; process
-itis	inflammation
-logist	specialist in the study and treatment of
-logy	study of
-megaly	large; enlargement
-oid	like; resembling
-oma	tumor; mass
-osis	abnormal condition
-pathy	disease
-phagia	eating; swallowing
-tomy	incision; cut into

Matching Prefixes, Combining Forms, and Suffixes

Directions: In each exercise that follows, match the word element in Column A with its meaning in Column B. Some meanings may be used more than once.

Prefixes

Column A

D	1. poly-
E	2. para-
A	3. hyper-
B	4. endo-
C	5. hypo-

Column B

A. above; above normal
B. within
C. below; below normal
D. many; much
E. beside; near

Combining Forms

Column A

D	1. glyc/o
A	2. acr/o
D	3. glycos/o
H	4. thym/o
B	5. aden/o
C	6. carcin/o
J	7. thyroid/o
I	8. crin/o
E	9. dips/o
F	10. ur/o
D	11. gluc/o
G	12. adren/o
J	13. thyr/o

Column B

A. extremity
B. gland
C. cancer
D. glucose; sugar
E. thirst
F. urine; urinary tract
G. adrenal gland
H. thymus gland
I. to secrete
J. thyroid gland

Suffixes

Column A

__A__	1. -megaly
__L__	2. -al
__E__	3. -oid
__L__	4. -ic
__M__	5. -phagia
__N__	6. -e
__B__	7. -logist
__P__	8. -emia
__C__	9. -logy
__O__	10. -ia
__I__	11. -itis
__H__	12. -ism
__J__	13. -ectomy
__F__	14. -pathy
__G__	15. -tomy
__D__	16. -osis
__K__	17. -oma

Column B

A. large; enlargement

B. specialist in the study and treatment of

C. study of

D. abnormal condition

E. like; resembling

F. disease

G. incision; cut into

H. condition; process

I. inflammation

J. surgical removal; excision

K. tumor; mass

L. pertaining to

M. eating; swallowing

N. noun suffix with no meaning

O. condition

P. blood condition

SCORECARD: How Did You Do?

Number correct (_____), divided by 35 (_____), multiplied by 100 equals _____ (your score)

Breaking Down and Building Endocrine System Terms

Now that you have mastered the prefixes, combining forms, and suffixes for medical terminology pertaining to the endocrine system, you have the ability to dissect and build a large number of terms related to this body system.

The chart that appears on the next two pages contains a list of medical terms commonly used in pulmonology, the medical specialty involving the study, diagnosis, and treatment of the endocrine system. For each term, a dissection has been provided, along with the meaning of each word element and the definition of the term as a whole.

Term	Dissection	Word Part/Meaning	Term Meaning
Note: *For simplification, combining vowels have been omitted from the Word Part/Meaning column.*			
1. **acromegaly** (ĂK-rō-MĔG-ă-lē)	acr/o/megaly	**acr** = extremity **megaly** = large; enlargement	large extremity; enlargement of an extremity
2. **adenocarcinoma** (ĂD-ĕ-nō-KĂR-sĭ-NŌ-mă)	aden/o/carcin/oma	**aden** = gland **carcin** = cancer **oma** = tumor; mass	cancerous tumor of a gland
3. **adenoid** (ĂD-ĕ-noyd)	aden/oid	**aden** = gland **oid** = like; resembling	resembling a gland
4. **adenoma** (ĂD-ĕ-NŌ-mă)	aden/oma	**aden** = gland **oma** = tumor; mass	tumor of a gland
5. **adenomegaly** (ĂD-ĕ-nō-MĔG-ă-lē)	aden/o/megaly	**aden** = gland **megaly** = large; enlargement	enlargement of a gland
6. **adrenal** (ă-DRĒ-năl)	adren/al	**adren** = adrenal gland **al** = pertaining to	pertaining to the adrenal gland
7. **adrenalectomy** (ă-DRĒ-năl-ĔK-tō-mē)	adrenal/ectomy	**adrenal** = adrenal gland **ectomy** = surgical removal; excision	excision of the adrenal gland
8. **adrenalopathy** (ă-DRĒ-nă-LŎP-ă-thē)	adrenal/o/pathy	**adrenal** = adrenal gland **pathy** = disease	disease of the adrenal gland
9. **endocrinologist** (ĔN-dō-krĭ-NŎL-ō-jĭst)	endo/crin/o/logist	**endo** = within **crin** = to secrete **logist** = specialist in the study and treatment of	specialist in the study and treatment of to secrete within
10. **endocrinology** (ĔN-dō-krĭ-NŎL-ō-jē)	endo/crin/o/logy	**endo** = within **crin** = to secrete **logy** = study of	the study of to secrete within
11. **endocrinopathy** (ĔN-dō-krĭ-NŎP-ă-thē)	endo/crin/o/pathy	**endo** = within **crin** = to secrete **pathy** = disease	disease of to secrete within
12. **glycemia** (glī-SĒ-mē-ă)	glyc/emia	**glyc** = glucose; sugar **emia** = blood condition	blood condition of glucose (condition of glucose in the blood)
13. **hyperglycemia** (HĪ-pĕr-glī-SĒ-mē-ă)	hyper/glyc/emia	**hyper** = above normal **glyc** = glucose; sugar **emia** = blood condition	blood condition of above-normal glucose

Prefixes = Green   Root Words = Red   Suffixes = Blue

Term	Dissection	Word Part/Meaning	Term Meaning
14. **hyperthyroidism** (hī-per-THĪ-royd-ĭzm)	hyper/thyroid/ism	**hyper** = above normal **thyroid** = thyroid gland **ism** = condition; process	condition of above-normal thyroid gland
15. **hypoglycemia** (HĪ-pō-glī-SĒ-mē-ă)	hypo/glyc/emia	**hypo** = below normal **glyc** = glucose; sugar **emia** = blood condition	blood condition of below-normal glucose
16. **hypothyroidism** (HĪ-pō-THĪ-royd-ĭzm)	hypo/thyroid/ism	**hypo** = below normal **thyroid** = thyroid gland **ism** = condition; process	condition of below-normal thyroid gland
17. **polydipsia** (pŏl-ē-DĬP-sē-ă)	poly/dips/ia	**poly** = many; much **dips** = thirst **ia** = condition	condition of much (excessive) thirst
18. **polyphagia** (PŎL-ē-FĀ-jē-ă)	poly/phag/ia	**poly** = many; much **phag** = eat; swallow **ia** = condition	condition of much (excessive) eating
19. **polyuria** (pŏl-ē-YŪ-rē-ă)	poly/ur/ia	**poly** = many; much **ur** = urine; urinary tract **ia** = condition	condition of much (excessive) urine
20. **thymectomy** (thī-MĔK-tō-mē)	thym/ectomy	**thym** = thymus gland **ectomy** = surgical removal; excision	excision of the thymus gland
21. **thymic** (THĪ-mĭk)	thym/ic	**thym** = thymus gland **ic** = pertaining to	pertaining to the thymus gland
22. **thymoma** (thī-MŌ-mă)	thym/oma	**thym** = thymus gland **oma** = tumor; mass	tumor of the thymus gland
23. **thyroidectomy** (thī-roy-DĔK-tō-mē)	thyroid/ectomy	**thyroid** = thyroid gland **ectomy** = surgical removal; excision	excision of the thyroid gland
24. **thyroiditis** (THĪ-roy-DĪ-tĭs)	thyroid/itis	**thyroid** = thyroid gland **itis** = inflammation	inflammation of the thyroid gland
25. **thyromegaly** (THĪ-rō-MĔG-ă-lē)	thyr/o/megaly	**thyr** = thyroid gland **megaly** = large; enlargement	enlargement of the thyroid gland

Prefixes = Green   Root Words = Red   Suffixes = Blue

Using the pronunciation guide in the Breaking Down and Building chart, practice saying each medical term aloud. To hear the pronunciation of each term, go to the Pronounce It activity at the G-W companion website.

Audio Activity: Pronounce It

Directions: At the companion website, listen as each medical term listed below is pronounced. Practice pronouncing the terms until you are comfortable saying them aloud.

acromegaly
(ĂK-rō-MĔG-ă-lē)

adenocarcinoma
(ĂD-ĕ-nō-KĂR-sĭ-NŌ-mă)

adenoid
(ĂD-ĕ-noyd)

adenoma
(ĂD-ĕ-NŌ-mă)

adenomegaly
(ĂD-ĕ-nō-MĔG-ă-lē)

adrenal
(ă-DRĒ-năl)

adrenalectomy
(ă-DRĒ-năl-ĔK-tō-mē)

adrenalopathy
(ă-DRĒ-nă-LŎP-ă-thē)

endocrinologist
(ĔN-dō-krĭ-NŎL-ō-jĭst)

endocrinology
(ĔN-dō-krĭ-NŎL-ō-jē)

endocrinopathy
(ĔN-dō-krĭ-NŎP-ă-thē)

glycemia
(glī-SĒ-mē-ă)

hyperglycemia
(HĪ-pĕr-glī-SĒ-mē-ă)

hyperthyroidism
(hī-per-THĪ-royd-ĭzm)

hypoglycemia
(HĪ-pō-glī-SĒ-mē-ă)

hypothyroidism
(HĪ-pō-THĪ-royd-ĭzm)

polydipsia
(pŏl-ē-DĬP-sē-ă)

polyphagia
(PŎL-ē-FĀ-jē-ă)

polyuria
(pŏl-ē-YŪ-rē-ă)

thymectomy
(thī-MĔK-tō-mē)

thymic
(THĪ-mĭk)

thymoma
(thī-MŌ-mă)

thyroidectomy
(thī-roy-DĔK-tō-mē)

thyroiditis
(THĪ-roy-DĪ-tĭs)

thyromegaly
(THĪ-rō-MĔG-ă-lē

Audio Activity: Spell It

Directions: Cover the medical terms in the Pronounce It activity with a sheet of paper. At the companion website, listen as the terms are read aloud. Correctly spell each term below.

1. acromegaly
2. adenocarcinoma
3. adenoid
4. adenoma
5. adenomegaly
6. adrenal
7. adrenalectomy
8. adrenalopathy
9. endocrinologist
10. endocrinology
11. endocrinopathy
12. glycemia
13. hyperglycemia
14. hyperthyroidism
15. hypoglycemia
16. hypothyroidism
17. polydipsia
18. polyphagia
19. polyuria
20. thymectomy
21. thymic
22. thymoma
23. thyroidectomy
24. thyroiditis
25. thyromegaly

Break It Down

Directions: Dissect each medical term into its word elements by placing a slash between each word part (prefix, root word, combining vowel, and suffix). Then define each term.

Example:

Medical Term: adenomegaly

Dissection: aden/o/megaly

Definition: enlargement of a gland

Medical Term	Dissection
1. thyromegaly	t h y r /o /m e g a l y

Definition: enlargement of the thyroid gland

2. glycemia	g l y c /e m i a

Definition: blood condition of glucose (condition of glucose in the blood)

3. hyperglycemia	h y p e r /g l y c /e m i a

Definition: blood condition of above-normal glucose

4. thyroiditis	t h y r o i d /i t i s

Definition: inflammation of the thyroid gland

5. adenoid	a d e n /o i d

Definition: resembling a gland

Medical Term	Dissection
6. thyroidectomy	t h y r o i d / e c t o m y

Definition: excision of the thyroid gland

| 7. hyperthyroidism | h y p e r / t h y r o i d / i s m |

Definition: condition of above-normal thyroid gland

| 8. polyuria | p o l y / u r / i a |

Definition: condition of much (excessive) urine

| 9. adrenal | a d r e n / a l |

Definition: pertaining to the adrenal gland

| 10. endocrinologist | e n d o / c r i n / o / l o g i s t |

Definition: specialist in the study and treatment of to secrete within

| 11. acromegaly | a c r / o / m e g a l y |

Definition: large extremity; enlargement of an extremity

| 12. polyphagia | p o l y / p h a g / i a |

Definition: condition of much (excessive) eating

SCORECARD: How Did You Do?

Number correct (_____), divided by 12 (_____), multiplied by 100 equals _____ (your score)

Build It

Directions: Build the medical term that matches each definition below by supplying the correct word elements.

P (Prefixes) = Green
RW (Root Words) = Red
S (Suffixes) = Blue
CV (Combining Vowel) = Purple

1. specialist in the study and treatment of to secrete within

endo	crin	o	logist
P	RW	CV	S

2. enlargement of the thyroid gland

thyr	o	megaly
RW	CV	S

3. condition of much (excessive) urine

poly	ur	ia
P	RW	S

4. cancerous tumor of a gland

aden	o	carcin	oma
RW	CV	RW	S

5. blood condition of below-normal glucose

hypo	glyc	emia
P	RW	S

6. enlargement of a gland

aden	o	megaly
RW	CV	S

7. excision of the thyroid gland

thyroid	ectomy
RW	S

8. excision of the adrenal gland

adrenal	ectomy
RW	S

9. large extremity; enlargement of an extremity

acr	o	megaly
RW	CV	S

10. disease of the adrenal gland

adrenal	o	pathy
RW	CV	S

11. inflammation of the thyroid gland

thyroid	itis
RW	S

12. disease of to secrete within

endo	crin	o	pathy
P	RW	CV	S

13. blood condition of glucose

glyc	emia
RW	S

14. blood condition of above-normal glucose

hyper	glyc	emia
P	RW	S

15. resembling a gland

aden	oid
RW	S

16. condition of above-normal thyroid gland

hyper	thyroid	ism
P	RW	S

17. condition of much (excessive) thirst

poly	dips	ia
P	RW	S

18. tumor of a gland

aden	oma
RW	S

SCORECARD: How Did You Do?

Number correct (_____), divided by 18 (_____), multiplied by 100 equals _____ (your score)

Interpret the Pronunciation

Directions: Write the correct spelling of the medical term beside each pronunciation.

1. ĂD-ĕ-noyd   adenoid
2. glī-SĒ-mē-ă   glycemia
3. HĪ-pō-THĪ-royd-ĭzm   hypothyroidism
4. ĔN-dō-krĭ-NŎL-ō-jĭst   endocrinologist
5. pŏl-ē-DĬP-sē-ă   polydipsia
6. ĔN-dō-krĭ-NŎL-ō-jē   endocrinology
7. ă-DRĒ-nă-LŎP-ă-thē   adrenalopathy
8. THĪ-roy-DĪ-tĭs   thyroiditis
9. ĂD-ĕ-nō-KÄR-sĭ-NŌ-mă   adenocarcinoma
10. HĪ-pō-glī-SĒ-mē-ă   hypoglycemia
11. ĔN-dō-krĭ-NŎP-ă-thē   endocrinopathy
12. thī-MŌ-mă   thymoma
13. ă-DRĒ-năl   adrenal
14. PŎL-ē-FĀ-jē-ă   polyphagia
15. thī-MĔK-tō-mē   thymectomy
16. ĂD-ĕ-NŎP-ă-thē   adenopathy
17. THĪ-mĭk   thymic
18. hī-per-THĪ-royd-ĭzm   hyperthyroidism
19. pŏl-ē-YŪ-rē-ă   polyuria
20. THĪ-rō-MĔG-ă-lē   thyromegaly
21. ă-DRĒ-năl-ĔK-tō-mē   adrenalectomy

SCORECARD: How Did You Do?

Number correct (_____), divided by 21 (_____), multiplied by 100 equals _____ (your score)

Diseases and Disorders

Diseases and disorders of the endocrine system run the spectrum of the mild to the severe. Some of them are congenital (present at birth); others are rooted in autoimmune dysfunction. In this section, we will briefly explore the major characteristics and causes of some common pathological conditions of the endocrine system.

Acromegaly

Acromegaly (ĂK-rō-MĔG-ă-lē) is a rare disorder that develops when the pituitary gland produces too much growth hormone (Figure 11.2). The result is increased bone growth and enlarged internal organs. A benign (noncancerous) tumor of the pituitary gland is the most common cause of acromegaly.

In adults, common signs of acromegaly include abnormally enlarged hands and feet, a broadened head, and a deepened, husky voice. In children, acromegaly is called *gigantism*. A common sign of acromegaly in children is excessive height caused by abnormally fast growth, unlike that which may occur during normal adolescent development.

Addison's Disease

When the adrenal glands produce an insufficient amount of the hormone cortisol, the result is **Addison's disease** (also called *Addison disease*). Cortisol affects almost every organ system and is vital for a normal metabolism. Its most important job is to help the body respond to stress.

Symptoms of Addison's disease develop slowly and may include fatigue, low blood pressure, loss of appetite, weight loss, and hyperpigmentation (above-normal darkening of the skin) (Figure 11.3 on the next page). Patients with Addison's disease are treated with hormone replacement therapy.

Perhaps the most famous example of a person with Addison's disease was President John F. Kennedy, who also was diagnosed with hypothyroidism (discussed later in this section) after his 1960 election. Kennedy's well-known, year-round "tan" is probably attributable to Addison's hyperpigmentation.

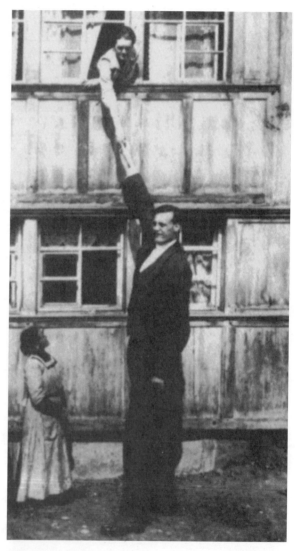

Science Source

Figure 11.2 When the pituitary gland secretes an excessive amount of growth hormone, the result is acromegaly, a rare disorder.

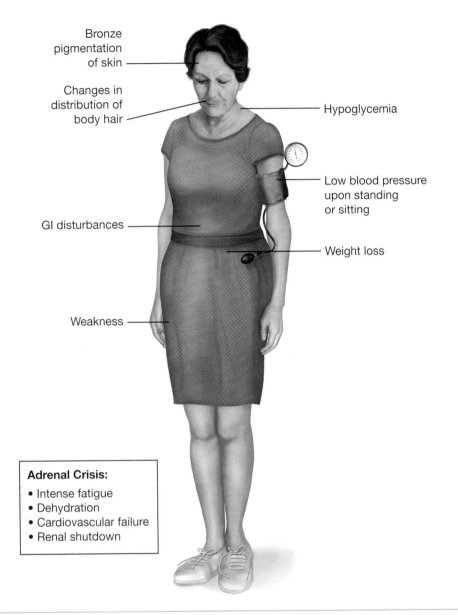

Bronze
pigmentation
of skin

Changes in
distribution of
body hair

Hypoglycemia

Low blood pressure
upon standing
or sitting

GI disturbances

Weight loss

Weakness

Adrenal Crisis:
- Intense fatigue
- Dehydration
- Cardiovascular failure
- Renal shutdown

Figure 11.3 Common signs and symptoms of Addison's disease, the result of a deficiency in cortisol secretion by the adrenal glands.

Cretinism

Cretinism (krĕ-tĭn-ĭzm), also known as *congenital hypothyroidism*, is a loss of thyroid function that is present from birth. The thyroid gland either is absent or fails to secrete thyroid hormones that are vital for brain development, physical growth, and metabolism. The result is a severe disruption in mental and physical growth in the infant.

Not all cases of cretinism are congenital in nature. This severe form of hypothyroidism may be acquired later in life. Cretinism that develops during childhood or adulthood is called *myxedema* (MĬKS-ĕ-DĒ-mă).

Cushing's Syndrome

Cushing's syndrome (also called *Cushing syndrome*) is a disorder resulting from prolonged bodily exposure to high levels of the hormone cortisol. The hallmark signs of Cushing's syndrome include a fatty hump between the shoulders, obesity in the upper body, and a rounded face that is often described as a "moon face" (Figure 11.4).

Weight gain in Cushing's syndrome stretches the already thin and weakened skin to hemorrhage, producing purple or red stretch marks called *striae* (STRĪ-ē). Cushing's syndrome may also develop from excessive use of steroids.

Diabetes Mellitus

Diabetes mellitus (MĚL-ĭ-tŭs), or **DM**, is a disorder characterized by hyperglycemia due to a dysfunctional pancreas. The pancreas secretes both glucose and insulin. DM is a result of insulin deficiency or insulin ineffectiveness.

Physiological Overview

Insulin is the only hormone in the body that lowers blood sugar. Insulin helps transport glucose, the body's major source of energy, to the cells. Without glucose, the cells of the body cannot function or survive. Without insulin, they cannot absorb glucose. Insulin deficiency causes problems with metabolism of carbohydrates, proteins, and fats.

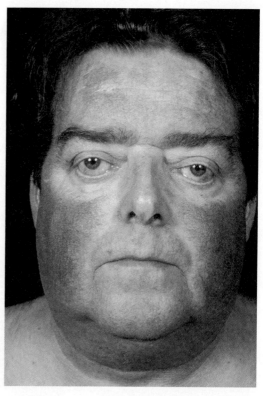

Biophoto Associates/Photo Researchers, Inc

Figure 11.4 A rounded face, typically described as a "moon face," is a hallmark characteristic of Cushing's syndrome.

The physiological effects of insulin deficiency include polyuria (excessive urination), polydipsia (excessive thirst), and polyphagia (overeating) with unexplained weight loss (Figure 11.5 on the next page). Long-term complications of DM may include peripheral neuropathy (numbness and tingling in the feet and/or hands) and diabetic retinopathy (vision problems due to retinal disease). Uncontrolled diabetes may result in *gangrene*, death of tissues caused by a blood-supply decrease or absence. This metabolic disease is the leading cause of blindness, renal failure, and gangrene of the lower extremities.

Major Types of Diabetes Mellitus

There are two major types of diabetes mellitus. **Type 1 diabetes mellitus**, formerly known as *juvenile-onset diabetes* or *insulin-dependent diabetes mellitus (IDDM)*, typically occurs before the age of 25 and is characterized by little to no insulin secretion. (The term *type 1 diabetes mellitus* is usually shortened to *type 1 diabetes*.)

Type 2 diabetes mellitus, formerly known as *adult-onset diabetes* or *non-insulin-dependent diabetes mellitus (NIDDM)*, occurs predominantly in adults.

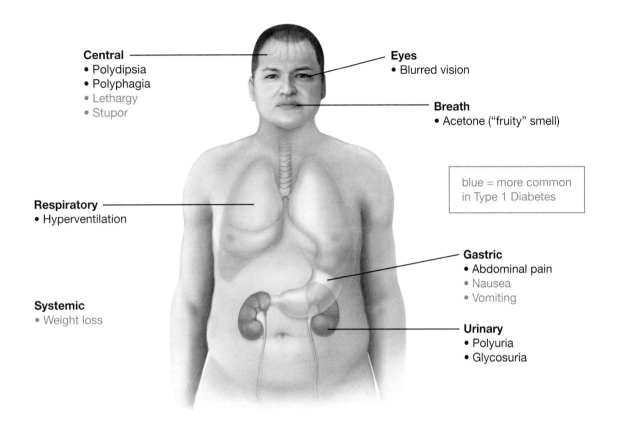

Central
- Polydipsia
- Polyphagia
- Lethargy
- Stupor

Eyes
- Blurred vision

Breath
- Acetone ("fruity" smell)

blue = more common in Type 1 Diabetes

Respiratory
- Hyperventilation

Gastric
- Abdominal pain
- Nausea
- Vomiting

Systemic
- Weight loss

Urinary
- Polyuria
- Glycosuria

Figure 11.5 Major signs and symptoms of diabetes mellitus

Insulin secretion is insufficient to meet bodily needs. Type 2 DM may be controlled by diet and oral medications. In some cases, however, insulin therapy may be required. The term *type 2 diabetes mellitus* is typically shortened to *type 2 diabetes*.

Diabetic patients who require insulin must monitor their blood glucose levels daily using a glucose meter (Figure 11.6). A small drop of blood is obtained by pricking the skin with a very small needle called a *lancet*. The blood drop is placed on a disposable test strip, which is read by the meter and used to calculate the patient's blood glucose level. Modern glucose meters are about the size of the palm of the hand and are battery-operated.

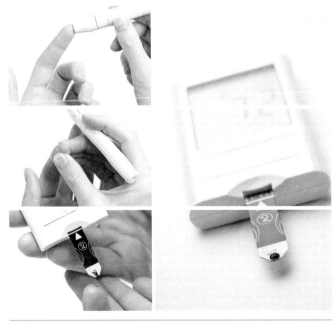

Figure 11.6 A patient performs a blood sugar test with a glucose meter.

Diabetes Insipidus

Diabetes insipidus (ĭn-SĬP-ĭ-dŭs), or **DI**, is not to be confused with diabetes mellitus. Diabetes insipidus is a rare disease in which the posterior pituitary gland produces an insufficient amount of antidiuretic hormone (ADH). DI is characterized by polyuria and polydipsia, which can lead to dehydration.

Graves' Disease

Graves' disease is an autoimmune disease in which the thyroid gland produces and releases excessive amounts of thyroid hormone into the blood, resulting in hyperthyroidism. Symptoms of Graves' disease include *exophthalmos* (ĔKS-ŏf-THĂL-mŏs), protruding or bulging of the eyes; a goiter (chronic enlargement of the thyroid gland); and edema in the lower extremities (Figure 11.7).

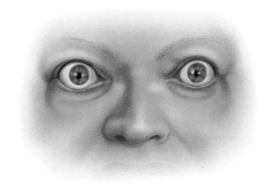

Hypothyroidism

Hypothyroidism, or *underactive thyroid*, is a disorder in which the thyroid gland does not produce a sufficient amount of thyroid hormone. Inadequate production of thyroid hormone decreases metabolism.

Symptoms of hypothyroidism, which develop gradually, may include weight gain, dry skin, bradycardia (slow heart rate), and lethargy (Figure 11.8 on the next page). Hormone replacement therapy, in the form of natural or synthetic thyroid hormone, is necessary.

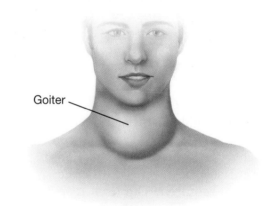

Goiter

Tests and Procedures

In this section, you will learn about tests and procedures used to help diagnose pathological conditions of the endocrine system.

Fasting Blood Sugar Test

The **fasting blood sugar (FBS) test** is a type of blood test that analyzes the amount of glucose in the blood after the patient has not eaten for at least eight

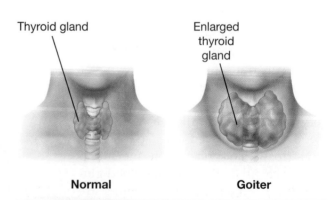

Thyroid gland

Enlarged thyroid gland

Normal

Goiter

Figure 11.7 Bulging eyes and a goiter (enlarged thyroid gland) are typical of Graves' disease.

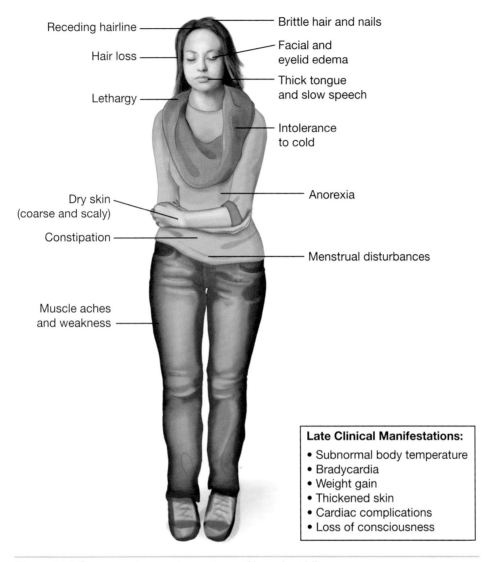

Figure 11.8 Common signs and symptoms of hypothyroidism

Late Clinical Manifestations:
- Subnormal body temperature
- Bradycardia
- Weight gain
- Thickened skin
- Cardiac complications
- Loss of consciousness

hours (called *fasting*). A needle is inserted into a vein in the arm, and blood is withdrawn for analysis. The process of withdrawing blood from a vein for laboratory analysis is called a *venipuncture*.

The fasting blood sugar test is a screening tool that aids in diagnosing diabetes. The FBS is also effective for the regular monitoring of diabetic patients' blood glucose levels.

Glucose Tolerance Test

The **glucose tolerance test (GTT)**, another type of fasting blood sugar test, determines how the body breaks down sugar. Like the fasting blood sugar test, the GTT requires a period of fasting, typically between eight and twelve hours.

Before the glucose tolerance test, a fasting blood sugar is drawn. Then the patient drinks a glucose (sugar) solution, and blood samples are drawn at timed intervals (Figure 11.9). An oral glucose tolerance test may take up to three hours to complete. This diagnostic test is often used to confirm a diagnosis of diabetes mellitus.

Thyroid Scan

A **thyroid scan** is a nuclear medicine imaging procedure that uses a radioactive iodine tracer to record the structure and function of the thyroid gland (Figure 11.10 on the next page). The scan shows the size and shape of the thyroid gland and is useful in detecting thyroid cysts or cancerous tumors.

Thyroid-Stimulating Hormone Test

The **thyroid-stimulating hormone test** is a laboratory test that measures the amount of thyroid-stimulating hormone (TSH) in the blood and the function of the thyroid gland. The TSH test is performed using venipuncture. It is given to patients with signs and symptoms of a thyroid disorder, such as hypothyroidism or hyperthyroidism.

Thyroid hormones control metabolism and regulate growth and development. TSH is manufactured by the pituitary gland, which "tells" the thyroid

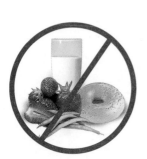

No food or drink
8 to 12 hours prior
to test

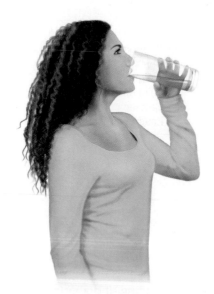

Drink glucose

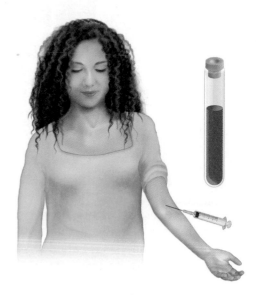

Blood tested at regular intervals

High glucose level = Potential diabetes

Figure 11.9 A glucose tolerance test is performed to confirm a diagnosis of diabetes. Before a glucose tolerance test, a fasting blood sugar is drawn. The patient drinks a sugar solution, and blood samples are taken at timed intervals.

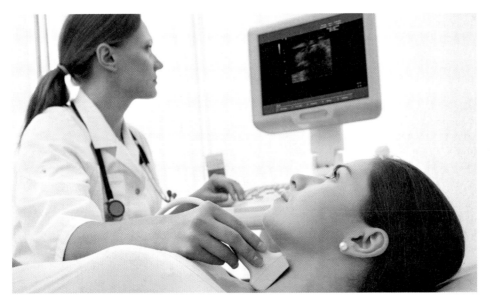

Figure 11.10 A technician performs a diagnostic thyroid scan on a patient.

gland to produce and release thyroid hormones (for example, thyroxine) into the blood (Figure 11.11). In other words, TSH controls production of the other thyroid hormones.

Thyroxine Test

Thyroxine (thī-RŎK-sēn or thī-RŎK-sĭn) is another hormone manufactured by the thyroid gland. It plays a vital role in brain development, bone health, metabolism, and cardiac, muscular, and digestive functions.

The **thyroxine test** analyzes thyroid function by measuring the amount of thyroxine in the blood. Like the thyroid-stimulating hormone (TSH) test, the thyroxine test is performed when a patient is suspected of having a disorder such as hyperthyroidism or hypothyroidism.

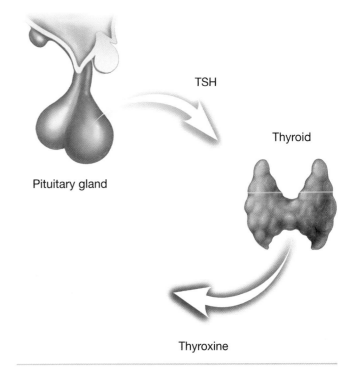

Figure 11.11 Thyroid-stimulating hormone, or TSH, is made by the pituitary gland, which "tells" the thyroid gland to manufacture and secrete thyroid hormones into the bloodstream.

Multiple Choice: Diseases and Disorders

Directions: Write the letter of the disease or disorder that matches each numbered definition.

_B_ 1. disorder characterized by hyperglycemia from a dysfunctional pancreas
  a. diabetes insipidus
  b. diabetes mellitus
  c. hypothyroidism
  d. cretinism

_B_ 2. rare hormonal disorder that develops when the pituitary gland produces excessive growth hormone
  a. Addison's disease
  b. acromegaly
  c. Cushing's syndrome
  d. Graves' disease

_B_ 3. rare disorder in which the pituitary gland produces too little antidiuretic hormone, leading to polyuria and polydipsia
  a. hypothyroidism
  b. diabetes insipidus
  c. diabetes mellitus
  d. Addison's disease

_A_ 4. disorder that arises when the adrenal glands produce an insufficient amount of cortisol
  a. Addison's disease
  b. acromegaly
  c. Graves' disease
  d. Cushing's syndrome

_A_ 5. congenital disorder characterized by loss of thyroid function
  a. hypothyroidism
  b. cretinism
  c. diabetes insipidus
  d. diabetes mellitus

_B_ 6. disorder characterized by a rounded face, upper-body obesity, and a fatty hump between the shoulders
  a. acromegaly
  b. Cushing's syndrome
  c. Addison's disease
  d. Graves' disease

_A_ 7. disorder in which the thyroid gland fails to produce enough thyroid hormone
  a. cretinism
  b. Graves' disease
  c. hypothyroidism
  d. diabetes mellitus

_A_ 8. disease marked by excessive secretion of thyroid hormone into the blood
  a. Graves' disease
  b. hypothyroidism
  c. Cushing's syndrome
  d. Addison's disease

SCORECARD: How Did You Do?

Number correct (_____), divided by 8 (_____), multiplied by 100 equals _____ (your score)

Multiple Choice: Tests and Procedures

Directions: Write the letter of the diagnostic test or procedure that matches each numbered definition.

_A_ 1. imaging procedure that uses a radioactive iodine tracer to detect cysts or cancerous tumors of the thyroid gland
  a. thyroid scan
  b. thyroxine test
  c. thyroid-stimulating hormone test
  d. glucose tolerance test

_A_ 2. test that measures the amount of the thyroid hormone that plays an important role in brain development, bone health, metabolism, and heart, muscle, and digestive functions
  a. thyroxine test
  b. fasting blood-sugar test
  c. thyroid scan
  d. glucose tolerance test

<u>D</u>   3. test that analyzes the amount of glucose in the blood
   a. glucose tolerance test
   b. fasting blood sugar test
   c. thyroxine test
   d. both a and b

<u>A</u>   4. laboratory test that measures the amount of the hormone produced and released into the bloodstream by the pituitary gland
   a. thyroid-stimulating hormone test
   b. thyroxine test
   c. thyroid scan
   d. glucose tolerance test

<u>B</u>   5. test that determines how the body breaks down sugar
   a. thyroxine test
   b. glucose tolerance test
   c. fasting blood sugar test
   d. thyroid-stimulating hormone test

SCORECARD: How Did You Do?

Number correct (_____), divided by 5 (_____), multiplied by 100 equals _____ (your score)

Assessment

Identifying Abbreviations

Directions: Write the abbreviation for each medical term listed below.

Medical Term	Abbreviation
1. diabetes mellitus	DM
2. non-insulin-dependent diabetes mellitus	NIDDM
3. diabetes insipidus	DI
4. insulin-dependent diabetes mellitus	IDDM
5. antidiuretic hormone	ADH
6. fasting blood sugar	FBS
7. glucose tolerance test	GTT
8. thyroid-stimulating hormone	TSH

SCORECARD: How Did You Do?

Number correct (_____), divided by 8 (_____), multiplied by 100 equals _____ (your score)

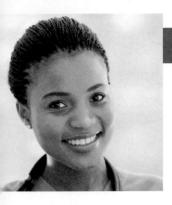

Analyzing the Intern Experience

In the Intern Experience described at the beginning of this chapter, we met Liza, who was assigned to an internship as a medical assistant with Stringfield Medical Associates. Liza listened and observed as the doctor talked with Mrs. Kathryn Noah, a 78-year-old patient with poor ambulation, fever, and sensations of numbness and tingling in her left big toe. The numbness and tingling were accompanied by a bluish discoloration and a foul-smelling discharge from the toe.

After examining Mrs. Noah, the physician made a diagnosis and a treatment plan. Later, he made a dictated recording of the patient's health information, which was subsequently transcribed into a chart note.

We will now learn more about Mrs. Noah's condition from a clinical perspective, interpreting the medical terms in her chart note as we analyze the scenario presented in the Intern Experience.

Audio Activity: Kathryn Noah's Chart Note

Directions: At the companion website, listen and read along as the physician dictates Kathryn Noah's chart note, shown below. Then do the exercise that appears after the chart note.

CHART NOTE

Patient Name: Noah, Kathryn
ID Number: 93654KN
Examination Date: February 12, 20xx

SUBJECTIVE
Kathryn is a 78-year-old patient who is here for a **diabetic** recheck. She rarely checks her blood sugars. She has not checked her sugar levels in the past 2 weeks and has lost 5–10 pounds since her last visit. Patient complains of numbness and tingling of the left great (big) toe with a foul-smelling discharge.

OBJECTIVE
She is inconsistent in taking her diabetic meds. **BP** is 140/98. Low-grade fever of 101. Eye exam is negative. Nose, mouth, neck, and **thyroid** exam are negative. Heart is without murmurs. Lungs are clear. Obese abdomen. Inflamed left great toe, bluish in color, with **purulent** discharge. The toe is cold to the touch with slight **sloughing** (falling off) of the skin.

ASSESSMENT
1. **Gangrene** of left great toe.
2. **Type 2 diabetes**, suboptimal control.
3. Obesity.

PLAN
Admit for amputation of left great toe due to gangrene.

Interpret Kathryn Noah's Chart Note

Directions: After listening to the dictated recording and reading the chart note on Kathryn Noah, provide the medical term that matches each definition below. You may encounter terms that were introduced in previous chapters.

Example: condition of below-normal thyroid gland   *Answer:* hypothyroidism

1. gland in the base of the neck; plays a vital role in metabolism and other life-sustaining functions

   thyroid

2. pertaining to pus

   purulent

3. disorder characterized by hyperglycemia from a dysfunctional pancreas

   type 2 diabetes

4. falling off

   sloughing

5. death of tissue due to deficient blood supply

   gangrene

6. pertaining to diabetes

   diabetic

7. blood pressure

   BP

SCORECARD: How Did You Do?

Number correct (_____), divided by 7 (_____), multiplied by 100 equals _____ (your score)

Working with Medical Records

In this activity, you will interpret the medical records (chart notes) of patients with health conditions related to the endocrine system. These examples illustrate typical medical records prepared in a real-world healthcare environment. To interpret these chart notes, you will apply your knowledge of word elements (prefixes, combining forms, and suffixes), diseases and disorders, and tests and procedures related to the endocrine system.

Audio Activity: Dorothy Frederick's Chart Note

Directions: At the companion website, listen and read along as the physician dictates Dorothy Frederick's chart note, shown on the next page. Then do the exercise that appears after the chart note.

CHART NOTE

Patient Name: Frederick, Dorothy
ID Number: 11472DR
Examination Date: November 23, 20xx

SUBJECTIVE
Dorothy is a 40-year-old music teacher here for follow-up of unusual irritability and fatigue over the past month. She also complains of anxiety and has noticed an intermittent rapid or irregular heartbeat. She said she always has a slight hand tremor, but it seems to be getting worse. She thinks the Paxil® (anti-anxiety medication) may be helping her sleep, but has not seen much of an improvement.

OBJECTIVE
Patient appears well. **HEENT** (head, eyes, ears, nose, and throat) are normal. A slightly enlarged **thyroid** is palpated. No **adenopathy**. There is a scar from a previous **lymphadenectomy**. Lungs are clear. **Tachycardia** noted. No **edema** of the lower extremities. Abdomen is soft and nontender. Lab report indicates a decreased **TSH** level. Other lab results were negative.

ASSESSMENT
Graves' disease

PLAN
Continue with Paxil for her anxiety and depression. She will be scheduled for a **thyroid scan** and **ECG**. I am referring her to an **endocrinologist** for further treatment.

Assessment

Interpret Dorothy Frederick's Chart Note

Directions: After listening to the dictated recording and reading the chart note on Dorothy Frederick, provide the medical term that matches each definition below.

Example: blood condition of above-normal glucose   *Answer:* hyperglycemia

1. excision of the lymph glands — lymphadenectomy

2. fast heartbeat — tachycardia

3. thyroid-stimulating hormone — TSH

4. autoimmune disease in which the thyroid gland secretes excessive amounts of thyroid hormone into the blood — Graves' disease

5. electrocardiogram — ECG

6. disease of the lymph glands — adenopathy

7. head, eyes, ears, nose, and throat — HEENT

8. nuclear medicine imaging procedure that records the structure and function of the thyroid gland

thyroid scan

9. swelling

edema

10. specialist in the study and treatment of endocrine system diseases and disorders

endocrinologist

11. gland in the base of the neck; plays a vital role in metabolism and other life-sustaining functions

thyroid

SCORECARD: How Did You Do?

Number correct (_____), divided by 11 (_____), multiplied by 100 equals _____ (your score)

Audio Activity: Ralph Dixon's Chart Note

Directions: At the companion website, listen and read along as the physician dictates Ralph Dixon's chart note, shown below. Then do the exercise that appears after the chart note.

CHART NOTE

Patient Name: Dixon, Ralph
ID Number: 87457RD
Examination Date: August 4, 20xx

SUBJECTIVE
This is a **diabetic**, 20-year-old male patient who requests medical clearance to renew his driver's license.

OBJECTIVE
The patient states that he checks his glucose levels twice daily, which run in the 100–200 range. Further questioning reveals intermittent glucose levels in the 275–300 range. He states that he had **hyperglycemia**-like symptoms of **polydipsia** and **polyuria** twice last month. He had **hypoglycemic** symptoms consisting of weakness and inability to concentrate once in the last month. Vital signs are normal. Eye exam is negative. Examination of the feet shows some slight callous formation on the heels bilaterally (pertaining to both sides) with some cracked skin. No evidence of fungal infection or ulceration. Examination of feet normal and symmetric.

ASSESSMENT
Type 1 diabetes with suboptimal control.

PLAN
The importance of good **glycemic** control was discussed in detail with the patient. He is scheduled to see a diabetic nutritionist next week and was given information about local diabetic support groups. Return for a follow-up in one month or sooner if needed.

Interpret Ralph Dixon's Chart Note

Directions: After listening to the dictated recording and reading the chart note on Ralph Dixon, provide the medical term that matches each definition below.

Example: tumor of the thymus gland   *Answer:* thymoma

1. condition of much (excessive) thirst   polydipsia

2. pertaining to glucose or sugar   glycemic

3. condition of above-normal glucose in the blood   hyperglycemia

4. disorder characterized by hyperglycemia from a dysfunctional pancreas   type 1 diabetes

5. condition of much (excessive) urine   polyuria

6. pertaining to diabetes   diabetic

7. pertaining to below-normal glucose in the blood   hypoglycemic

---

SCORECARD: How Did You Do?

Number correct (_____), divided by 7 (_____), multiplied by 100 equals _____ (your score)

Chapter Review

Word Elements Summary

Prefixes

Prefix	Meaning
endo-	within
hyper-	above; above normal
hypo-	below; below normal
para-	beside; near
poly-	many; much

Combining Forms

Root Word/Combining Vowel	Meaning
acr/o	extremity
aden/o	gland
adren/o, adrenal/o	adrenal gland
carcin/o	cancer
crin/o	to secrete
dips/o	thirst
gluc/o	glucose; sugar
glyc/o	glucose; sugar
glycos/o	glucose; sugar
thym/o	thymus gland
thyr/o, thyroid/o	thyroid gland
ur/o	urine; urinary tract

Suffixes

Suffix	Meaning
-al	pertaining to
-e	noun suffix with no meaning
-ectomy	surgical removal; excision
-emia	blood condition
-ia	condition
-ic	pertaining to

(Continued)

Suffix	Meaning
-ism	condition; process
-itis	inflammation
-logist	specialist in the study and treatment of
-logy	study of
-megaly	large; enlargement
-oid	like; resembling
-oma	tumor; mass
-osis	abnormal condition
-pathy	disease
-phagia	eating; swallowing
-tomy	incision; cut into

More Practice: Activities and Games

The activities on the following pages will help you reinforce your skills and check your mastery of the medical terminology that you learned in this chapter. Visit the companion website for More Practice games and activities.

Break It Down

Directions: Dissect each medical term into its word elements by placing a slash between each word part (prefix, root word, combining vowel, and suffix). Then define each term.

Example:
Medical Term: polydipsia
Dissection: poly/dips/ia
Definition: condition of much (excessive) thirst

Medical Term	Dissection
1. parathyroidectomy	p a r a/t h y r o i d/e c t o m y

Definition: surgical removal (of the area) near the thyroid gland

| 2. hypothymic | h y p o/t h y m/i c |

Definition: pertaining to below the thymus gland

Medical Term	Dissection

3. adenitis   a d e n / i t i s

Definition: inflammation of a gland
_____

4. hypothyroidism   h y p o / t h y r o i d / i s m

Definition: condition of below-normal thyroid gland
_____

5. adrenopathy   a d r e n / o / p a t h y

Definition: disease of the adrenal gland
_____

6. thyrotomy   t h y r / o / t o m y

Definition: incision of the thyroid gland
_____

7. hyperglycosuria   h y p e r / g l y c o s / u r / i a

Definition: condition of above-normal glucose in the urine
_____

8. polyadenitis   p o l y / a d e n / i t i s

Definition: inflammation of many glands
_____

9. hyperadrenalism   h y p e r / a d r e n a l / i s m

Definition: condition of above-normal adrenal gland
_____

10. endocrine   e n d o / c r i n / e

Definition: to secrete within (*e* = noun suffix with no meaning)
_____

Medical Term	Dissection
11. hyperglycemia	h y p e r / g l y c / e m i a

Definition: blood condition of above-normal glucose

| 12. thyromegaly | t h y r / o / m e g a l y |

Definition: enlargement of the thyroid gland

Identifying Abbreviations

Directions: Write the abbreviation for each medical term listed below.

Medical Term	Abbreviation
1. fasting blood sugar	FBS
2. thyroid-stimulating hormone	TSH
3. diabetes mellitus	DM
4. glucose tolerance test	GTT
5. diabetes insipidus	DI
6. antidiuretic hormone	ADH
7. head, eyes, ears, nose, and throat	HEENT

Spelling

Directions: Write the correct spelling beside each misspelled medical term below.

1. polidypsia	polydipsia	
2. thyramegaly	thyromegaly	
3. endacrinologist	endocrinologist	
4. adrenalapathy	adrenalopathy	
5. glycemea	glycemia	
6. thiroyditis	thyroiditis	
7. endochrinopathy	endocrinopathy	
8. polyphagea	polyphagia	
9. adinosis	adenosis	
10. endalcrinology	endocrinology	
11. hypoglysemia	hypoglycemia	
12. polyurea	polyuria	

Audio Activity: Pamela Rolf's Chart Note

Directions: At the companion website, listen and read along as the physician dictates Pamela Rolf's chart note, shown below. Then do the exercise that appears after the chart note.

CHART NOTE

Patient Name: Rolf, Pamela
ID Number: 54773EG
Examination Date: April 14, 20xx

SUBJECTIVE
Pamela has **edema** of the hands and legs. She complains of being constantly tired and cold. She still has problems with constipation and some weight gain. She has no hot flashes or depression. She has been on Synthroid® 110 mcg (micrograms) daily.

OBJECTIVE
BP is 124/76. Weight is 175 pounds, which is about 5 pounds heavier than a month ago. **HEENT** is normal. Chest, lungs, and heart rate are normal. **Thyroid** is clear to palpation. No **goiter** detected.

ASSESSMENT
Hypothyroidism

PLAN
Patient scheduled for **TSH test** next week. She will continue with Synthroid 110 mcg daily. She will return in 2 weeks to discuss her test results.

Assessment

Interpret Pamela Rolf's Chart Note

Directions: After listening to the dictated recording and reading the chart note on Pamela Rolf, provide the medical term that matches each definition below. You may encounter terms that were introduced in previous chapters.

Example: inflammation of the thyroid gland   *Answer:* thyroiditis

1. disorder in which the thyroid gland does not produce a sufficient amount of thyroid hormone

   hypothyroidism

2. lab test performed via venipuncture to measure the amount of thyroid-stimulating hormone in the blood

   TSH test

3. gland in the base of the neck; plays a vital role in metabolism and other life-sustaining functions

   thyroid

4. swelling

   edema

5. head, eyes, ears, nose, and throat

   HEENT

Chapter 12

The Urinary System

ur / o / logy: the study of urine and the urinary system

Chapter Organization

- Intern Experience
- Overview of Urinary System Anatomy and Physiology
- Word Elements
- Breaking Down and Building Urinary System Terms
- Diseases and Disorders
- Procedures and Treatments
- Analyzing the Intern Experience
- Working with Medical Records
- Chapter Review

Chapter Objectives

After completing this chapter, you will be able to

1. label an anatomical diagram of the urinary system;
2. dissect and define common medical terminology related to the urinary system;
3. build terms used to describe urinary system diseases and disorders and diagnostic procedures;
4. pronounce and spell common medical terminology related to the urinary system;
5. understand that the processes of building and dissecting a medical term based on its prefix, word root, and suffix enable you to analyze an extremely large number of medical terms beyond those presented in this chapter;
6. interpret the meaning of abbreviations associated with the urinary system; and
7. interpret medical records containing terminology and abbreviations related to the urinary system.

You will see this icon ![icon] at various points throughout this chapter. The icon indicates that you will find interactive activities and games on the Medical Terminology Companion Website. These activities and games will help you learn, practice, and expand your medical terminology knowledge and skills. Some of these activities are also available on the Medical Terminology Mobile Website.

Companion Website
www.g-wlearning.com/healthsciences

Mobile Site
www.m.g-wlearning.com/5800

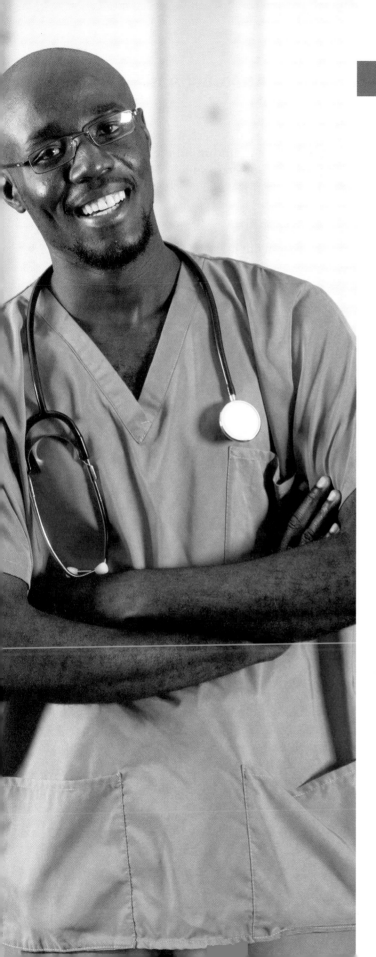

Intern Experience

Thomas O'Connor, an intern with Middletown Clinic, has been assigned this week to assist Dr. Nefron, a general practitioner. Their first patient is Shara, a college freshman with a complaint of bodily discomfort and fatigue. Thomas escorts Shara to exam room 4. "I've been feeling extremely tired," she says. Her roommate had suggested that she visit the campus doctor; however, Shara did not go because she had to study for final exams. The symptoms did not go away, so after her exams she came to the clinic.

Shara informs Thomas that, besides fatigue and a general feeling of unwellness, her urine has been red for three days, she has been urinating frequently, there is a burning sensation with urination, and she has lower back pain. She reveals that her family doctor has treated her for similar symptoms on several other occasions. Thomas notes these symptoms in Shara's chart and tells her that the doctor will want to do a urinalysis to help determine the cause of her symptoms.

As you will learn later in this chapter, Shara is suffering from a condition that has affected her urinary tract. To help you understand her health problem, this chapter will present word elements (combining forms, prefixes, and suffixes) that make up medical terms related to the urinary system. As you learn these terms, you will recognize many common word elements from your study of body systems covered in previous chapters—particularly prefixes and suffixes, which are universal word elements.

We will begin our study of the urinary system with a brief overview of its anatomy and physiology. Later in the chapter you will learn about some common urinary conditions, diagnostic tests and procedures, and treatment methods.

Overview of Urinary System Anatomy and Physiology

The **urinary system** is involved in several processes necessary for maintaining homeostasis, a state of physiological equilibrium in the body. The urinary system removes waste products of metabolism from the blood in the form of urine, which is excreted from the body.

Main Functions of the Urinary System

The primary functions of the urinary system are to
1. remove nitrogenous (nī-TRŎJ-ĕ-nŭs) waste products such as urea, uric acid, ammonia, and creatinine (krē-ĂT-ĭ-nēn), chemical substances that are toxic to the human body;
2. help regulate the electrolyte content of the blood;
3. maintain normal pH levels—the acid/base balance of the blood; and
4. assist in the regulation of blood pressure and red blood cell production.

Major Organs and Structures of the Urinary System

The primary organs of the urinary system are
- the kidneys (2);
- the ureters (2);
- the urinary bladder (1); and
- the urethra (1)

The urinary system, or **urinary tract**, is composed of the kidneys, ureters (ū-RĒ-tĕrs), bladder, and urethra (ū-RĒ-thră) (Figure 12.1). The **kidneys** filter waste products from our blood but also return substances that the body needs back into the circulatory (cardiovascular) system.

Nephrons (NĚF-rŏns) are the fundamental units within the kidneys that perform this filtration function. Each kidney contains nearly one million of these microscopic structures! After the nephrons have formed urine, the urine drains into the **renal pelvis**, a large, funnel-shaped cavity that narrows to form a pair of ureters.

The **ureters** are tube-like structures that carry urine from each kidney to the urinary bladder. Located at the floor of the pelvic cavity, the **urinary bladder** (more commonly called the **bladder**) is a hollow, muscular organ that temporarily stores urine. Just like the stomach, it has the ability to stretch. Its elastic walls expand to accommodate those four glasses of soda that you consume at a party, and they shrivel when the bladder is empty.

The **urethra** is a muscular tube that drains urine from the bladder and transports it out of the body. It has both voluntary and involuntary, circular-shaped muscles called *sphincter muscles* that allow you to control your bladder function. At the end of the urethra is an opening called the **urinary meatus** (mē-Ā-tŭs) that expels urine to the outside of the body.

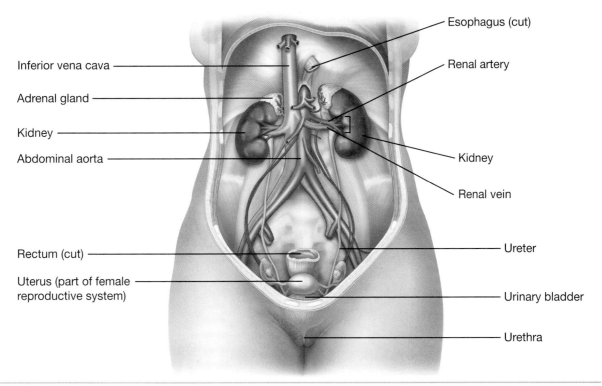

Inferior vena cava

Adrenal gland

Kidney

Abdominal aorta

Rectum (cut)

Uterus (part of female reproductive system)

Esophagus (cut)

Renal artery

Kidney

Renal vein

Ureter

Urinary bladder

Urethra

Figure 12.1 Organs and structures of the urinary system.

The act of excreting urine is called **urination**, **voiding**, or **micturition** (mĭk-tū-RĬ-shŭn). Sometimes a concentration of mineral salts forms a stone called a **calculus**, which blocks the passage of urine through the ureters. This condition is more commonly known as a "kidney stone." Kidney stones cause intense **flank** (lower back) pain accompanied by spasms, medically described as **renal colic**. Another common symptom of a kidney stone is urinary **frequency**—urinating often and usually in small amounts. (Urinary frequency may also be the result of any of a number of other health conditions, such as a urinary tract infection.

Urology (yū-RŎL-ō-jē) is the branch of medicine involving the study of the urine and the urinary system, and the diagnosis and treatment of **urological** (yū-rō-LŎJ-ĭ-kăl) conditions. A **urologist** (yū-RŎL-ō-jĭst) is a physician who specializes in the study, diagnosis, and treatment of urinary system diseases and disorders.

Anatomy and Physiology Vocabulary

Now that you have been introduced to the basic structure and functions of the urinary system, let's explore in more detail the key terms presented in the introduction.

Key Term	Definition
bladder	expandable pouch that stores urine; *urinary bladder*
calculus	stone
renal colic	painful spasms in the lower back that are associated with calculus (kidney stone) formation
flank	lower back (area between the ribs and hips)
frequency	urinating often, usually in small amounts
kidney	organ of the urinary system that produces urine
micturition	act of expelling urine
nephron	microscopic, fundamental working unit of the kidney
renal pelvis	funnel-shaped structure that collects urine and sends it to the ureter
ureter	tube that carries urine from the kidneys to the bladder
urethra	tube that transports urine to the outside of the body
urinary meatus	opening at the end of the urethra
urination	act of expelling urine
urine	water and waste products excreted by the kidneys
urologist	physician who specializes in the study, diagnosis, and treatment of urinary system diseases and disorders
urology	study of urine and the urinary system
voiding	act of expelling urine

E-Flash Card Activity: Anatomy and Physiology Vocabulary

Directions: After you have reviewed the anatomy and physiology vocabulary related to the urinary system, practice with the e-flash cards until you are comfortable with the spelling and definition of each term.

Identifying Major Organs and Structures of the Urinary System

Directions: Label the anatomical diagram of the urinary system.

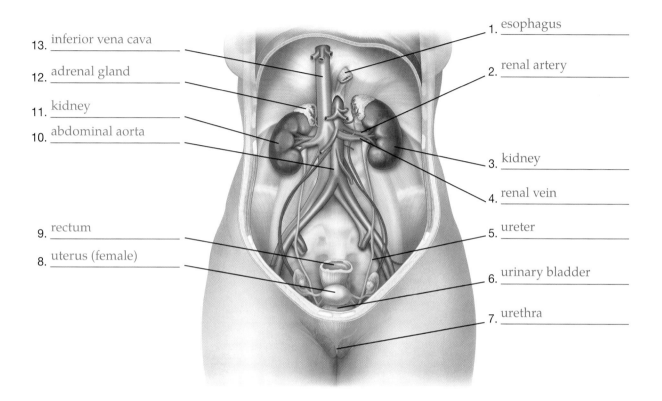

13. inferior vena cava

12. adrenal gland

11. kidney

10. abdominal aorta

9. rectum

8. uterus (female)

1. esophagus

2. renal artery

3. kidney

4. renal vein

5. ureter

6. urinary bladder

7. urethra

Number correct (_____), divided by 13 (_____), multiplied by 100 equals _____ (your score)

Matching Anatomy and Physiology Vocabulary

Directions: Match the vocabulary term in Column A with its meaning in Column B. Some meanings may be used more than once.

Column A

F   1. micturition

I   2. urine

G   3. urethra

M   4. kidney

H   5. bladder

F   6. voiding

C   7. nephron

E   8. ureter

D   9. renal pelvis

K   10. calculus

B   11. urinary meatus

J   12. renal colic

A   13. frequency

P   14. urology

N   15. flank

F   16. urination

O   17. urologist

Column B

A. urinating often

B. opening at the end of the urethra

C. microscopic, fundamental working unit of the kidney

D. funnel-shaped structure that collects urine and sends it to the ureter

E. tube that carries urine from the kidneys to the bladder

F. act of expelling urine

G. tube that transports urine to the outside of the body

H. expandable pouch that stores urine

I. water and waste products excreted by the kidneys

J. painful spasm

K. stone

M. organ of the urinary system that produces urine

N. lower back (area between the ribs and hips)

O. physician who specializes in the study, diagnosis, and treatment of urinary system diseases and disorders

P. study of urine and the urinary system

SCORECARD: How Did You Do?

Number correct (_____), divided by 17 (_____), multiplied by 100 equals _____ (your score)

Word Elements

In this section you will learn word elements—prefixes, combining forms, and suffixes—that are common to the urinary system. By learning these word elements and understanding how they are combined to build medical terms, you will be able to analyze Shara's health condition (described in the Intern Experience at the beginning of this chapter) and identify a large number of terms associated with the urinary system.

E-Flash Card Activity: Word Elements

Directions: Review the word elements in the tables that follow. Then, practice with the e-flash cards until you are able to quickly recognize the different word parts (prefixes, combining forms, and suffixes) and their meanings. The e-flash cards are grouped together by prefixes, combining forms, and suffixes, followed by a cumulative review of all the word elements that you learned in this chapter.

Prefixes

Let's start our study of urinary system word elements by reviewing the prefixes listed in the table below.

Prefix	Meaning
a-	not; without
an-	not; without
dys-	painful; difficult
intra-	within
peri-	around
poly-	many; much

Combining Forms

Listed below are combining forms that appear in medical terms used to describe the urinary system. Which of these are you already familiar with?

Root Word/Combining Vowel	Meaning
cyst/o	bladder; sac containing fluid
glyc/o	sugar; glucose
glycos/o	sugar; glucose
hem/o, hemat/o	blood
hydr/o	water
lith/o	stone
meat/o	opening
nephr/o	kidney
noct/o	night
olig/o	scanty; few
py/o	pus
pyel/o	renal pelvis
ren/o	kidney
son/o	sound
sten/o	narrow; constricted
ur/o	urine; urinary tract

(Continued)

Root Word/Combining Vowel	Meaning
ureter/o	ureter
urethr/o	urethra
urin/o	urine
vesic/o	bladder

Suffixes

Listed below are suffixes used in medical terms pertaining to the urinary system. You have also encountered these suffixes in your study of terms related to other body systems.

Suffix	Meaning
-al	pertaining to
-algia	pain
-cele	hernia; swelling; protrusion
-dipsia	thirst
-ectomy	surgical removal; excision
-emia	blood condition
-gram	record; image
-ia	condition
-iasis	abnormal condition
-itis	inflammation
-logist	specialist in the study and treatment of
-logy	study of
-lysis	destruction
-megaly	large; enlargement
-oma	tumor; mass
-osis	abnormal condition
-pexy	surgical fixation
-plasty	surgical repair
-ptosis	drooping; downward displacement
-rrhaphy	suture
-scope	instrument used to observe
-scopy	process of observing
-stomy	new opening
-tomy	incision; cut into
-tripsy	process of crushing

Matching Prefixes, Combining Forms, and Suffixes

Directions: In each exercise that follows, match the word element in Column A with its meaning in Column B. Some meanings may be used more than once.

Prefixes

Column A

__B__ 1. a-
__D__ 2. dys-
__C__ 3. poly-
__E__ 4. peri-
__B__ 5. an-
__A__ 6. intra-

Column B

A. within
B. not; without
C. many; much
D. painful; difficult
E. around

Combining Forms

Column A

__K__ 1. ureter/o
__D__ 2. py/o
__M__ 3. lith/o
__E__ 4. hem/o
__B__ 5. hydr/o
__G__ 6. glyc/o
__O__ 7. nephr/o
__N__ 8. urin/o
__A__ 9. sten/o
__H__ 10. son/o
__L__ 11. cyst/o
__O__ 12. ren/o
__G__ 13. glycos/o
__P__ 14. urethr/o
__N__ 15. ur/o
__L__ 16. vesic/o
__E__ 17. hemat/o
__J__ 18. pyel/o
__I__ 19. meat/o
__F__ 20. olig/o
__C__ 21. noct/o

Column B

A. narrow; constricted
B. water
C. night
D. pus
E. blood
F. scanty; few
G. sugar; glucose
H. sound
I. opening
J. renal pelvis
K. ureter
L. bladder
M. stone
N. urine; urinary tract
O. kidney
P. urethra

Suffixes

Column A

_M_ 1. -ia
_X_ 2. -iasis
_S_ 3. -pexy
_Q_ 4. -ptosis
_X_ 5. -osis
_R_ 6. -rrhaphy
_P_ 7. -dipsia
_O_ 8. -tripsy
_K_ 9. -emia
_N_ 10. -plasty
_I_ 11. -stomy
_W_ 12. -cele
_B_ 13. -lysis
_D_ 14. -al
_C_ 15. -algia
_T_ 16. -itis
_J_ 17. -logy
_E_ 18. -megaly
_H_ 19. -tomy
_G_ 20. -oma
_L_ 21. -logist
_F_ 22. -scope
_U_ 23. -gram
_V_ 24. -ectomy
_A_ 25. -scopy

Column B

A. process of observing
B. destruction
C. pain
D. pertaining to
E. large; enlargement
F. instrument used to observe
G. tumor; mass
H. incision; cut into
I. new opening
J. study of
K. blood condition
L. specialist in the study and treatment of
M. condition
N. surgical repair
O. process of crushing
P. thirst
Q. drooping; downward placement
R. suture
S. surgical fixation
T. inflammation
U. record; image
V. surgical removal; excision
W. hernia; swelling; protrusion
X. abnormal condition

SCORECARD: How Did You Do?

Number correct (_____), divided by 52 (_____), multiplied by 100 equals _____ (your score)

Breaking Down and Building Urinary System Terms

Now that you have mastered the prefixes, combining forms, and suffixes for medical terminology pertaining to the urinary system, you have the ability to dissect and build a large number of terms related to this body system.

Below is a list of medical terms commonly used in urology, the medical specialty concerned with the study, diagnosis, and treatment of the urinary system. For each term, a dissection has been provided, along with the meaning of each word element and the definition of the term as a whole.

Term	Dissection	Word Part/Meaning	Term Meaning
Note: For simplification, combining vowels have been omitted from the Word Part/Meaning column.			
1. **anuria** (ăn-YŪ-rē-ă)	an/ur/ia	an = not; without ur = urine; urinary tract ia = condition	condition of without urine
2. **cystectomy** (sĭs-TĔK-tō-mē)	cyst/ectomy	cyst = bladder; sac containing fluid ectomy = surgical removal; excision	excision of the bladder
3. **cystitis** (sĭs-TĪ-tĭs)	cyst/itis	cyst = bladder; sac containing fluid itis = inflammation	inflammation of the bladder
4. **cystocele** (SĬS-tō-sēl)	cyst/o/cele	cyst = bladder; sac containing fluid cele = hernia; swelling; protrusion	hernia/swelling of the bladder
5. **cystolithiasis** (SĬS-tō-lĭ-THĪ-ă-sĭs)	cyst/o/lith/iasis	cyst = bladder; sac containing fluid lith = stone iasis = abnormal condition	abnormal condition of a stone in the bladder
6. **cystolithotomy** (SĬS-tō-lĭ-THŎT-ō-mē)	cyst/o/lith/o/tomy	cyst = bladder; sac containing fluid lith = stone tomy = incision; cut into	incision to the bladder for a stone
7. **cystoplasty** (SĬS-tō-PLĂS-tē)	cyst/o/plasty	cyst = bladder; sac containing fluid plasty = surgical repair	surgical repair of the bladder

Prefixes = Green   Root Words = **Red**   Suffixes = Blue

Term	Dissection	Word Part/Meaning	Term Meaning
8. **cystoscope** (SĬS-tō-skōp)	cyst/o/scope	**cyst** = bladder; sac containing fluid **scope** = instrument used to observe	instrument used to observe the bladder
9. **cystoscopy** (sĭs-TŎS-kō-pē)	cyst/o/scopy	**cyst** = bladder; sac containing fluid **scopy** = process of observing	process of observing the bladder
10. **cystotomy** (sĭs-TŎT-ō-mē)	cyst/o/tomy	**cyst** = bladder; sac containing fluid **tomy** = incision; cut into	incision to the bladder
11. **dysuria** (dĭs-YŪ-rē-ă)	dys/ur/ia	**dys** = painful; difficult **ur** = urine; urinary tract **ia** = condition	condition of painful/difficult urination
12. **glycosuria** (GLĪ-kōs-YŪ-rē-ă)	glycos/ur/ia	**glycos** = glucose; sugar **ur** = urine; urinary tract **ia** = condition	condition of sugar in the urine
13. **hematuria** (HĒ-mă-TŪ-rē-ă)	hemat/ur/ia	**hemat** = blood **ur** = urine; urinary tract **ia** = condition	condition of blood in the urine
14. **hydronephrosis** (HĪ-drō-nĕ-FRŌ-sĭs)	hydr/o/nephr/osis	**hydro** = water **nephr** = kidney **osis** = abnormal condition	abnormal condition of water in the kidney
15. **lithotripsy** (LĬTH-ō-TRĬP-sē)	lith/o/tripsy	**lith** = stone **tripsy** = process of crushing	process of crushing a stone
16. **nephrectomy** (nĕ-FRĔK-tō-mē)	nephr/ectomy	**nephr** = kidney **ectomy** = surgical removal; excision	excision of the kidney
17. **nephritis** (nĕ-FRĪ-tĭs)	nephr/itis	**nephr** = kidney **itis** = inflammation	inflammation of the kidney
18. **nephrolithiasis** (NĔF-rō-lĭ-THĪ-ă-sĭs)	nephr/o/lith/iasis	**nephr** = kidney **lith** = stone **iasis** = abnormal condition	abnormal condition of a stone in the kidney
19. **nephroma** (nĕ-FRŌ-mă)	nephr/oma	**nephr** = kidney **oma** = tumor; mass	tumor of the kidney
20. **nephropexy** (NĔF-rō-PĔKS-ē)	nephr/o/pexy	**nephr** = kidney **pexy** = surgical fixation	surgical fixation of the kidney
21. **nephroplasty** (NĔF-rō-PLĂS-tē)	nephr/o/plasty	**nephr** = kidney **plasty** = surgical repair	surgical repair of the kidney

Prefixes = Green   Root Words = Red   Suffixes = Blue

Term	Dissection	Word Part/Meaning	Term Meaning
22. **nephroptosis** (NĔF-rŏp-TŌ-sĭs)	nephr/o/ptosis	**nephr** = kidney **ptosis** = drooping; downward displacement	drooping or downward displacement of the kidney
23. **nephrorrhaphy** (nĕf-ROR-ă-fē)	nephr/o/rrhapy	**nephr** = kidney **rrhaphy** = suture	suture of the kidney
24. **nephrostomy** (nĕ-FRŎS-tō-mē)	nephr/o/stomy	**nephr** = kidney **stomy** = new opening	new opening in the kidney
25. **nephrotomy** (nĕ-FRŎT-ō-mē)	nephr/o/tomy	**nephr** = kidney **tomy** = incision; cut into	incision to the kidney
26. **nocturia** (nŏkt-YŪ-rē-ă)	noct/ur/ia	**noct** = night **ur** = urine; urinary tract **ia** = condition	condition of (producing) urine at night
27. **oliguria** (ŎL-ĭg-YŪ-rē-ă)	olig/ur/ia	**olig** = scanty; few **ur** = urine; urinary tract **ia** = condition	condition of scanty urine
28. **periurethral** (PĔR-ē-yū-RĒ-thrăl)	peri/urethr/al	**peri** = around **urethr** = urethra **al** = pertaining to	pertaining to around the urethra
29. **polydipsia** (PŎL-ē-DĬP-sē-ă)	poly/dips/ia	**poly** = many; much **dips** = thirst **ia** = condition	condition of much thirst
30. **pyelogram** (PĪ-ĕ-lō-GRĂM)	pyel/o/gram	**pyel** = renal pelvis **gram** = record; image	record/image of the renal pelvis
31. **pyelonephritis** (PĪ-ĕ-lō-nĕ-FRĪ-tĭs)	pyel/o/nephr/itis	**pyel** = renal pelvis **nephr** = kidney **itis** = inflammation	inflammation of the kidney and renal pelvis
32. **pyelonephrosis** (PĪ-ĕ-lō-nĕ-FRŌ-sĭs)	pyel/o/nephr/osis	**pyel** = renal pelvis **nephr** = kidney **osis** = abnormal condition	abnormal condition of the kidney and renal pelvis
33. **pyonephritis** (PĪ-ō-nĕf-RĪ-tĭs)	py/o/nephr/itis	**py** = pus **nephr** = kidney **itis** = inflammation	inflammation and pus in the kidney
34. **pyuria** (pī-YŪ-rē-ă)	py/ur/ia	**py** = pus **ur** = urine; urinary tract **ia** = condition	condition of pus in the urine
35. **uremia** (yū-RĒ-mē-ă)	ur/emia	**ur** = urine; urinary tract **emia** = blood condition	blood condition of urine (waste products of urine in the blood)

Prefixes = **Green**   Root Words = **Red**   Suffixes = **Blue**

Term	Dissection	Word Part/Meaning	Term Meaning
36. **ureterolithiasis** (yū-RĒ-tĕr-ō-lĭth-Ī-ă-sĭs)	ureter/o/lith/iasis	**ureter** = ureter **lith** = stone **iasis** = abnormal condition	abnormal condition of a stone in the ureter
37. **ureteropyelonephritis** (yū-RĒ-tĕr-ō-PĪ-ĕl-ō-nĕf-RĪ-tĭs)	ureter/o/pyel/o/ nephr/itis	**ureter** = ureter **pyel** = renal pelvis **nephr** = kidney **itis** = inflammation	inflammation of the ureter, renal pelvis, and kidney
38. **ureterostenosis** (yū-RĒ-tĕr-ō-stĕn-Ō-sĭs)	ureter/o/sten/osis	**ureter** = ureter **sten** = narrow; constricted **osis** = abnormal condition	abnormal condition of a narrow or constricted ureter
39. **ureterovesicostomy** (yū-RĒ-tĕr-ō-vĕs-ĭ-KŎS-tō-mē)	ureter/o/vesic/o/ stomy	**ureter** = ureter **vesic** = bladder **stomy** = new opening	new opening in the ureter and bladder
40. **urethral** (yū-RĒ-thrăl)	urethr/al	**urethr** = urethra **al** = pertaining to	pertaining to the urethra
41. **urethralgia** (yū-rē-THRĂL-jē-ă)	urethr/algia	**urethr** = urethra **algia** = pain	pain in the urethra
42. **urethrocystitis** (yū-RĒ-thrō-sĭs-TĪ-tĭs)	urethr/o/cyst/itis	**urethr** = urethra **cyst** = bladder; sac containing fluid **itis** = inflammation	inflammation of the urethra and bladder
43. **urethroscope** (yū-RĒ-thrō-skōp)	urethr/o/scope	**urethr** = urethra **scope** = instrument used to observe	instrument used to observe the urethra
44. **urogram** (YŪ-rō-grăm)	ur/o/gram	**ur** = urine; urinary tract **gram** = record; image	record/image of the urinary tract
45. **urologist** (yū-RŎL-ō-jĭst)	ur/o/logist	**ur** = urine; urinary tract **logist** = specialist in the study and treatment of	specialist in the study and treatment of the urinary tract
46. **urology** (yū-RŎL-ō-jē)	ur/o/logy	**ur** = urine; urinary tract **logy** = study of	study of the urine and urinary tract

Prefixes = Green   Root Words = Red   Suffixes = Blue

Using the pronunciation guide in the Breaking Down and Building chart, practice saying each medical term aloud. To hear the pronunciation of each term, go to the Pronounce It activity at the G-W companion website.

Audio Activity: Pronounce It

Directions: At the companion website, listen as each medical term listed below is pronounced. Practice pronouncing the terms until you are comfortable saying them aloud.

anuria
(ăn-YŪ-rē-ă)

cystectomy
(sĭs-TĔK-tō-mē)

cystitis
(sĭs-TĪ-tĭs)

cystocele
(SĬS-tō-sēl)

cystolithiasis
(SĬS-tō-lĭ-THĪ-ă-sĭs)

cystolithotomy
(SĬS-tō-lĭ-THŎT-ō-mē)

cystoplasty
(SĬS-tō-PLĂS-tē)

cystoscope
(SĬS-tō-skōp)

cystoscopy
(sĭs-TŎS-kō-pē)

cystotomy
(sĭs-TŎT-ō-mē)

dysuria
(dĭs-YŪ-rē-ă)

glycosuria
(GLĪ-kōs-YŪ-rē-ă)

hematuria
(HĒ-mă-TŪ-rē-ă)

hydronephrosis
(HĪ-drō-nĕ-FRŌ-sĭs)

lithotripsy
(LĬTH-ō-TRĬP-sē)

nephrectomy
(nĕ-FRĔK-tō-mē)

nephritis
(nĕ-FRĪ-tĭs)

nephrolithiasis
(NĔF-rō-lĭ-THĪ-ă-sĭs)

nephroma
(nĕ-FRŌ-mă)

nephropexy
(NĔF-rō-PĔKS-ē)

nephroplasty
(NĔF-rō-PLĂS-tē)

nephroptosis
(NĔF-rŏp-TŌ-sĭs)

nephrorrhaphy
(nĕf-ROR-ă-fē)

nephrostomy
(nĕ-FRŎS-tō-mē)

nephrotomy
(nĕ-FRŎT-ō-mē)

nocturia
(nŏkt-YŪ-rē-ă)

oliguria
(ŎL-ĭg-YŪ-rē-ă)

periurethral
(PĔR-ē-yū-RĒ-thrăl)

polydipsia
(PŎL-ē-DĬP-sē-ă)

pyelogram
(PĪ-ĕ-lō-GRĂM)

pyelonephritis
(PĪ-ĕ-lō-nĕ-FRĪ-tĭs)

pyelonephrosis
(PĪ-ĕ-lō-nĕ-FRŌ-sĭs)

pyonephritis
(PĪ-ō-nĕf-RĪ-tĭs)

pyuria
(pī-YŪ-rē-ă)

uremia
(yū-RĒ-mē-ă)

ureterolithiasis
(yū-RĒ-tĕr-ō-lĭth-Ī-ă-sĭs)

ureteropyelonephritis
(yū-RĒ-tĕr-ō-PĪ-ĕl-ō-nĕf-RĪ-tĭs)

ureterostenosis
(yū-RĒ-tĕr-ō-stĕn-Ō-sĭs)

ureterovesicostomy
(yū-RĒ-tĕr-ō-vĕs-ĭ-KŎS-tō-mē)

urethral
(yū-RĒ-thrăl)

urethralgia
(yū-rē-THRĂL-jē-ă)

urethrocystitis
(yū-RĒ-thrō-sĭs-TĪ-tĭs)

urethroscope
(yū-RĒ-thrō-skōp)

urogram
(YŪ-rō-grăm)

urologist
(yū-RŎL-ō-jĭst)

urology
(yū-RŎL-ō-jē)

Audio Activity: Spell It

Directions: Cover the medical terms in the Pronounce It activity with a sheet of paper. At the companion website, listen as the terms are read aloud. Correctly spell each term below.

1. anuria
2. cystectomy
3. cystitis
4. cystocele
5. cystolithiasis

6. cystolithotomy
7. cystoplasty
8. cystoscope
9. cystoscopy
10. cystotomy

11. dysuria _____
12. glycosuria _____
13. hematuria _____
14. hydronephrosis _____
15. lithotripsy _____
16. nephrectomy _____
17. nephritis _____
18. nephrolithiasis _____
19. nephroma _____
20. nephropexy _____
21. nephroplasty _____
22. nephroptosis _____
23. nephrorrhaphy _____
24. nephrostomy _____
25. nephrotomy _____
26. nocturia _____
27. oliguria _____
28. periurethral _____

29. polydipsia _____
30. pyelogram _____
31. pyelonephritis _____
32. pyelonephrosis _____
33. pyonephritis _____
34. pyuria _____
35. uremia _____
36. ureterolithiasis _____
37. ureteropyelonephritis _____
38. ureterostenosis _____
39. ureterovesicostomy _____
40. urethral _____
41. urethralgia _____
42. urethrocystitis _____
43. urethroscope _____
44. urogram _____
45. urologist _____
46. urology _____

Assessment

Break It Down

Directions: Dissect each medical term below into its word elements by placing a slash between each word part (prefix, root word, combining vowel, and suffix). Then define each term.

Example:

Medical Term: nephropyelogram

Dissection: nephr/o/pyel/o/gram

Definition: record/image of the kidney and renal pelvis

Medical Term	Dissection
1. urogram	u r/o/g r a m

Definition: record or image of the urinary tract _____

2. polydipsia	p o l y/d i p s/i a

Definition: condition of much thirst _____

Medical Term	Dissection
3. nephrotomy	n e p h r / o / t o m y

Definition: incision to the kidney

4. nephroplasty	n e p h r / o / p l a s t y

Definition: surgical repair of the kidney

5. cystoplasty	c y s t / o / p l a s t y

Definition: surgical repair of the bladder

6. pyelonephritis	p y e l / o / n e p h r / i t i s

Definition: inflammation of the kidney and renal pelvis

7. nephrolithiasis	n e p h r / o / l i t h / i a s i s

Definition: abnormal condition of a stone in the kidney

8. cystitis	c y s t / i t i s

Definition: inflammation of the bladder

9. urethrocystitis	u r e t h r / o / c y s t / i t i s

Definition: inflammation of the urethra and bladder

10. anuria	a n / u r / i a

Definition: condition of without urine

Medical Term	Dissection

11. hydronephrosis

h y d r/o/n e p h r/o s i s

Definition: abnormal condition of water in the kidney

_____

12. cystoscopy

c y s t/o/s c o p y

Definition: process of observing the bladder

_____

13. nephropexy

n e p h r/o/p e x y

Definition: surgical fixation of the kidney

_____

14. urology

u r/o/l o g y

Definition: study of the urine and urinary tract

_____

15. cystotomy

c y s t/o/t o m y

Definition: incision to the bladder

_____

16. cystectomy

c y s t/e c t o m y

Definition: excision of the bladder

_____

17. nocturia

n o c t/u r/i a

Definition: condition of (producing) urine at night

_____

18. cystolithotomy

c y s t/o/l i t h/o/t o m y

Definition: incision to the bladder for a stone

_____

Medical Term	Dissection
19. glycosuria	g l y c o s/u r/i a

Definition: condition of sugar in the urine

20. nephritis	n e p h r/i t i s

Definition: inflammation of the kidney

21. cystoscope	c y s t/o/s c o p e

Definition: instrument used to observe the bladder

22. nephrorrhaphy	n e p h r/o/r r h a p h y

Definition: suture of the kidney

23. pyelonephrosis	p y e l/o/n e p h r/o s i s

Definition: abnormal condition of the kidney and renal pelvis

24. nephroma	n e p h r/o m a

Definition: tumor of the kidney

25. urethralgia	u r e t h r/a l g i a

Definition: pain in the urethra

SCORECARD: How Did You Do?

Number correct (_____), divided by 25 (_____), multiplied by 100 equals _____ (your score)

Build It

Directions: Build the medical term that matches each definition below by supplying the correct word elements.

P (Prefixes) = Green
RW (Root Words) = Red
S (Suffixes) = Blue
CV (Combining Vowel) = Purple

1. abnormal condition of a narrow or constricted ureter

ureter	o	sten	osis
RW	CV	RW	S

2. condition of without urine

an	ur	ia
P	RW	S

3. new opening in the ureter and bladder

ureter	o	vesic	o	stomy
RW	CV	RW	CV	S

4. process of crushing a stone

lith	o	tripsy
RW	CV	S

5. abnormal condition of a stone in the kidney

nephr	o	lith	iasis
RW	CV	RW	S

6. incision to the bladder for a stone

cyst	o	lith	o	tomy
RW	CV	RW	CV	S

7. new opening in the kidney

nephr	o	stomy
RW	CV	S

8. abnormal condition of a stone in the ureter

ureter	o	lith	iasis
RW	CV	RW	S

9. incision to the kidney

$$\underset{\text{RW}}{\text{nephr}} \quad \underset{\text{CV}}{\text{o}} \quad \underset{\text{S}}{\text{tomy}}$$

10. blood condition of urine (waste products of urine in the blood)

$$\underset{\text{RW}}{\text{ur}} \quad \underset{\text{S}}{\text{emia}}$$

11. hernia/swelling of the bladder

$$\underset{\text{RW}}{\text{cyst}} \quad \underset{\text{CV}}{\text{o}} \quad \underset{\text{S}}{\text{cele}}$$

12. incision to the bladder

$$\underset{\text{RW}}{\text{cyst}} \quad \underset{\text{CV}}{\text{o}} \quad \underset{\text{S}}{\text{tomy}}$$

13. inflammation and pus in the kidney

$$\underset{\text{RW}}{\text{py}} \quad \underset{\text{CV}}{\text{o}} \quad \underset{\text{RW}}{\text{nephr}} \quad \underset{\text{S}}{\text{itis}}$$

14. abnormal condition of a stone in the bladder

$$\underset{\text{RW}}{\text{cyst}} \quad \underset{\text{CV}}{\text{o}} \quad \underset{\text{RW}}{\text{lith}} \quad \underset{\text{S}}{\text{iasis}}$$

15. inflammation of the urethra and bladder

$$\underset{\text{RW}}{\text{urethr}} \quad \underset{\text{CV}}{\text{o}} \quad \underset{\text{RW}}{\text{cyst}} \quad \underset{\text{S}}{\text{itis}}$$

16. excision of the kidney

$$\underset{\text{RW}}{\text{nephr}} \quad \underset{\text{S}}{\text{ectomy}}$$

17. inflammation of the ureter, renal pelvis, and kidney

$$\underset{\text{RW}}{\text{ureter}} \quad \underset{\text{CV}}{\text{o}} \quad \underset{\text{RW}}{\text{pyel}} \quad \underset{\text{CV}}{\text{o}} \quad \underset{\text{RW}}{\text{nephr}} \quad \underset{\text{S}}{\text{itis}}$$

SCORECARD: How Did You Do?

Number correct (_____), divided by 17 (_____), multiplied by 100 equals _____ (your score)

Diseases and Disorders

Diseases and disorders of the urinary system run the spectrum of the mild to the severe. In this section, we will briefly explore the major characteristics and causes of some common pathological conditions of this body system.

Urinary Tract Infection

When bacteria invade the urinary tract, they can cause a **urinary tract infection (UTI)**. Bacteria typically enter the bladder via the urethra. Cystitis and urethritis are two common types of lower urinary tract infections. Inflammation of the urethra is called **urethritis** (yū-rē-THRĪ-tĭs). Inflammation of the bladder is called **cystitis** (sĭs-TĪ-tĭs). Bladder inflammation caused by a bacterial infection is known as *bacterial cystitis*.

Symptoms of a UTI include fever, lower back pain, urinary frequency, and a sensation of burning during urination. The urine may appear dark yellow or even pink if blood is present. A urinalysis is often performed to determine the presence of bacteria and white blood cells in the urine.

If a bladder infection (cystitis) is left untreated, the infection can spread upward through the ureters and into the pelvis of the kidney, causing **pyelitis** (PĪ-ĕ-LĪ-tĭs). Thus, an infection of the kidneys that also involves the renal pelvis is called *pyelonephritis* (PĪ-ĕ-lō-nĕ-FRĪ-tĭs).

Cystitis

Cystitis (sĭs-TĪ-tĭs) is an inflammation of the urinary bladder, usually due to an ascending urinary tract infection. An ascending UTI is one in which the bacteria travel from the bladder up through the ureter and into the kidney. Most cases of cystitis are caused by *Escherichia coli* (ĕsh-ĕr-ĪK-ē-ă KŌ-lī), a bacillus (type of bacteria) found in the lower gastrointestinal tract (stomach and intestines).

Cystitis is a common problem, especially in females. Because the urethra in the female is shorter than that in the male, bacteria do not have to travel very far to enter the bladder of a female. Urinary frequency, painful urination, chills, and fever are common symptoms of cystitis. A burning sensation during urination, which may or may not be accompanied by pyuria (pī-YŪ-rē-ă) (pus in the urine), may also be experienced.

Urinary Incontinence

Urinary incontinence is a disorder involving loss of bladder control. It can result in **enuresis** (ĕn-yū-RĒ-sĭs), commonly known as *bedwetting*.

Urinary incontinence (often shortened to the term *incontinence*), may be a symptom of an underlying medical condition or the result of everyday habits. Certain medications, foods, and beverages (such as caffeinated coffee, tea, and soda) can cause excessive urination and temporary urinary incontinence. Urinary tract infections often produce a strong urge to urinate, which can result in incontinence. Aging, pregnancy, and certain cancers can irritate the bladder, leading to urinary incontinence.

Urinary Retention

Urinary retention is the abnormal, involuntary holding of urine in the bladder, which leads to incomplete emptying of the bladder. Neurological dysfunction or an obstruction in the urinary tract can contribute to urinary retention. When a problem interferes with the nerve impulses reaching the bladder, a person is not aware that his or her bladder is full. Weak bladder muscles can also result in urinary retention. Other factors that can cause urinary retention include surgery, certain medications, and enlargement of the prostate gland.

Hydronephrosis

Hydronephrosis (HĪ-drō-nĕ-FRŌ-sĭs) is a condition that causes *distension* (inflation) and *dilation* (expansion) of the renal pelvis, resulting in enlargement of the kidney (Figure 12.2). It is usually caused by an obstructing stone or stricture (narrowing) in the ureter. It often leads to progressive atrophy (wasting away) of the kidney.

Kidney Stones

Kidney stones, also known as *renal calculi*, are small "pebbles" of salt and minerals that form inside the kidney. They can affect any part of the urinary tract from the kidneys to the bladder. Kidney stones are classified by their location in the kidney (*nephrolithiasis*), ureter (*ureterolithiasis*), or bladder (*cystolithiasis*).

Stones that obstruct the ureter or renal pelvis produce excruciating, intermittent pain that radiates from the flank to the groin. As described in the Overview of Urinary System Anatomy and Physiology earlier in this chapter, this phenomenon is clinically characterized as *renal colic*. Renal colic is commonly accompanied by urinary urgency, hematuria (blood in the urine), painful urination, fever, nausea, and vomiting.

A diagnosis of nephrolithiasis is made based on information obtained from a physical examination, personal and family health history, urinalysis, and radiographic studies. In addition, blood tests and ultrasound studies may aid in the diagnosis. Kidney stones occur more often in men than in women.

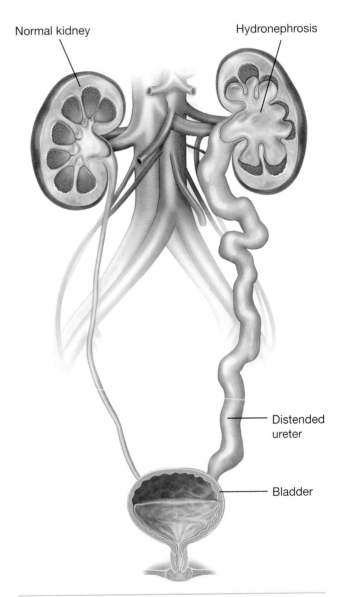

Normal kidney

Hydronephrosis

Distended ureter

Bladder

Figure 12.2 Hydronephrosis, typically caused by an obstruction or a stricture in the ureter, causes the kidney to become enlarged.

Pyelonephritis

Pyelonephritis (PĪ-ĕ-lō-nĕ-FRĪ-tĭs) is an inflammation of the renal pelvis and kidney (Figure 12.3). It is often caused by a bacterial infection. Pyelonephritis can be described as an *ascending urinary tract infection* because the bacteria in the bladder ascend (travel up) the ureters to the kidneys.

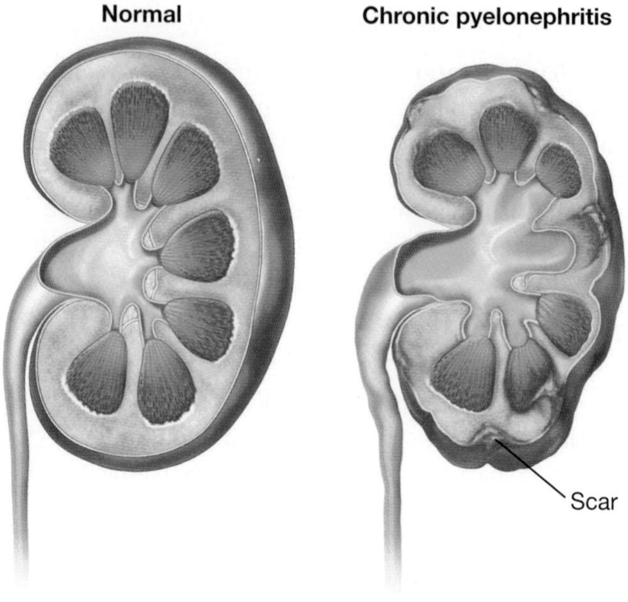

Uremia

Uremia (yū-RĒ-mē-ă) is a condition associated with renal (kidney) failure. In uremia, the kidneys do not remove *urea* (yū-RĒ-ă), a waste product, from the blood. Thus, the blood is not completely cleansed of toxins and other substances that should have been excreted in the urine.

Uremia is a life-threatening condition that produces symptoms of low urine production (oliguria), tachycardia (rapid heart rate), edema (swelling), polydipsia (excessive thirst), dry mouth, fatigue, weakness, pallor (pale skin), confusion, and possible loss of consciousness.

Normal   **Chronic pyelonephritis**

Scar

Figure 12.3 Pyelonephritis, an inflammation of the renal pelvis and the kidney, is frequently caused by a bacterial infection.

Cystocele

Cystocele (SĬS-tō-sēl) occurs when the urinary bladder *herniates* (protrudes) through the wall of the vagina (Figure 12.4). Doctors may refer to a cystocele as a *prolapsed bladder* because the vaginal wall has collapsed, causing the bladder to bulge downward into the vagina.

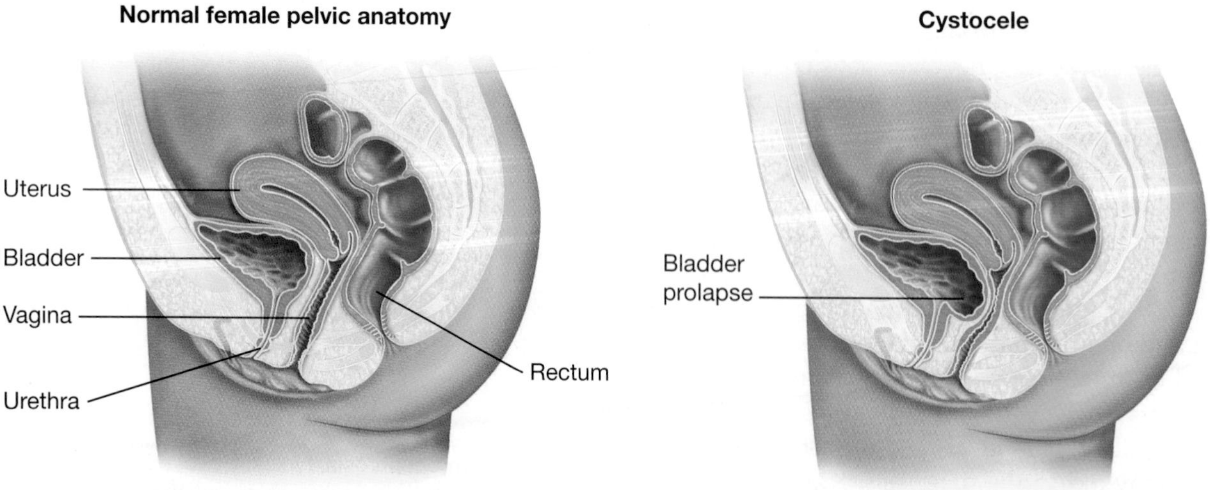

Normal female pelvic anatomy   **Cystocele**

Uterus

Bladder

Vagina

Urethra

Rectum

Bladder prolapse

Figure 12.4 When the bladder protrudes through the vaginal wall, the result is a cystocele, or prolapsed bladder.

A cystocele is also known as a **vesicocele** (VĔS-ĭ-kō-SĒL). Patients with this condition may experience difficulty emptying their bladder, urinary incontinence, and repeated bladder infections.

Procedures and Treatments

In this section, we will briefly describe some diagnostic tests and procedures used to help identify disorders and diseases of the urinary system, as well as some common therapeutic procedures used to treat certain conditions.

Urinalysis

Urinalysis (YŪR-ĭ-NĂL-ĭ-sĭs), or **UA**, is a laboratory analysis of the urine, often performed in a doctor's office using a dipstick and/or microscopy. A *dipstick* is a plastic stick filled with squares of many different colors (Figure 12.5). Each square contains a reagent, a chemical substance used to detect and measure other substances.

A dipstick is placed in a patient's urine specimen. When the urine interacts with the reagent, it changes color. All the reagent squares on the dipstick are compared to those on a color chart located on the container. The resulting color indicates any of various types of urinary problems. A dipstick urinalysis can help diagnose a urinary condition based on pH (acidity or alkalinity), specific gravity, or the content of substances such as blood, protein, glucose, ketones (a by-product of the breakdown of fat instead of glucose), or bilirubin (a substance produced when the liver breaks down old red blood cells).

Microscopic urinalysis provides more detailed information about a urine specimen when dipstick results are abnormal. The specimen is viewed under a high-magnification microscope (one with a high-powered field of view). More than four erythrocytes (red blood cells) seen in a high-powered field is an abnormal finding.

Culture and Sensitivity Test

A **culture and sensitivity (C&S)** (Figure 12.6) involves a *culture test*, in which microorganisms from a sample of a patient's urine are placed in a culture medium in a petri dish, and a *sensitivity test* to determine what medicine (typically an antibiotic) will effectively treat a urinary tract infection (UTI).

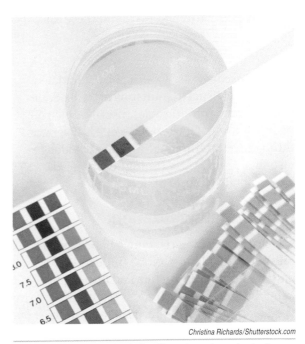

Christina Richards/Shutterstock.com

Figure 12.5 A urinalysis is often done in a doctor's office using a dipstick that contains chemical reagents, which help detect and measure the presence of other chemical substances.

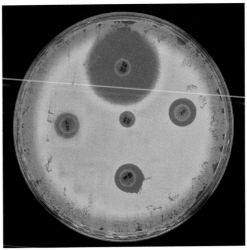

Corbis Images

Figure 12.6 In this culture and sensitivity test, the clear rings around the antibiotic disks indicate that the antibiotic will be effective in treating an infection caused by the bacteria cultivated in the petri dish.

In a manual sensitivity test, disks with various antibiotics are placed on a culture plate along with a suspension of the isolated bacteria. If the infection is bacterial, the antibiotics most effective in treating the UTI will inhibit bacterial growth near the disks, and there will be larger zones of inhibition around these disk.

Cystoscopy

Cystoscopy (sĭs-TŎS-kō-pē), abbreviated as **cysto**, is a visual examination of the bladder using a very thin, flexible, tube-like instrument (Figure 12.7). The optic scope is inserted through the urethra and into the bladder to visualize the mucosa (lining) of the bladder and to obtain a biopsy if necessary.

Urinary Catheterization

Urinary catheterization (abbreviated as **cath**) involves placing a tube through the urinary meatus into the urethra and then manipulating the tube into the bladder (Figure 12.8). Urinary catheterization is commonly used for continuous drainage of the bladder. It may also be used to obtain a sterile urine sample or to *instill* (introduce) medications into the bladder.

An *indwelling catheter* drains urine from the bladder to a bag outside the body. It is held in place by a balloon tip filled with water and can be left inside the body for a longer period of time than a standard urinary catheter.

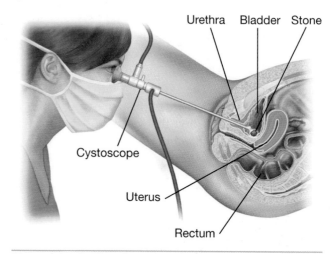

Figure 12.7 Cystoscopy is the visual examination of the bladder using a cystoscope.

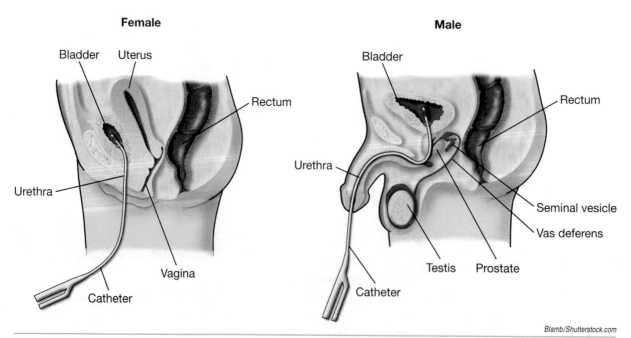

Figure 12.8 Urinary catheterization in the female and in the male.

Blamb/Shutterstock.com

Intravenous Pyelogram

Intravenous pyelogram (PĪ-ĕ-lō-grăm), or **IVP**, is a radiographic procedure in which a contrast agent is injected into the body to visualize the urinary tract (Figure 12.9). A contrast agent, sometimes referred to as a *dye*, is often used in radiographic procedures. It allows visualization of bodily structures that are not dense enough to show up on routine X-rays.

Once the contrast agent has been injected into a vein, a rapid series of radiographs captures the visual progress of the agent through the kidneys, ureters, and bladder, providing information about their structure and function. Intravenous pyelogram is also called a *urogram*.

Renal Scan

A **renal scan** is a nuclear medicine imaging procedure that reveals the size, shape, position, and function of the kidneys. In this procedure, a radioactive isotope is injected intravenously into the patient. The isotope is absorbed by the kidneys and emits radioactive particles that are captured by a scanner. The scanner transforms the data collected into an image.

A renal scan is particularly useful when a person is allergic to the contrast material (dye) used in an intravenous pyelogram (IVP). Abnormal results of a renal scan are a sign of impaired kidney function.

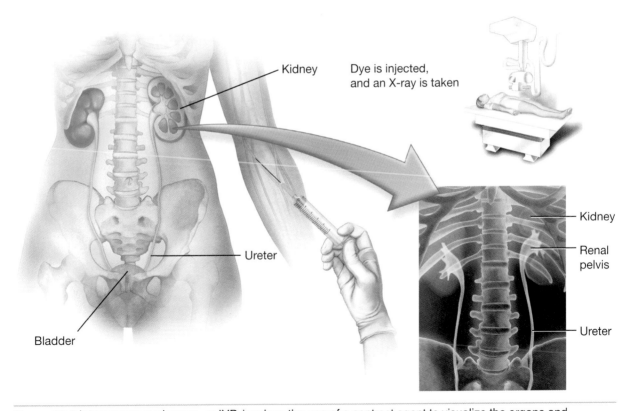

Figure 12.9 Intravenous pyelogram, or IVP, involves the use of a contrast agent to visualize the organs and structures of the urinary tract.

Renal Ultrasound

A **renal ultrasound** is an imaging technique that uses high-frequency sound waves and a computer to generate images of the kidneys. It is used to detect abnormal masses or blockages.

The renal ultrasound is a painless, noninvasive (does not pierce the skin) procedure that requires little preparation on the part of the patient. Because it does not involve exposure to radiation, it is an ideal diagnostic imaging method for the pregnant patient. A renal ultrasound is also called a *renal sonogram*.

Renal Dialysis

Renal dialysis is an artificial method of filtration used to remove waste products and excess water from the body when the kidneys fail to perform this function (Figure 12.10).

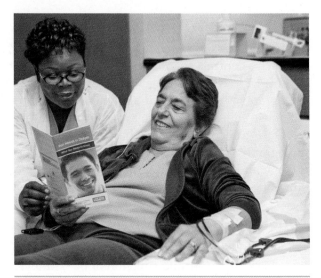

Figure 12.10 A patient with kidney failure undergoes renal dialysis to remove waste products and excess water from her body.

There are two main types of dialysis: *hemodialysis* and *peritoneal dialysis*. Both methods rid the body of harmful wastes by filtering the blood.

Hemodialysis, the more common dialysis method for renal failure, accomplishes the task of filtration using a machine called a *dialyzer* (Figure 12.11). In peritoneal dialysis, the lining of the patient's own abdomen (the *peritoneal membrane*) is used to filter the blood.

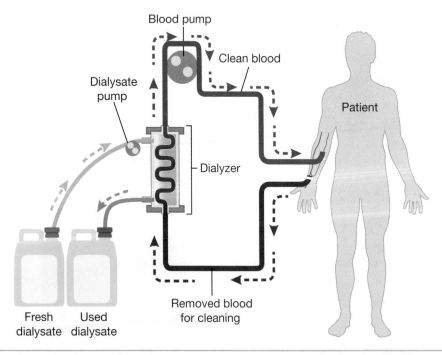

Figure 12.11 In hemodialysis, the more common treatment method for kidney failure, a dialyzer cleanses the patient's blood and returns clean blood back into the body.

Multiple Choice: Diseases and Disorders

Directions: Write the letter of the disease or disorder that matches each numbered definition.

_B_ 1. the abnormal, involuntary holding of urine in the bladder
  a. urinary incontinence
  b. urinary retention
  c. polyuria
  d. oliguria

_C_ 2. inflammation of the kidney and renal pelvis
  a. hydronephrosis
  b. pyonephrosis
  c. pyelonephritis
  d. nephrolithiasis

_A_ 3. disorder characterized by loss of bladder control
  a. urinary incontinence
  b. urinary frequency
  c. nocturia
  d. polyuria

_C_ 4. inflammation of the bladder due to an ascending urinary tract infection
  a. hydronephrosis
  b. hydronephritis
  c. cystitis
  d. uremia

_A_ 5. condition that causes distension and dilation of the renal pelvis, resulting in enlargement of the kidney
  a. hydronephrosis
  b. pyelonephritis
  c. uremia
  d. polyuria

_A_ 6. condition in which the bladder herniates, or protrudes, through the vaginal wall
  a. cystocele
  b. vesicocele
  c. hypercystocele
  d. both a and b

_C_ 7. cystitis and urethritis are two common types of
  a. renal pelvis infections
  b. hernial conditions of the bladder
  c. urinary tract infections
  d. diseases that require renal dialysis treatment

SCORECARD: How Did You Do?

Number correct (_____), divided by 7 (_____), multiplied by 100 equals _____ (your score)

Multiple Choice: Procedures and Treatments

Directions: Write the letter of the diagnostic test or therapeutic procedure that matches each numbered definition.

_A_ 1. visual examination of the bladder using a very thin, flexible, tube-like instrument
  a. cystoscopy
  b. cystogram
  c. cystourethrogram
  d. intravenous pyelogram

_D_ 2. radiographic procedure in which a contrast agent is injected into the body to visualize the urinary tract
  a. cystogram
  b. urethrogram
  c. catheterization
  d. intravenous pyelogram

_C_ 3. test used to determine the most effective antibiotic for treating a urinary tract infection
  a. urinalysis
  b. cystoscopy
  c. culture and sensitivity test
  d. renal scan

_A_ 4. nuclear medicine imaging procedure that shows the size, shape, position, and function of the kidneys
  a. renal scan
  b. intravenous pyelogram
  c. cystoscopy
  d. cystogram

<u>B</u> 5. lab analysis of urine that may be performed
using a dipstick or a microscope
    a. culture and sensitivity test
    b. urinalysis
    c. urinary catheterization
    d. intravenous pyelogram

<u>A</u> 6. procedure in which a tube is inserted through
the urinary meatus of the urethra and then
manipulated into the bladder
    a. urinary catheterization
    b. cystoscopy
    c. intravenous pyelogram
    d. renal dialysis

<u>C</u> 7. artificial method of filtration used to remove
excess waste and water from the body
    a. hemodialysis
    b. peritoneal dialysis
    c. both (a) and (b)
    d. neither (a) nor (b)

<u>D</u> 8. imaging technique in which high-frequency
sound waves and a computer are used to
generate images of the kidneys
    a. cystogram
    b. intravenous pyelogram
    c. renal scan
    d. renal ultrasound

SCORECARD: How Did You Do?

Number correct (_____), divided by 8 (_____), multiplied by 100 equals _____ (your score)

Assessment

Identify Abbreviations

Directions: Write the abbreviation for each medical term listed below.

Medical Term	Abbreviation
1. urinalysis	UA
2. cystoscopy	cysto
3. urinary tract infection	UTI
4. intravenous pyelogram	IVP
5. urinary catheterization	cath
6. culture and sensitivity (test)	C&S test

SCORECARD: How Did You Do?

Number correct (_____), divided by 6 (_____), multiplied by 100 equals _____ (your score)

Analyzing the Intern Experience

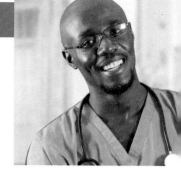

In the Intern Experience described at the beginning of this chapter, we met Thomas, an intern who was assigned to assist Dr. Nefron, a general practitioner with the Middletown Clinic. Thomas listened and observed as Dr. Nefron met with Shara, a college student who came to the clinic because of symptoms that included fatigue, general bodily discomfort, lower back pain, urinary frequency, and a burning sensation upon urination.

Dr. Nefron obtained Shara's personal and family health history, performed a physical examination, and ordered a urinalysis. He then made a diagnosis and formulated a treatment plan for Shara. Later, he made a dictated recording of the patient's health information, which was subsequently transcribed into a chart note.

We will now learn more about Shara's condition from a clinical perspective, interpreting the medical terms in her chart note as we analyze the scenario presented in the Intern Experience.

Audio Activity: Shara Brown's Chart Note

Directions: At the companion website, listen and read along as the physician dictates Shara Brown's chart note, shown below. Then do the exercise that appears after the chart note.

CHART NOTE

Patient Name: Brown, Shara
ID Number: 89736
Examination Date: October 1, 20xx

SUBJECTIVE
Shara presents with **frequency**, urgency, fever, and burning upon urination for 3–5 days accompanied by malaise, **flank** pain, **hematuria**, and **renal colic**. She delayed care until completion of final exams. Patient has a history of multiple bladder infections.

OBJECTIVE
BP (blood pressure) 120/80, pulse 76, respirations 22/min. Dipstick **urinalysis** showed yellow urine, cloudy with 80–100 WBCs (white blood cells), and many bacteria.

ASSESSMENT
UTI and **cystitis**.

TREATMENT PLAN
Cephalexin 500 mg p.o. t.i.d. x 10 days (take one 500-mg tablet of the antibiotic cephalexin by mouth 3 times a day for 10 days). Recommend follow-up with **urologist**. Chronic cystitis vs. **pyelonephritis**.

Interpret Shara Brown's Chart Note

Directions: After listening to the dictated recording and reading the chart note on Shara Brown, provide the medical term that matches each definition below.

Example: inflammation of the kidney   *Answer:* nephritis

1. specialist in the study and treatment of diseases and disorders of the urinary tract

   urologist

2. urinating often

   frequency

3. painful spasms in the lower back

   renal colic

4. bacterial infection in the urinary tract

   cystitis

5. chemical analysis of the urine

   urinalysis

6. infection in the urinary tract

   UTI

7. lower back

   flank

8. condition of blood in the urine

   hematuria

9. inflammation of the kidney and renal pelvis

   pyelonephritis

SCORECARD: How Did You Do?

Number correct (_____), divided by 9 (_____), multiplied by 100 equals _____ (your score)

Working with Medical Records

In this activity, you will interpret the medical records (chart notes) of patients with health conditions related to the urinary system. These examples illustrate typical medical records prepared in a real-world healthcare environment. To interpret these chart notes, you will apply your knowledge of word elements (prefixes, combining forms, and suffixes), diseases and disorders, and procedures and treatments related to the urinary system.

Audio Activity: Elizabeth Townsend's Chart Note

Directions: At the companion website, listen and read along as the physician dictates Elizabeth Townsend's chart note, shown on the next page. Then do the exercise that appears after the chart note.

CHART NOTE

Patient Name: Townsend, Elizabeth
ID Number: 12333
Examination Date: February 23, 20xx

SUBJECTIVE
This 14-year-old female presents with urinary **frequency** and **incontinence** for the past 2 days. She has had pain on urination for the past 3–5 days; no **hematuria** noted. No **flank** pain. Patient did complain that her stomach hurt. Fever of 101° for the past 24 hours. No vomiting. Patient has a history of a urinary tract infection several months ago; however, no repeat **urinalysis** was performed. She has not had an **intravenous pyelogram** or **renal ultrasound**. Family history is significant; paternal grandmother had a **nephrectomy**.

OBJECTIVE
Alert and in no distress. Abdomen is soft with no masses, tenderness, or hepatosplenomegaly (enlargement of the liver and spleen). No guarding (a reflexive response to protect an area of pain).

LABORATORY
Urinalysis shows 60–80 WBCs (white blood cells) and 80–100 RBCs (red blood cells) and positive nitrates.

ASSESSMENT
Recurrent **UTI**.

TREATMENT PLAN
Ciprofloxacin 500 mg b.i.d. x 10 days (take 500 mg of ciprofloxacin twice a day for 10 days). Obtain urine **C&S**. Repeat urinalysis and urine culture 2 days after completion of antibiotics. Follow up with renal ultrasound.

Assessment

Interpret Elizabeth Townsend's Chart Note

Directions: After listening to the dictated recording and reading the chart note on Elizabeth Townsend, provide the medical term that matches each definition below.

Example: suture of the kidney   *Answer:* nephrorrhaphy

1. excision of the kidney — nephrectomy

2. lower back — flank

3. procedure in which high-frequency sound waves are used to study the kidneys — renal ultrasound

4. urinary tract infection — UTI

5. lab test used to determine the most effective antibiotic for treating a urinary tract infection — C&S

6. chemical analysis of the urine — urinalysis

7. urinating often — frequency

8. loss of bladder control

9. condition of blood in the urine

10. radiographic procedure used to visualize the urinary tract

incontinence _____

hematuria _____

intravenous pyelogram _____

SCORECARD: How Did You Do?

Number correct (_____), divided by 10 (_____), multiplied by 100 equals _____ (your score)

Audio Activity: Brian Simmons's Chart Note

Directions: At the companion website, listen and read along as the physician dictates Brian Simmons's chart note, shown below. Then do the exercise that appears after the chart note.

CHART NOTE

Patient Name: Simmons, Brian
ID Number: 53589
Examination Date: March 13, 20xx

HISTORY OF PRESENT ILLNESS
Patient had onset 2 hours ago of **colicky**, right **flank** pain that radiates around to the right lower quadrant and into the **urethra**. Patient states urine seems to have blood in it along with the **dysuria**. Pain becomes more severe for 1–10 minutes and then eases off. When pain is severe, he rates it at 8 on a scale of 1–10. Patient denies fever, chills, nausea, vomiting, or diarrhea.

PAST MEDICAL HISTORY
Denies history of **nephrolithiasis** or **cholelithiasis**. Denies prior, similar episodes. No drug allergies.

EXAMINATION
Patient is a 52-year-old male, appearing intermittently uncomfortable. There is mild tenderness noted to the lower portion of the right kidney upon palpation (examination using the hands or fingers). Lungs are clear. Abdomen is soft and nontender. No suprapubic (above the pubic bone) tenderness. Extremities have good pulses without edema.

LABORATORY
Clean-catch urinalysis showed **hematuria** and **pyuria**.

DIAGNOSIS
Right **ureterolithiasis**.

TREATMENT PLAN
Pain subsided. However, shortly after examination severe pain returned in right flank and right lower quadrant. Patient was given ketorolac tromethamine 60 mg and sent for an **IVP**.

Interpret Brian Simmons's Chart Note

Directions: After listening to the dictated recording and reading the chart note on Brian Simmons, provide the medical term that matches each definition below. You may encounter terms that were introduced in previous chapters.

Example: excision of the kidney   *Answer:* nephrectomy

1. condition of blood in the urine — hematuria

2. tube that carries urine to the outside of the body — urethra

3. abnormal condition of a stone in the kidney — nephrolithiasis

4. lower back — flank

5. characterized by painful spasms — colicky

6. painful or difficult urination — dysuria

7. abnormal condition of a stone in the ureter — ureterolithiasis

8. intravenous pyelogram; radiographic procedure used to visualize the urinary tract — IVP

9. condition of pus in the urine — pyuria

10. abnormal condition of a stone in the gallbladder — cholelithiasis

SCORECARD: How Did You Do?

Number correct (_____), divided by 10 (_____), multiplied by 100 equals _____ (your score)

Chapter Review

Word Elements Summary

Prefixes

Prefix	Meaning
a-	not; without
an-	not; without
dys-	painful; difficult
intra-	within
peri-	around
poly-	many; much

Combining Forms

Root Word/Combining Vowel	Meaning
cyst/o	bladder; sac containing fluid
glyc/o	sugar; glucose
glycos/o	sugar; glucose
hem/o, hemat/o	blood
hydr/o	water
lith/o	stone
meat/o	opening
nephr/o	kidney
noct/o	night
olig/o	scanty; few
py/o	pus
pyel/o	renal pelvis
ren/o	kidney
son/o	sound
sten/o	narrow; constricted
ur/o	urine; urinary tract
ureter/o	ureter
urethr/o	urethra
urin/o	urine
vesic/o	bladder

Suffixes

Suffix	Meaning
-al	pertaining to
-algia	pain
-cele	hernia; swelling; protrusion
-dipsia	thirst
-ectomy	surgical removal; excision
-emia	blood condition
-gram	record; image
-ia	condition
-iasis	abnormal condition
-itis	inflammation
-logist	specialist in the study and treatment of
-logy	study of
-lysis	destruction
-megaly	large; enlargement
-oma	tumor; mass
-osis	abnormal condition
-pexy	surgical fixation
-plasty	surgical repair
-ptosis	drooping; downward displacement
-rrhaphy	suture
-scope	instrument used to observe
-scopy	process of observing
-stomy	new opening
-tomy	incision; cut into
-tripsy	process of crushing

More Practice: Activities and Games

The activities on the following pages will help you reinforce your skills and check your mastery of the medical terminology that you learned in this chapter. Visit the companion website for More Practice games and activities.

Medical Term Identification

Directions: For each item below, fill in the blank with the correct term.

1. Laboratory analysis of the urine: <u>urinalysis</u>.

2. Condition that causes distension and dilation of the renal pelvis, resulting in enlargement of the kidney: <u>hydronephrosis</u>.

3. Condition associated with renal failure in which the kidneys do not remove urea and other waste products from the blood: <u>uremia</u>.

4. Inflammation of the urinary bladder: <u>cystitis</u>.

5. Inflammation of the urethra: <u>urethritis</u>.

6. Artificial method of filtration for removing waste products and excess water from the body when the kidneys fail to perform this function: <u>renal dialysis</u>.

7. Procedure that involves placing a tube through the urinary meatus into the urethra: <u>urinary catheterization</u>.

8. Nephrolithiasis is the formation of stones in the <u>kidney</u>.

9. When a person has had a nephrectomy, his or her <u>kidney</u> has been surgically removed.

10. The urinary tract is composed of the kidneys, ureters, bladder, and <u>urethra</u>.

11. At the end of the urethra is an opening called the <u>urinary meatus</u>, which expels urine to the outside of the body.

12. A physician who specializes in the study, diagnosis, and treatment of urinary tract diseases and disorders is called a <u>urologist</u>.

True or False

Directions: Indicate whether each statement below is true or false.

True or False?

<u>T</u>   1. The prefix **dys-** means "painful" or "difficult."

<u>F</u>   2. The root word **nephr** means "night."

<u>T</u>   3. The root words **glyc** and **glycos** both mean "sugar."

<u>F</u>   4. The root word **ureter** means "urethra."

<u>T</u>   5. The suffix **-lysis** means "destruction."

<u>F</u>   6. The suffix **-iasis** means "normal condition."

<u>T</u>   7. The suffix **-dipsia** means "thirst."

<u>F</u>   8. The term *hydronephrosis* contains a prefix, a root word, and a suffix.

<u>T</u>   9. The term *ureterostenosis* contains two root words and one suffix.

True or False?

___T___ 10. We have close to one million nephrons in each kidney.

___T___ 11. The act of excreting urine is called *micturition*.

___F___ 12. Frequency is urinating often and usually in large amounts.

___T___ 13. A dipstick is a chemical stick used in urinalysis.

___F___ 14. Cystitis is an inflammation of the kidney and renal pelvis.

___F___ 15. Urinary retention is the voluntary holding of urine.

___T___ 16. An intravenous pyelogram is a radiographic procedure in which a contrast agent is injected into the body to visualize the urinary tract.

Break It Down

Directions: Dissect each medical term below into its word elements by placing a slash between each word part (prefix, root word, combining vowel, and suffix). Then define each term.

Example:

Medical Term: pyuria

Dissection: py/ur/ia

Definition: condition of pus in the urine

Medical Term	Dissection
1. hematocele	h e m a t / o / c e l e

Definition: swelling of blood

_____

Medical Term	Dissection
2. urogram	u r / o / g r a m

Definition: image of the urinary tract

_____

Medical Term	Dissection
3. perirenal	p e r i / r e n / a l

Definition: pertaining to around the kidney

_____

Medical Term	Dissection
4. meatorrhaphy	m e a t / o / r r h a p h y

Definition: suture of an opening

_____

Medical Term	Dissection

5. hydrocele

h y d r/o/c e l e

Definition: swelling of water

---

6. lithotomy

l i t h/o/t o m y

Definition: cut into stone

---

7. meatoscope

m e a t/o/s c o p e

Definition: instrument used to observe an opening

---

8. urolithiasis

u r/o/l i t h/i a s i s

Definition: abnormal condition of a stone in the urinary tract

---

9. renogram

r e n/o/g r a m

Definition: image of the kidney

---

10. intrarenal

i n t r a/r e n/a l

Definition: pertaining to within the kidney

---

11. cystopyelonephritis

c y s t/o/p y e l/o/n e p h r/i t i s

Definition: inflammation of the bladder, renal pelvis, and kidney

---

12. uronephrosis

u r/o/n e p h r/o s i s

Definition: abnormal condition of urine in the kidney

Audio Activity: Mara Rodriguez's Chart Note

Directions: At the companion website, listen and read along as the physician dictates Mara Rodriquez's chart note, shown below. Then do the exercise that appears after the chart note.

CHART NOTE

Patient Name: Rodriguez, Mara
ID Number: 65588
Examination Date: August 29, 20xx

SUBJECTIVE
This 43-year-old female presents with **subcostal** pain and episodes of gross (visible to the naked eye) **hematuria**. She was seen in the ER approximately 3 weeks ago for similar symptoms. At that time a **renal ultrasound** was performed. It showed no evidence of **hydronephrosis** or renal mass. Today patient complains of some nausea and vomiting. She denies fever, chills, **dysuria**, or **frequency**. There is no previous history of urinary tract infections, **calculus** formation, or genitourinary (reproductive and urinary system) surgery.

OBJECTIVE
On physical examination, the abdomen appears relatively soft but diffusely tender (not limited to one location), particularly in the left upper and left lower quadrants. Some guarding was noted with no clearly elicited rebound tenderness. (When the areas were palpated, no rebound tenderness occurred when the physician's palpating hand was withdrawn.) **Urinalysis** today shows 6–10 erythrocytes (red blood cells) per high power field. There is no suggestion of infection with leukocytes or bacteria.

ASSESSMENT
The **etiology** of the pain remains unclear, although possibilities include a calculus, cholecystitis (inflammation of the gallbladder), or ovarian cyst. With absence of obstruction on the renal ultrasound, the cause of pain is not suggestive of a stone. Negative urinalysis also mitigates against **pyelonephritis**, and the pain is clearly abdominal. The etiology of the gross hematuria remains unclear.

TREATMENT PLAN
A surgical consultation for further evaluation of the abdomen is advised.

Interpret Mara Rodriquez's Chart Note

Directions: After listening to the dictated recording and reading the chart note on Mara Rodriquez, provide the medical term that matches each definition below. You may encounter terms that were introduced in previous chapters.

Example: inflammation of the bladder   *Answer:* cystitis

1. condition of blood in the urine   hematuria
2. abnormal condition of water in the kidney   hydronephrosis
3. a stone composed of mineral salts, which can block passage of urine through the ureters   calculus
4. cause   etiology
5. procedure that uses high-frequency sound waves to study the kidneys   renal ultrasound
6. chemical analysis of the urine   urinalysis
7. painful or difficult urination   dysuria
8. below the ribs   subcostal
9. urinating often   frequency
10. inflammation of the renal pelvis and kidney   pyelonephritis

Spelling

Directions: Write the correct spelling beside each misspelled medical term below.

1. cistoplasty   cystoplasty
2. hydranephrosis   hydronephrosis
3. haematuria   hematuria
4. nocturea   nocturia
5. cistytis   cystitis
6. periurrethral   periurethral
7. nephrolithiosis   nephrolithiasis
8. polydipsea   polydipsia
9. urethrascope   urethroscope
10. lythotripsy   lithotripsy
11. cystosele   cystocele
12. urrologist   urologist
13. oligurea   oliguria
14. pyalonephritis   pyelonephritis
15. nerphoma   nephroma

Cumulative Review

Chapters 11–12: Endocrine System and Urinary System

Directions: Check your mastery of common word elements used in medical terminology related to the endocrine system and the urinary system. Write the definition of each prefix, combining form, and suffix listed below. For more cumulative review practice, visit the companion website.

Prefixes

a-	not; without
an-	not; without
dys-	painful; difficult
endo-	within
hyper-	above; above normal
hypo-	below; below normal
intra-	inside; within
para-	near; beside
poly-	many; much

Combining Forms

acr/o	extremity
aden/o	gland
adren/o, adrenal/o	adrenal gland
carcin/o	cancerous; cancer
crin/o	to secrete
cyst/o	sac containing fluid; bladder
dips/o	thirst
gluc/o	glucose; sugar
glyc/o	glucose; sugar
glycos/o	glucose; sugar

hem/o, hemat/o	blood
hydr/o	water
lith/o	stone
meat/o	opening
nephr/o	kidney
noct/o	night
olig/o	scanty; few
py/o	pus
pyel/o	renal pelvis
ren/o	kidney
son/o	sound
sten/o	narrow; constricted
thym/o	thymus gland
thyr/o, thyroid/o	thyroid gland
ur/o	urine; urinary tract
ureter/o	ureter
urethr/o	urethra
urin/o	urine
vesic/o	bladder

Suffixes

-al	pertaining to
-algia	pain
-cele	hernia; swelling; protrusion
-dipsia	thirst
-e	noun suffix with no meaning
-ectomy	surgical removal; excision
-emia	blood condition
-gram	record; radiographic image

-ia	condition
-iasis	abnormal condition
-ic	pertaining to
-ism	condition; process
-itis	inflammation
-logist	specialist in the study and treatment of
-logy	study of
-lysis	breakdown; loosening; dissolving
-megaly	large; enlargement
-oid	like; resembling
-oma	tumor; mass
-osis	abnormal condition
-pathy	disease
-pexy	surgical fixation
-phagia	condition of eating or swallowing
-plasty	surgical repair
-ptosis	drooping; downward displacement
-rrhaphy	suture
-scope	instrument used to observe
-scopy	process of observing
-stomy	new opening
-tomy	incision; cut into
-tripsy	crushing

Appendix A

Medical Word Elements

Prefixes

Prefix	Meaning
a-	not; without
ad-	toward
an-	not; without
anti-	against
auto-	self
brady-	slow
dia-	through; complete
dys-	painful; difficult
endo-	within
epi-	upon; above
extra-	outside
hemi-	half
hyper-	above; above normal
hypo-	below; below normal
inter-	between

Prefix	Meaning
intra-	inside; within
meta-	change; beyond
pan-	all; everything
para-	near; beside
per-	through
peri-	around
poly-	many; much
quadri-	four
retro-	back; behind
sub-	beneath; below
supra-	above
sym-, syn-	together; with
tachy-	fast
trans-	across

Combining Forms

Root Word/ Combining Vowel	Meaning
acr/o	extremity
aden/o	gland
adenoid/o	adenoids
adren/o, adrenal/o	adrenal gland
angi/o	blood vessel; lymph vessel
anter/o	front
arteri/o	artery
arthr/o	joint
articul/o	joint
ather/o	fatty substance
audi/o	hearing
blephar/o	eyelid
bronch/o, bronchi/o	bronchial tube; bronchus
burs/a, burs/o	bursa; sac
carcin/o	cancerous; cancer
cardi/o	heart
carp/o	carpals (wrist bones)
celi/o	abdomen
cephal/o	head
cerebell/o	cerebellum
cerebr/o	cerebrum
cervic/o	cervix; neck
chol/e	bile; gall
cholecyst/o	gallbladder
chondr/o	cartilage
clavicul/o	clavicle (collarbone)
coccyg/o	coccyx (tailbone)
col/o, colon/o	colon; large intestine
colp/o	vagina

Root Word/ Combining Vowel	Meaning
coron/o	heart
cost/o	rib
cran/o, crani/o	skull; cranium
crin/o	to secrete
cry/o	cold
contus/o	bruising
cutane/o	skin
cyan/o	blue
cyst/o	sac containing fluid; bladder
cyt/o	cell
derma/a, derm/o, dermat/o	skin
dips/o	thirst
dist/o	away from the point of origin
diverticul/o	diverticulum
dors/o	along the back (of the body)
duoden/o	duodenum
ecchym/o	blood in the tissues
electr/o	electrical activity
embol/o	plug; embolus
encephal/o	brain
enter/o	intestines
erythemat/o	redness
erythr/o	red
esophag/o	esophagus
femor/o	femur (thigh bone)
fibul/o	fibula
gastr/o	stomach

(Continued)

Root Word/ Combining Vowel	Meaning
gingiv/o	gums
gloss/o	tongue
gluc/o	glucose; sugar
glyc/o	glucose; sugar
glycos/o	glucose; sugar
gynec/o	woman; female
hem/o	blood
hemat/o	blood
hepat/o	liver
herni/o	hernia; rupture; protrusion
humer/o	humerus (upper arm bone)
hydr/o	water
hyster/o	uterus
ile/o	ileum
ili/o	ilium
immune/o	protection
infer/o	below; beneath
ir/o	iris
irid/o	iris
isch/o	to keep back
ischi/o	ischium (part of the hip bone)
jejun/o	jejunum
kerat/o	cornea
kines/o, kinesi/o	movement
kyph/o	hump
lapar/o	abdomen
later/o	side
leuk/o	white
lip/o	fat

Root Word/ Combining Vowel	Meaning
lith/o	stone
lob/o	lobe (a defined portion of an organ or structure)
lord/o	curve
lymph/o	lymph
malign/o	causing harm, cancer
mamm/o	breast
mast/o	breast
meat/o	opening
medi/o	middle
melan/o	black
mening/o, meningi/o	meninges (membranes covering the brain and spinal cord)
men/o	menstruation
metacarp/o	metacarpals (bones of the hand)
metatars/o	metatarsals (bones of the foot)
metr/o, metri/o	uterus
muscul/o	muscle
my/o	muscle
myc/o	fungus
myel/o	bone marrow; spinal cord
myring/o	tympanic membrane; eardrum
necr/o	death
nephr/o	kidney
neur/o	nerve
noct/o	night
ocul/o	eye
olig/o	scanty; few
onych/o	nail

(Continued)

Root Word/ Combining Vowel	Meaning
oophor/o	ovary
ophthalm/o	eye
opt/o	eye; vision
optic/o	eye; vision
or/o	mouth
orchid/o	testes
organ/o	organ
orth/o	straight
oste/o	bone
ot/o	ear
ox/o	oxygen
pancreat/o	pancreas
patell/a, patell/o	patella (kneecap)
path/o	disease
peps/o	digestion
phag/o	eat; swallow; engulf
phalang/o	phalanges (bones of fingers or toes)
pharyng/o	pharynx; throat
phleb/o	vein
pleg/o	paralysis
pleur/o	pleura
pneum/o, pneumon/o	lung; air
polyp/o	polyp; small growth
por/o	pore; duct; small opening
poster/o	back of the body
presby/o	old age
proct/o	anus and rectum
prostat/o	prostate gland
proxim/o	nearest the point of origin

Root Word/ Combining Vowel	Meaning
prurit/o	itching
psych/o	mind
pub/o	pubis (part of the hip bone)
pulmon/o	lung
py/o	pus
pyel/o	renal pelvis
radi/o	radius (bone of the forearm); X-ray
radicul/o	nerve root
rect/o	rectum
ren/o	kidney
retin/o	retina
rhin/o	nose
sacr/o	sacrum (bone at base of the spine)
salping/o	uterine tube; fallopian tube
scapul/o	scapula (shoulder blade)
schiz/o	split
scler/o	sclera (white of the eye)
scoli/o	crooked; bent
scrot/o	scrotum
seb/o	oil or sebum
sial/o	saliva
sigmoid/o	sigmoid colon
son/o	sound
spin/o	spine; backbone
spir/o	breathe; breathing
splen/o	spleen
spondyl/o	vertebra; spine
squam/o	scale-like

(Continued)

Root Word/ Combining Vowel	Meaning
sten/o	narrow; constricted
stern/o	sternum (breastbone)
tars/o	ankle bones
ten/o	tendon
tendin/o, tendon/o	tendon
tens/o	pressure; tension
testicul/o	testes
thorac/o	chest
thromb/o	clot
thym/o	thymus gland
thyr/o, thyroid/o	thyroid gland
tibi/o	tibia (shin bone)
tonsil/o	tonsils
topic/o	place
trache/o	trachea; windpipe

Root Word/ Combining Vowel	Meaning
trich/o	hair
tympan/o	tympanic membrane; eardrum
uln/o	ulna (bone of the forearm)
ur/o	urine; urinary tract
ureter/o	ureter
urethr/o	urethra
urin/o	urine
vagin/o	vagina
vas/o	vessel; duct
vascul/o	blood vessel
ven/o, ven/i	vein
vertebr/o	vertebra; spine
vesic/o	bladder
xer/o	dry

Suffixes

Suffix	Meaning
-ac	pertaining to
-al	pertaining to
-algia	pain
-ancy	state of
-ar	pertaining to
-ary	pertaining to
-asthenia	weakness
-atic	pertaining to
-ation	process; condition; state of being or having
-cele	hernia; swelling; protrusion
-centesis	surgical puncture to remove fluid
-clasia	surgical breaking
-cyte	cell
-desis	to bind or tie together surgically
-dipsia	thirst
-dynia	pain
-e	noun suffix with no meaning
-eal	pertaining to
-ectasis	dilatation; dilation; expansion
-ectomy	surgical removal; excision
-edema	swelling
-ema	condition
-emesis	vomiting
-emia	blood condition
-esthesia	sensation; feeling
-gen	producing; originating; causing
-gram	record; radiographic image

Suffix	Meaning
-graph	instrument used to record an image
-graphy	process of recording an image
-ia	condition
-iasis	abnormal condition
-ic	pertaining to
-ical	pertaining to
-ion	condition; process
-ior	pertaining to
-ism	condition; process
-itis	inflammation
-kinesia	movement
-kinesis	movement
-logist	specialist in the study and treatment of
-logy	study of
-lysis	breakdown; loosening; dissolving
-malacia	softening
-megaly	large; enlargement
-meter	instrument used to measure
-metry	process of measuring; measurement
-oid	like; resembling
-oma	tumor; mass
-opia	vision
-osis	abnormal condition
-ous	pertaining to
-pathy	disease
-penia	deficiency; abnormal reduction
-pexy	surgical fixation

(Continued)

Suffix	Meaning
-phagia	condition of eating or swallowing
-pharynx	pharynx; throat
-phasia	speech
-plasty	surgical repair
-pnea	breathing
-ptosis	drooping; downward displacement
-rrhage	bursting forth (of blood)
-rrhagia	bursting forth (of blood)
-rrhaphy	suture
-rrhea	flow; discharge
-rrhexis	rupture
-sclerosis	hardening
-scope	instrument used to observe

Suffix	Meaning
-scopy	process of observing
-spasm	involuntary muscle contraction
-stasis	stop; stand still
-stomy	new opening
-thorax	chest; pleural cavity
-tic	pertaining to
-tome	instrument used to cut
-tomy	incision; cut into
-tripsy	crushing
-trophy	development
-us	structure; thing
-y	condition; process

Appendix B

Medical Abbreviations and Acronyms

acquired immunodeficiency syndrome	AIDS	implantable cardioverter defibrillator	ICD
		incision and drainage	I&D
anterior cruciate ligament	ACL	inflammatory bowel disease	IBD
antidiuretic hormone	ADH	insulin-dependent diabetes mellitus	IDDM
arterial blood gas	ABG	intravenous pyelogram	IVP
autoimmune hemolytic anemia	AIHA	lateral collateral ligament	LCL
automated external defibrillator	AED	lower gastrointestinal	LGI
benign prostatic hypertrophy	BPH	lumbar puncture	LP
biopsy	Bx	magnetic resonance angiogram	MRA
cardiopulmonary resuscitation	CPR	magnetic resonance imaging	MRI
cerebral palsy	CP	medial collateral ligament	MCL
cerebral vascular attack	CVA	mononucleosis	mono
cerebrospinal fluid	CSF	multiple sclerosis	MS
chest X-ray	CXR	myocardial infarction	MI
chronic obstructive pulmonary disease	COPD	non-insulin-dependent diabetes mellitus	NIDDM
computerized tomography	CT		
congestive heart failure	CHF	nuclear medicine imaging	NMI
continuous positive airway pressure	CPAP	pelvic inflammatory disease	PID
coronary artery disease	CAD	physical therapy	PT
culture and sensitivity test	C&S	premenstrual syndrome	PMS
cystoscopy	cysto	pulmonary function test	PFT
diabetes insipidus	DI	rest, ice, compression, and elevation	RICE
diabetes mellitus	DM	rheumatoid arthritis	RA
dilation and curettage	D&C	sexually transmitted disease	STD
Duchenne muscular dystrophy	DMD	systemic lupus erythematosus	SLE
electrocardiogram	ECG	thyroid-stimulating hormone	TSH
electroencephalogram	EEG	transient ischemic attack	TIA
electromyogram	EMG	transurethral resection of the prostate	TURP
enzyme-linked immunosorbent assay	ELISA	traumatic brain injury	TBI
esophagogastroduodenoscopy	EDG	ultraviolet light	UV
fasting blood sugar	FBS	upper gastrointestinal	UGI
gastroesophageal reflux disease	GERD	upper respiratory infection	URI
glucose tolerance test	GTT	urinalysis	UA
head, eyes, ears, nose, and throat	HEENT	urinary catheterization	cath
herpes simplex virus 1	HSV-1	urinary tract infection	UTI
human immunodeficiency virus	HIV	ventilation/perfusion scan	VPS

Photo Credits

Chapter 2

Intern Experience: M. Thatcher/Shutterstock.com

Figure 2.3 Suzanne Tucker/Shutterstock.com

Figure 2.5A Suzanne Tucker/Shutterstock.com

Figure 2.5B JTeffects/Shutterstock.com

Figure 2.5C Naiyyer/Shutterstock.com

Figure 2.6 Librakv/Shutterstock.com

Figure 2.7 carroteater/Shutterstock.com

Figure 2.8 lekcej/Shutterstock.com

Figure 2.9 Levent Konuk/Shutterstock.com

Figure 2.10 Stephen VanHorn/Shutterstock.com

Figure 2.11 Kenxro/Shutterstock.com

Chapter 3

Intern Experience: Karin Hildebrand Lau/
Shutterstock.com

Figure 3.6 Hubert Raguet/Science Source

Figure 3.9 Living Art Enterprises, LLC/Science Source

Figure 3.12 Santibhavank P/Shutterstock.com

Chapter 4

Intern Experience: Stuart Jenner/Shutterstock.com

Figure 4.4 English/Custom Medical Stock Photo

Figure 4.11 Mediscan/Visuals Unlimited, Inc.

Figure 4.12 Mediscan/Visuals Unlimited, Inc.

Figure 4.13 GRei/Shutterstock.com

Figure 4.17 SNEHIT/Shutterstock.com

Chapter 5

Intern Experience: Stuart Jenner/Shutterstock.com

Figure 5.4 Alila Medical Media/Shutterstock.com

Figure 5.5 Alila Medical Media/Shutterstock.com

Chapter 6

Intern Experience: iodrakon/Shutterstock.com

Figure 6.5 Alila Medical Media/Shutterstock.com

Figure 6.6 Smereka/Shutterstock.com.

Concept adapted from Lighthouse International;
http://lighthouse.org/about-low-vision-blindness/vision-disorders/age-related-macular-degeneration-amd/.

Figure 6.9 Radu Bercan/Shutterstock.com

Figure 6.12 Maica/istockphoto.com

Chapter 7

Intern Experience: Paul Matthew Photography/
Shutterstock.com

Figure 7.11B AJ Photo/sciencesource.com

Chapter 8

Intern Experience: imging/Shutterstock.com

Chapter 9

Intern Experience: michaeljung/Shutterstock.com

Figure 9.10 Santibhavank P/Shutterstock.com

Figure 9.11 Brian Chase/Shutterstock.com

Figure 9.12 Life in View/Science Source

Chapter 10

Intern Experience: Geo Martinez/Shutterstock.com

Figure 10.3 kalewa/Shutterstock.com

Figure 10.6 Body Scientific International, LLC.
Adapted from US Department of Health and Human
Services. Office on Women's Health.Washington,
DC: available at http://womenshealth.gov/heart-health-stroke/signs-of-a-heart-attack/.

Figure 10.7 Dr. Barry Slaven/Visuals Unlimited, Inc.

Figure 10.10 epstock/Shutterstock.com

Figure 10.11 Ouellette Theroux/Publiphoto/Science
Source

Figure 10.14 AJPfilm /Custom Medical Stock Photo

Figure 10.15 khuruzero/Shutterstock.com

Chapter 11

Intern Experience: michaeljung/Shutterstock.com

Figure 11.2 Science Source

Figure 11.4 Biophoto Associates/Photo Researchers, Inc

Figure 11.10 Alexander Raths/www.123RF.com

Chapter 12

Intern Experience: michaeljung/Shutterstock.com

Figure 12.5 Christina Richards/Shutterstock.com

Figure 12.6 Corbis Images

Figure 12.8 Blamb/Shutterstock.com

Index

cardiac arrhythmia, 426
cardiac catheterization, 424
cardiac hypertrophy, 422
cardiologist, 16, 405, 412, 414
cardiology, 405, 412, 414
cardiomegaly, 412, 414, 431
cardiomyopathy, 412, 414
cardiopulmonary, 412, 414
cardiopulmonary resuscitation (CPR),
    387, 424
cardiorrhaphy, 148, 151
cardiorrhexis, 148, 151
cardiovascular, 404
cardiovascular system, 37, 402–439
    anatomical diagram, 404, 406
    anatomy and physiology vocabulary,
        405
    breaking down and building terms,
        412–413
    diseases and disorders, 420–423
    overview, 404
    procedures and treatments, 423–426
    word elements, 407
    working with medical records, 430
carpal, 148, 151
cartilage, 139
cataract, 260
cath lab, 424
cath. See catheterization
catheterization lab, 424
caudal, 27
celiectomy, 100, 103
central nervous system (CNS), 280, 282
cephalalgia, 289, 291
cephalic, 27, 289, 291
cerebellum, 281–282
cerebral, 289, 291
cerebral aneurysm, 296
cerebral angiography, 301
cerebral embolism, 296
cerebral palsy (CP), 297
cerebral vascular attack (CVA), 297
cerebrospinal, 289, 291
cerebrospinal fluid (CSF), 299, 303
cerebrovascular, 289, 291
cerebrum, 280, 282
cervical, 333, 335
cervicitis. 344
chancres. See syphilis
chest X-ray (CXR), 387
chlamydia, 343
cholecystitis, 100, 103
cholelithiasis, 100, 103
chondrocostal, 148, 151
chondrogenic, 148, 151
chondromalacia, 148, 151
chronic bronchitis, 383–385
chronic obstructive pulmonary disease
    (COPD), 384–385
circulatory system, 196, 404, 405
circumcision, 347
cirrhosis, 112
closed fracture. See fracture
CNS. See central nervous system (CNS)

coccygeal, 148, 151
cold sores, 72
colitis, 100, 103
collapsed lung. See pneumothorax
colon, 91
colonoscopy, 100, 103, 116
colostomy, 100, 103, 115
colposcope, 347
colposcopy, 333, 335, 347–348
combining form, 5, 10
combining vowel, 11
comedo, 69
compound or open fracture. See
    fracture
computed tomography. See
    computerized tomography
computerized tomography (CT), 169,
    299, 301
computerized tomography (CT) scan,
    167
concussion, 297–298
congenital hypothyroidism, 463
congestive heart failure (CHF),
    421–422
contact dermatitis, 71–72, 74
continuous positive airway pressure
    (CPAP), 387
contrast agent, 169. Also see
    intravenous pyelogram
contusion, 55, 58
COPD. See chronic obstructive
    pulmonary disease (COPD)
cornea, 238, 240
coronal plane, 25
coronary, 412, 414
coronary artery disease (CAD), 422
CPAP. See continuous positive airway
    pressure (CPAP)
CPR. See cardiopulmonary
    resuscitation (CPR)
cranial, 148, 151, 289, 291
cranial cavity, 32
craniotomy, 148, 151, 289, 291
cranium, 281
cretinism, 463
Crohn's disease, 110
croup, 385
cryosurgery, 74, 75
CT scanning. See computerized
    tomography
culture and sensitivity (C&S) test, 388,
    507–508
culture test, 388, 507
Cushing syndrome. See Cushing's
    syndrome
Cushing's syndrome, 464
cutaneous, 46, 48
CVA. See cerebral vascular attack (CVA)
CXR. See chest X-ray (CXR)
cyanodermal, 55, 58
cyanosis, 55, 58
cyanotic, 86
cystectomy, 84, 493, 497
cystic, 55, 58

cystitis, 493, 497, 504
cysto, 508
cystocele, 493, 497, 506–507
cystolithiasis, 493, 497, 505
cystolithotomy, 493, 497
cystoplasty, 493, 497
cystoscope, 494, 497
cystoscopy, 494, 497, 508
cystotomy, 497

D

D&C. See dilation and curettage
debridement, 74, 75
defibrillation, 424
dementia, 298
dermal, 46, 48, 55, 58
dermatitis, 55, 58
dermatologic, 85
dermatologist, 47, 48, 55, 58
dermatology, 17, 47, 48, 55, 58
dermatopathology, 86
dermis, 47, 48
descending colon, 92
diabetes insipidus (DI), 466
diabetes mellitus (DM), 464–465
    major types, 464–465
    physiological overview, 464
diabetes, complications affecting vision.
    See diabetic retinopathy
diabetic retinopathy, 261
dialyzer, 510
diarrhea, 100, 103
diencephalon, 281–282
digestive system, 37, 88–131
    anatomical diagram, 90, 92
    anatomy and physiology vocabulary,
        91
    breaking down and building terms,
        100–102
    diseases and disorders, 110
    main functions, 90–91
    major organs, 90, 92
    overview, 90
    procedures and treatments, 114–117
    word elements, 94
    working with medical records, 121
digestive tract, 90, 91, 93
digital rectal exam, 348
dilatation, 420
dilation, 420, 505
dilation and curettage (D&C), 348
dipstick. See urinalysis
distal, 27
distension, 505
diverticula, 115
diverticulitis, 100, 103, 115
diverticulosis, 100, 103
dizziness or sensation of spinning. See
    vertigo
DMD. See Duchenne muscular
    dystrophy (DMD)
Doppler sonography, 425
dorsal, 27, 148, 151

H

H. pylori, 114
hardening of the arteries. See arteriosclerosis
headache, recurring. See migraine headache
heart, 405
heart attack. See myocardial infarction (MI)
Helicobacter pylori (H. pylori), 113
Helper T cells. See T lymphocytes, 197
hematemesis, 102, 103
hematoma, 56, 58
hematuria, 494, 497
hematuria. See kidney stones
hemiplegia, 290, 291
hemodialysis, 510
hemorrhage, 413, 414
hemostasis, 413, 414
hemothorax, 374, 376
hepatitis, 102, 103, 112
hepatomegaly, 102, 103
herniated disk, 162–163
herpes, 72, 75
herpes simplex, 72
herpes simplex virus (HSV), 345
herpes simplex virus 1 (HSV-1), 72
herpes zoster, 72
hiatal hernia, 111
HIV infection, symptoms of, 215
HIV. See human immunodeficiency virus (HIV)
Hodgkin lymphoma, 218
Hodgkin's disease, 218
holter monitor, 425
homeostasis, 238, 280, 447
hormones, 446, 447
human immunodeficiency virus (HIV), 215
hydrocephalus, 290, 291
hydronephrosis, 494, 497, 505
hyperglycemia, 454, 456
hyperopia, 259
hyperopia. See farsightedness
hyperpigmentation. See Addison's disease
hyperpnea, 374, 376
hypersecretion, 446
hypertension, 413, 414, 420
hyperthyroidism, 455, 456
hypertrophy, 148, 151, 413-414, 422
hypodermic, 56, 58
hypogastric region, 34
hypoglycemia, 455, 456
hypoliposis, 86
hypopnea, 374, 376
hyposecretion, 446
hypotension, 413, 414
hypothalamus, 281, 447
hypothyroidism, 455, 456, 466–467
  late clinical manifestations, 467
hypotrichosis, 86
hysterectomy, 333, 335
hysterosalpingogram, 333, 335
hysterosalpingo-oophorectomy, 333, 335

I

ICD. See implantable cardioverter defibrillator (ICD)
idiopathic, 299
ileum, 91, 93
immune system, 197–198
immunization, 220
immunologist, 197, 198, 206, 208
immunology, 197, 198, 206, 208
implantable cardioverter defibrillator (ICD), 426
incision and drainage (I&D), 74
incontinence, 504
indwelling catheter. See urinary catheterization
Infarct, 422
inferior, 27
inflammatory autoimmune disease. See multiple sclerosis
inflammatory bowel disease (IBD), 110
inflammatory bowel disease. See Crohn's disease
ingrown toenail, 74
inspiration, 366
insulin-dependent mellitus (IDDM), 464
integumentary, 46, 48
integumentary system, 36, 44–87
  anatomical diagram, 47, 49
  anatomy and physiology vocabulary, 48
  breaking down and building terms, 54–59
  diseases and disorders, 69–73
  main functions, 46
  major structures, 46–49
  medical records, 78–80
  overview, 46
  procedures and treatments, 73–76
  working with medical records, 78
intensity. See audiometry
intercostal, 148, 151
internal, 27
internal ear, 239–240
intervertebral, 148, 151
intestinal blockages, 115
intracystic, 85
intradermal, 56, 58
intragastric, 8
intraocular pressure (IOP). See glaucoma
intravenous pyelogram (IVP), 509
invasive, 342
involuntary muscle, 139
iridectomy, 249, 252
iridopexy, 249, 252
iridoplasty, 249, 252
iridoplegia, 249, 252
iris, 240
iritis, 249, 252
ischemia, 420

J

jejunum, 91, 93
joint, 139
joint effusion, 163
juvenile-onset diabetes, 464

K

keratometer, 249, 252
keratometry, 252
Kernig's sign, 303
kidney stone. Also see calculus
kidney stones, 505
kidneys, 484, 486
kinesiology, 149, 151
kissing disease. See mononucleosis
knee injuries, 163–164
knee joint, injury. See ACL tear
kyphosis, 149, 151

L

lancet. See diabetes mellitus
laparoscope, 102, 103, 117, 221
laparoscopic hysterectomy, 349
laparoscopic splenectomy, 221
laparoscopy, 102, 103, 221, 333, 335
large intestine, 91, 93
laser eye surgery, 265
laser surgery, 74, 75
laser vision correction, 265
laser-assisted in situ keratomileusis (LASIK), 265
LASIK, 265
lateral, 27, 149, 151
lateral collateral ligament, 163
lateral epicondyle, 164
lateral epicondylitis, 164
lateral meniscus, 163
left hypochondriac region, 34
left iliac region, 34
left lower quadrant (LLQ), 33
left lumbar region, 34
left upper quadrant (LUQ), 33
lens, 240
leukocytes, 196
ligament, 139
lipocyte, 56, 58
lipoid, 56, 58
lipoma, 56, 58
lithotripsy, 494, 497
liver disease, 112
liver fibrosis, 112
lobule, 342
lordosis, 149, 151
lower gastrointestinal (LGI) series, 114
lumbar puncture (LP), 302
lungs, 366, 367
  inflammatory disease affects. See sarcoidosis
lymph, 196, 198
lymph nodes, 73
lymphadenitis, 206, 208

lymphadenopathy, 206, 208
lymphadenosis, 206, 208
lymphangiopathy, 206, 208
lymphatic, 206, 208
lymphatic and immune systems, 194–235
    anatomy and physiology vocabulary, 198–199
    breaking down and building terms, 205–208
    combining forms, 202–203
    diseases and disorders, 215–219
    overview, 196–201
    word elements, 202
    working with medical records, 225
lymphatic system, 37, 196, 199
    anatomical diagram, 196, 200
    major organs of, 200
lymphedema, 206, 208
lymphocyte, 196, 199, 206, 208
lymphocytoma, 206, 208
lymphoid, 206, 208
lymphoma, 206, 208
    malignant. *See* Hodgkin's disease

M

macular area. *See* macular degeneration
macular degeneration, 261
magnetic resonance angiogram (MRA), 303
magnetic resonance imaging (MRI) scan, 167, 170–171, 299
male contraception, vasectomy, 350
male reproductive system, 37
male-pattern baldness, 69
malignancy, 56, 58
malignant, 71
malignant melanoma, 71, 75
mammary glands, 324
mammography, 333, 335, 343
Mantoux test, 388
mastectomy, 333, 335
McMurray test, 171
medial, 27
medial meniscus, 163
median plane, 25
medical abbreviations, anatomical terms of position, direction, location, 34–35
medical records, integumentary system, 78–80
medical terminology,
    analyzing and breaking down terms, 14–17
    analyzing and defining medical terms, 6–9
    anatomical positions, planes, directions, and locations, 24–34
    building plural forms, 21–22
    introduction, 2–43
    mastering, 37

medical word parts, 9–10
    overview, 4–6
    pronunciation, 22–23
    spelling medical terms, 24
medical word parts, 9–14
    prefixes, 9–10
    root words and combining forms, 10–11
    suffixes, 11–14
medulla oblongata, 281
melanin, 47, 48
melanocytes, 47, 48, 56, 58
melanoma, 56, 58
Mèniére's disease, 262
meningeal, 290, 291
meninges, 281
meningitis, 290, 291, 299
meniscus, 139, 163–164
meniscus tears. *See* knee injuries
menorrhagia, 334
menorrhea, 334, 335
MI. *See* myocardial infarction (MI)
micturition, 485, 486
midbrain, 281
middle ear, 239, 240
middle ear bacterial/viral infection. *See* otitis media
midsagittal plane, 25
migraine headache, 299
mono. *See* mononucleosis
mononucleosis, 218
MS. *See* multiple sclerosis (MS)
multiple sclerosis (MS), 218
muscle degeneration. *See* muscular dystrophy
muscle tissue, three types, 137
muscular disorders. *See* muscular dystrophy
muscular dystrophy, 165
muscular system, 36, 139
musculoskeletal system, 132–193
    anatomical diagram, 134–135
    anatomy and physiology vocabulary, 135–136
    breaking down and building terms, 146
    diseases and disorders, 162–167
    major structures of muscular system, 134
    major structures of skeletal system, 135
    overview, 134
    procedures and treatments, 168–172
    word elements, 140
    working with medical records, 176
myalgia, 149, 151
myasthenia, 149, 151
mycotic, 17, 56, 58
myelogram, 290, 291
myitis, 149, 151
myocardial, 413, 414
myocardial infarction (MI), 422, 424
myocardial ischemia, 420

myopia, 259
myringectomy, 249, 252
myringitis, 249, 252
myringoplasty, 249, 252
myringotomy, 249, 252, 267
myxedema. *See* cretinism

N

nearsightedness. *See* myopia
necrogenic, 86
necrosis, 149, 151
necrotic, 56, 58
needle biopsy, 73
nephrectomy, 494, 497
nephritis, 494, 497
nephrolithiasis, 494, 497, 505
nephroma, 494, 497
nephrons, 484, 486
nephropexy, 494, 497
nephroplasty, 494, 497
nephroptosis, 495, 497
nephrorrhaphy, 495, 497
nephrostomy, 495, 497
nephrotomy, 497
nervous system, 36, 278–321
    anatomical diagram, 280, 283
    anatomy and physiology vocabulary, 282–284
    breaking down and building terms, 289–291
    definition, 280, 282
    diseases and disorders, 296–300
    functions and structures, 280–282
    major parts of brain, 284
    major structures, 283
    overview, 280
    procedures and treatments, 300–303
    word elements, 285
    working with medical records, 308
neural, 290, 291
neuralgia, 290, 291
neurologist, 282, 290, 291
neurology, 282, 290, 291
neurons, 281–282
neuropathy, 290, 291
neurotransmitters, 282
NIDDM. *See* diabetes mellitus
NMI. *See* nuclear imaging (NMI) test
nocturia, 342, 495, 497
non-insulin-dependent mellitus (NIDDM), 464
noninvasive, 342
nonspecific immunity, 197, 199
nuclear imaging (NMI) test, 168–169

O

obstructive sleep apnea, 386
ocular, 249, 252
oculomycosis, 249, 252
oliguria, 495, 497
onychectomy, 56, 58, 74, 75

regulation of acid-base (pH) levels, 367

word elements, 369

working with medical records, 393

rest, ice, compression, and elevation (RICE), 172

retina, 239, 241

retinal, 251, 252

retinitis, 251, 252

rheumatoid arthritis (RA), 217

rhinitis, 375, 376

RICE, 172

right hypochondriac region, 34

right iliac region, 34

right lower quadrant (RLQ), 33

right lumbar region, 34

right upper quadrant (RUQ), 33

Romberg sign. See Romberg test

Romberg test. See Romberg's sign

Romberg's sign, 303

root word, 10

root words and combining forms, general rules, 11

rotator cuff tear, 167

S

sagittal plane, 25

salpingitis, 334, 335

sarcoidosis, 218–219

scalp hair, acute loss. See alopecia

schizotrichia, 57, 58

sclera, 239, 241, 252

scleral, 251

scleritis, 251, 252

sclerotomy, 251, 252

scoliosis, 150, 151

scratch test, 220

scrotum, 324, 326

sebaceous, 46, 48

sebaceous glands. See acne

seborrhea, 57, 58

seborrheic, 85

sebum, 46, 48

second-degree burns, 70

seizures. See epilepsy

semicircular canals, 239, 241

seminal vesicles, 324, 326

sensitivity test, 388, 507

sensory ataxia, 303

sensory organs

anatomy and physiology vocabulary, 240–241

breaking down and building terms related to eye and ear, 248

diseases and disorders
ear, 262–263
eye, 259–262

ear, anatomical diagram, 240, 242

eye, anatomical diagram, 239, 241

eye and ear, 236–277

overview, 238

procedures and treatments
ear, 266–267

eye, 263–266

word elements, 243

working with medical records, 271

sexually transmitted disease (STD), 343

sexually transmitted diseases,
chlamydia, 343–344
genital herpes, 345
gonorrhea, 344
syphilis, 346

Shaken Baby Syndrome, 298

shingles, 72

sialorrhea, 102, 103

sigmoid, 91, 93

sigmoid colon, 91

sigmoidoscopy, 102, 103, 116

simple fracture. See fracture

skeletal system, 36, 139

skeletal system, major bones of, 138

skin cancer, 71

skin cancer. See malignant melanoma

SLE. See systemic lupus erythematosus (SLE)

sleep apnea. See obstructive sleep apnea

slipped disk, 163

slit lamp. See tonometry

small intestine, 91, 93

Snellen chart, 264

sound waves. See Doppler sonography

specific immunity, 199

speculum, 349

sperm, 324, 326

sphincter muscles, 484

spinal cavity, 32

spinal disks, 162

spinal fusion, 172

spinal tap. See lumbar puncture

spirometer, 375, 376, 388

spleen, 197, 199

splenectomy, 207, 208, 221

splenic, 207, 208

splenitis, 207, 208

splenoid, 207, 208

splenoma, 207, 208

splenomalacia, 207, 208

splenomegaly, 207, 208

splenopexy, 207, 208

splenorrhaphy, 207, 208

spondylarthritis, 150, 151

spondylodesis, 150, 151, 172

spondylolysis, 150, 151

spondylosis, 150, 151

sprain, 172

sputum, 383

sputum culture and sensitivity (C&S) test, 388

squamous, 57, 58

staging, 343

STD. See sexually transmitted disease (STD)

stenotic, 413, 414, 420

sternal, 150, 151

sternocostal, 150, 151

stimulus, 300

stoma. See colostomy

stomach, 90, 91, 93

stomach acid. See gastroesophageal reflux disease

stomach protrudes through abdomen. See hiatal hernia

strain, 172

Streptococcus, 219

striae, 464

stroke. See cerebral vascular attack (CVA)

subcostal, 150, 151

subcutaneous, 47, 48, 57

subdermal, 85

sudoriferous, 46, 48

suffixes, 11–14
associated with diagnostic procedures, 12
associated with diseases and disorders, 12
associated with surgical procedures, 13
definition, 11
general rules for use of, 13–14

superior, 27

supine, 27

suprapharyngeal, 16

synaptic cleft, 282

synkinesis, 150, 151

synovial compartment of joint. See joint effusion

syphilis, 346

systemic autoimmune disease. See rheumatoid arthritis,

systemic lupus erythematosus (SLE), 217

T

T cells. See T lymphocytes

T lymphocytes, 197

tachycardia, 17, 413, 414

tachypnea, 375, 376

TB skin test, 388

tendinitis, 150, 151

tendon, 139

tennis elbow. See lateral epicondylitis

testes, 324, 326, 447

testicles, 324

testosterone, 324

thalamus, 281

third-degree burns, 71

thoracentesis, 389

thoracic cavity, 32

thrombophlebitis, 413, 414

thrombosis, 413, 414

thrombus, 296

thymectomy, 207, 208, 455, 456

thymic, 207, 208, 455, 456

thymoma, 207, 208, 455, 456

thymus, 197, 199

thymus gland, 197, 447

thyroid gland, 447

thyroid scan, 468
thyroidectomy, 455, 456
thyroiditis, 455, 456
thyroid-stimulating hormone (TSH), 469
thyroid-stimulating hormone test,
    468–469
thyromegaly, 455, 456
thyroxine test, 469
TIA. *See* transient ischemic attack (TIA)
tinnitus, 262
tone. *See* audiometry
tonometry, 265–266
tonsillar, 207, 208
tonsillectomy, 207, 208, 221
tonsillitis, 207, 208, 219
tonsils, 196, 199
tonsils and throat, symptoms of
    tonsillitis, 219
tonsils, inflammation. *See* tonsillitis
topical, 57
trachea, 366–367
tracheal, 375, 376
tracheitis, 375, 376
tracheostenosis, 375, 376
tracheotomy, 375, 376
transcutaneous, 85
transdermal, 57
transient ischemic attack (TIA), 300
transport of oxygen, 366
transurethral resection of the prostate
    (TURP), 350
transverse colon, 92
transverse plane, 26
traumatic brain injury (TBI), 297
trichoid, 86
trichomycosis, 57, 58
TSH test. *See* thyroid-stimulating
    hormone test
tubal ligation, 351
tuberculin skin test, 388
TURP. *See* transurethral resection of
    the prostate
tympanectomy, 251, 252
tympanic, 251, 252
tympanic membrane, 239, 241, 267
tympanometer, 251, 252
tympanometry, 251, 252
tympanoplasty, 251, 252, 267
tympanorrhexis, 251, 252
tympanostomy, 251, 252, 267
Type 1 diabetes, 464
Type 1 diabetes mellitus, 464
Type 2 diabetes, 465
Type 2 diabetes mellitus, 465

U

UGI. *See* upper gastrointestinal (UGI)
    series
ulcers, 113–114
umbilical region, 34
underactive thyroid. *See*
    hypothyroidism
upper arm inflammation of lateral part.
    See lateral epicondylitis
upper gastrointestinal (UGI) series, 117
upper GI and small bowel series, 117
urea, 506
uremia, 495, 497, 506
ureter, 486
ureterolithiasis, 496, 497, 505
ureteropyelonephritis, 496, 497
ureterostenosis, 496, 497
ureterovesicostomy, 496, 497
ureters, 484
urethra, 324, 326, 484, 486
urethral, 496, 497
urethralgia, 496, 497
urethritis, 344, 594
urethrocystitis, 496, 497
urethroscope, 496, 497
urinalysis (UA), 507
urinary bladder, 484
urinary catheterization, 508
urinary incontinence, 504
urinary meatus, 484, 486
urinary retention, 342, 505
urinary system, 37, 482–527
    anatomical diagram, 485, 487
    anatomy and physiology vocabulary,
        485–486
    breaking down and building terms,
        493
    diseases and disorders, 504–507
    main functions, 484
    major organs and structures, 484–485
    overview, 484
    procedures and treatments, 507–510
    word elements, 488
    working with medical records, 514
urinary tract, 325, 484
urinary tract infection (UTI), 504
urination, 485, 486
urine, 486
urogram, 496, 497. *See* also
    intravenous pyelogram
urological, 485
urologist, 325, 334, 335, 485, 486, 496,
    497

urology, 325, 335, 485, 486, 496, 497
uterine tubes, 324, 326
uterus, 324, 326
UTI. *See* urinary tract infection (UTI)
UV damage, 71
UVA rays, 71
UVB rays, 71
uvula, 219

V

V/Q scan, 389
vaccination, 220
vaccine, 220
vagina, 324, 326
vaginitis, 334, 335
varicose veins, 423
vas deferens, 324, 326
vasculitis, 150, 151
vasectomy, 334, 335, 350
veins, 404, 405
venipuncture, 467
venous, 413, 414
ventilation, 366
ventilation/perfusion scan (VPS), 389
ventral, 27
ventral cavity, 32
venules, 404
vertebrae, 162
vertebral, 150–151
vertebral cavity, 32
vertebral column, 281
vertebral disk, rupture. *See* herniated
    disk
vertebral disks. *See* spinal disks
vertebrectomy, 150, 151
vertigo, 262
vesicocele, 507
viral infection. *See* mononucleosis
vision blurred. *See* astigmatism
visual acuity test, 263–264
voiding, 485, 486
voluntary muscle, 139

W

weight-loss surgery. *See* gastric bypass
    surgery
Western blot test, 220– 221
whitehead, 69

X

xeroderma, 57, 58